Will It Hurt the Baby?

Will It Hurt the Baby?

The Safe Use of Medications during Pregnancy and Breastfeeding

RICHARD S. ABRAMS, M.D.

Attending Physician
Rose Medical Center

Associate Clinical Professor of Medicine
Associate Clinical Professor of Obstetrics
University of Colorado School of Medicine
Denver, Colorado

 Addison-Wesley Publishing Company, Inc.
Reading, Massachusetts • Menlo Park, California • New York
Don Mills, Ontario • Wokingham, England • Amsterdam
Bonn • Sydney • Singapore • Tokyo • Madrid
San Juan

Many of the designations used by manufacturers and sellers to distinguish their products are claimed as trademarks. Where those designations appear in this book and Addison-Wesley was aware of a trademark claim, the designations have been printed in initial capital letters (e.g., Tylenol).

Library of Congress Cataloging-in-Publication Data

Abrams, Richard S. (Richard Stephen). 1946–
    Will it hurt the baby? : the safe use of medications during pregnancy and breastfeeding / Richard S. Abrams.
        p. cm.
    ISBN –201–51809–0
    1. Fetus—Effect of drugs on. 2 Pregnancy, Complications of--Chemotherapy—Safety measures. 3. Breast feeding—Safety measures.
    I. Title.
RG627.6.D79A27   1990   89–29434
618.3—dc20   CIP

Cover design by Hannus Design Associates
Text design by Joyce C. Weston
Set in 10-point Trump by Pine Tree Composition, Inc.

ABCDEFGHIJ-MW-9543210
First printing, May 1990

For Carol, Brian, and Katie

TO THE READER

This book profiles many of the most common prescription and over-the-counter (nonprescription) medications used in the United States. Like medications themselves, this information should be used with caution. *Will It Hurt the Baby?* is not intended to be a self-treatment manual. Read this information with the goal of supplementing what your physician has already told you, and use it to ask additional questions about why medication is being prescribed, what the possible side effects are, how safe the medication is during pregnancy and breastfeeding, and whether there is an appropriate alternative to taking a drug. It would be unthinkable for me or anyone else unfamiliar with your care to suggest specific medical therapy. Yet I believe that understanding your medications will allow you to participate more actively and confidently in medical decisions affecting you and your unborn child.

✺ ACKNOWLEDGMENTS

Single authorship of any book often belies the contributions of friends and colleagues whose ideas and critical review make the project successful. There are many people whom I wish to thank, some for specific help and others for acts of kindness and inspiration.

I deeply appreciate the critical comments of my colleagues at Rose Medical Center and the University of Colorado School of Medicine: Dorene Day, M.D.; Ronald Gibbs, M.D.; and Michele Velkoff, M.D. Susan Heitler, Ph.D. provided the psychological insight for non-pharmacologic alternatives to the use of sedatives, tranquilizers, and antidepressants. As I've done many times in the past, I relied heavily on the extraordinary expertise of Robert Wall, M.D. for his meticulous review of the entire manuscript. I am grateful to Nancy Simon for her library research skills. Her efforts helped ensure that the information in these pages is as accurate and up-to-date as possible. Bill Abrams and Julie Salamon lent their professional talents to help with style and content. Bill Clarke, a veteran newsman, taught me to communicate clearly and concisely. Energetic administrative assistance and wordprocessing were provided by Donna Forsberg, Michelle Miller, and Sandy Pierson.

A special thanks is due to my editor William Patrick for the substantial contribution he made to the planning and organization of this book. His gentle reminders about the book's purpose and tone kept me on track. The staff at Addison-Wesley turned my manuscript into a concise, readable book: Production Coordinator John Fuller, Copy Editor Rosemary Winfield, and Designer Joyce Weston. George Gibson, Nancy Fish, and Elizabeth Carduff directed the marketing efforts that got this book onto store shelves.

I remain forever grateful to my friend Curtis Vouwie for his encouragement, and for introducing me to Addison-Wesley. Finally, my wife Carol contributed her emotional support, insight, and writing skills to data that required constant translation from medical jargon to nontechnical, useful information. What I owe her cannot be adequately rewarded in print.

RSA

❧ CONTENTS

Hyperthermia
Hospital and Health Care Hazards
Solvents and Cleaners
Heavy Metals
Pesticides
Physical Exertion
Radiation, Microwaves, and Ultrasound

❧ FOREWORD

Nearly all women will take at least one medication during pregnancy. The average women takes three or four different drugs, excluding vitamins and mineral supplements, and patients with medical or obstetric complications may require even more. It is essential that unnecessary medications and those known to cause harm be avoided. But just as important, women should understand there are many medications that can be taken safely throughout pregnancy. An inappropriate fear of medications could lead to untreated illnesses that jeopardize both a mother and her developing baby. Thus, the goal is to balance the potential benefit of any medication and its possible risks.

My colleague and friend, Dr. Richard Abrams, has prepared an excellent resource about the safe use of medications during pregnancy and breastfeeding. Information is presented in nontechnical language and displayed in a well organized, easily readable format. Each drug profile provides detailed information on general usage, side effects, specific recommendations for use or avoidance during pregnancy and breastfeeding, and wherever possible, alternatives to the use of medications. The book also includes chapters on how drugs are tested for safety, the effects of common medical diseases, and the risks of environmental and occupational hazards during pregnancy.

Will It Hurt the Baby? is a timely and valuable resource for any pregnant woman and her family at this most exciting time in their lives.

Ronald S. Gibbs, M.D., Professor and Chairman
Department of Obstetrics and Gynecology
University of Colorado School of Medicine

First and foremost, do no harm
—Hippocrates

❧ INTRODUCTION

Few times in your life will be filled with greater anticipation than pregnancy. The care in choosing just the right name, the joy of informing future grandparents, and the endless discussions about child rearing are all part of the excitement couples share. Yet from the moment you discover you're pregnant, you will probably begin to worry. Hardly a day passes without wondering whether the baby will be all right. Worries grow even more intense if you need to take medication, work around chemicals or even if you've drunk a glass of wine or a cup of coffee. Will it hurt the baby?

Must nausea be endured, or is there safe medication for relief? If an infection occurs, can antibiotics be given without harm? Can medications taken for a chronic illness be continued throughout pregnancy? *Will It Hurt the Baby?* was inspired by many telephone calls from anxious mothers asking just such thoughtful questions about the safe use of medications during pregnancy and breastfeeding. The book is designed to help explain the need to treat certain medical illnesses during pregnancy, to offer reassurance about the safety of many medications, and to warn against the use of other drugs and chemicals that are clearly harmful to the baby. It is not a self-treatment manual. Your doctor is the only one who can properly diagnose and treat you during pregnancy. *Will It Hurt the Baby?* should, however, allow you to be more informed, to participate more actively in your care, and to be more confident about the safety of medications you need to take while pregnant.

Legitimate medication is used during pregnancy more than you might expect. A large survey conducted by the National Institutes of Health in Washington, D.C., compiled a list of 900 different drugs taken by women during pregnancy. Pregnant women take an average of almost four drugs (excluding nutritional supplements) during pregnancy, and only 20 percent abstain from all drug use. Perhaps even more significant is that 40 percent of the women in this survey took medication in the critical period of fetal development during the first trimester. Many were unaware they were pregnant.

1

Although it is true that most medications given to a pregnant woman do not harm the baby, unfortunately some do. It would be easy to recommend that no drugs be taken during pregnancy. This advice has been given to many women by friends and health-care professionals alike. The standard book of prescription medications, called the *Physician's Desk Reference*, advises doctors not to use any medication during pregnancy unless the potential benefit of that medication outweighs any risk. No one would disagree with this advice. Clearly, no drug should be taken during pregnancy unless it is absolutely necessary. Nevertheless, a blanket warning against the use of all drugs during pregnancy denies a woman relief from troublesome symptoms such as nausea and vomiting or subjects her and the baby to potentially dangerous consequences of curable illnesses like infections.

Can any medication be taken safely during pregnancy? What are the risks to a mother and her baby if a serious medical illness goes untreated? What should be done if a mother is exposed to a chemical or takes a medication during early pregnancy before she knows she is pregnant? None of these questions can be answered with 100 percent certainty. Yet it is the task of your physicians and counselors to guide you through these and other difficult questions that relate to the use of medications during pregnancy. *Will It Hurt the Baby?* is designed to give you more information about the risks and potential benefits of some of the most commonly used prescription and over-the-counter drugs. It also will help you prepare questions to ask your doctor.

How to Use the Book

Even though very few illnesses prevent pregnancy, virtually the entire spectrum of disease can complicate it. In the past many women with chronic medical problems were told never to attempt pregnancy. Others were told that no medications are safe during pregnancy. Today, we confront the occurrence of medical disorders during pregnancy with a decidedly more informed view. It is now clear that many common medical problems including diabetes, asthma, intestinal disorders, and even various heart diseases can be safely managed throughout pregnancy and result in a normal, healthy baby. Although many of these problems require daily medications, we now know that an ample number of medications have been used for years with a proven record of safety. *Will It Hurt the Baby?* begins with a discussion of some of the most common medical disorders encountered during pregnancy. Since a detailed description of each disorder is beyond the scope of this book, I have emphasized the special impact of medical illnesses on pregnancy and the effects of pregnancy on the usual course of an illness. It is clear that many illnesses require treatment with medications. If left untreated, many medical conditions may jeopardize both your health and your baby's. In the discussion of each illness some of the more frequently used medications are listed, but whenever possible suggestions are offered for the management of troublesome symptoms without drugs. Use this section of the book to become familiar with your particular illness and its unique interaction with pregnancy. In many cases you will find that there is minimal risk to the baby and that there is no need to change the way the problem is treated during pregnancy. Whenever the risk of an illness to your health or your baby's is significant, I have attempted to say so. Each time the use of a medication is considered during pregnancy, the risk of an untreated illness must be compared to the risk, if any, of taking a medication.

The majority of the book contains specific information about drugs—generic names, common brand names, FDA risk category, common use, possible side effects, appropriate adjustments in the dosage, safety during pregnancy and breastfeeding, and whenever possible, alternatives to medications. In many cases there may be a slight theoretical risk to using a drug during pregnancy, but that risk is thought to be insignificant and should not restrict its appropriate use. Some drugs should not be taken during early pregnancy when the baby's organs are being formed but can be safely used after the first trimester.

You can find information in the book by first consulting the index. If you have a particular medical illness and want to learn more about the effect of that illness on pregnancy, you can look up that illness in the index. Individual prescription or over-the-counter (nonprescription) drugs can be found by generic name or brand name. (Remember, *generic name* refers to the scientific or chemical name of a medication. The name the manufacturer gives to the drug is called the *brand name* or *trade name*.) Many drugs with the same generic name are marketed under a variety of brand names. The brand names Tylenol, Datril, Tempra, Anacin-3, and many others are all the same drug, generically known as acetaminophen.

Although it should not be necessary to warn pregnant women to avoid alcohol, tobacco, and illegal drugs, a staggering number of women continue to use these substances during pregnancy. This problem is so great that detailed information about the hazards of these substances is also included.

Finally, a growing body of scientific evidence has implicated chemical exposures in the environment and workplace to possible adverse effects on the outcome of pregnancy. Although there remain many unanswered questions about these hazards, reliable information now links some chemicals and toxins to fetal malformations. The section on environmental and chemical exposures identifies some of those risks and offers some suggestions for avoiding them.

Throughout your pregnancy you will make dozens of decisions weighing benefits against potential risks. Many of those decisions will involve the use of medications. Understanding the safe use of medications during pregnancy and breastfeeding will help you avoid inadvertently exposing your baby to potentially hazardous substances. Perhaps equally important, you should be reassured that many medications important for your good health are relatively safe and are unlikely to harm the baby.

Despite the deluge of modern media tales warning against everything from the air we breathe to the water we drink, there has never been a safer time to have a baby. Fears about the risks of most medications have been irrationally exaggerated. Clearly, a thoughtful approach to a healthy pregnancy includes avoiding any unnecessary medication, but if a medical condition arises that your physician feels should be treated with medication, consider the following advice:

- Ask your doctor for specific information about the risks versus the benefits of all medications (including over-the-counter drugs);
- Do your own research by consulting this book and others about the safety of medications during pregnancy;
- Understand the possible risks of not using a medication when you have a medical problem;
- Be aware of the proper way to take your medication and understand any possible side effects;
- Determine if there are safe alternatives to taking medications for your problem, especially during the first trimester;
- Finally, if you've already taken a medication or been exposed to a potentially harmful substance, consult your physician or genetic counselor to clearly understand the risks. In most cases the risks are less than you fear.

How Are Drugs Determined to Be Safe?

Technically, drugs are not determined to be safe. Some are proven to be harmful, and others are presumed to be safe when no evidence of harm can be demonstrated. The difference is subtle, but it means that no drug can be guaranteed to be 100 percent safe. Assuming that it is impossible to absolutely guarantee the safety of any drug or chemical during pregnancy, how do physicians balance benefit versus potential harm? To understand this important question, let's explore how medications are tested for their effect during pregnancy.

Official approval for the safety of a drug during pregnancy rests with the Food and Drug Administration (FDA). The responsibility of the FDA is enormous, and its task is extremely difficult. The FDA's information about the potential for a drug to cause birth defects comes largely from animal experiments.

Most, if not all, drugs and chemicals can cause birth defects in animals if enough of the drug is given during the early part of pregnancy. When researchers study a new drug in animals, they first determine the dosage of a drug that will predictably cause birth defects, called the *threshold level*. The threshold level may be 100 to 1,000 times the usual treatment dosage in humans. The dosage of any drug or amount of exposure to any chemical must be kept as far as possible below this level. After identifying the threshold level at which a drug predictably causes birth defects, researchers attempt to determine the *safe level* or *no observable effect level*. This level corresponds to the greatest amount of drug or chemical that consistently produces no recognizable birth defects in experimental animals. This information is included in the FDA's final recommendation about the safety of a drug during pregnancy.

Animal studies remain the only practical and ethical way to study the effects of new drugs during pregnancy, but animal research is far from perfect. Certain strains of animals (usually rats and mice) are known to be vulnerable to birth defects when exposed to a drug, while a human fetus exposed to the same drug may not have any ill effects. Unfortunately, it is also true that certain animals are resistant to the adverse effects of drugs that clearly cause malformations in humans. Tragically, a few drug-induced birth defects were discovered only *after* the birth of an affected child. The well-publicized story of the drug thalidomide provides one example.

During the 1950s thalidomide, a sedative, was given to many pregnant women in Europe. Before being used by patients, the drug had been tested in animals for its safety during pregnancy and approved for use by humans. It took several years before physicians realized that many of the infants born to women who took thalidomide had distinct, catastrophic birth defects.

Because animal studies cannot detect all possible hazards, the FDA and medical researchers are constantly looking for possible links between drugs or chemicals, and birth defects. This is no simple matter. At times the link between a drug taken during pregnancy and a subsequent birth defect can be very uncertain. When a birth defect is diagnosed in a newborn, it is always enticing to assume that a drug taken during early pregnancy was the direct cause of the malformation. Often this assumption of cause and effect is incorrect. For example, a drug may have been given to treat an illness that itself can cause birth defects. We know that some mothers with type I diabetes (juvenile diabetes) have a higher risk than other women of having a baby with a birth defect. Daily injections of insulin needed to treat diabetes might be mistakenly assumed to cause birth defects. We know, however, that this is not the case.

Another possibility is that a fetal malformation that occurred spontaneously during early pregnancy can produce symptoms in a pregnant woman. If a drug were prescribed to relieve the symptoms, it might later be incorrectly accused of causing the birth defect. Consider the following example: A pregnant woman whose fetus has a disorder of the esophagus called *esophageal atresia* often develops too much amniotic fluid around the baby, a condition called *polyhydramnios*. If a diuretic were used to reduce the mother's extra fluid, the drug might be blamed for the esophageal problem even though the defect was present before the drug was given.

How Common Are Birth Defects and What Causes Them?

A birth defect is an abnormality of structure, function, or body metabolism that often causes a physical or mental disability, shortened lifespan, or death during pregnancy or the newborn period. The severity of birth defects ranges from relatively minor malformations such as a misshapen toe to malformations of the heart or brain incompatible with life. Some birth defects may not become evident for months or even years. Learning difficulties, for example, may not show up for several years or until a child enters school.

Birth defects are the nation's most serious child health problem. They affect more than 250,000 babies in the United States each year. With more than 3,000 known birth defects, it's a wonder that the vast majority of babies are born normal. Fortunately, fewer than 3 percent of babies born to healthy mothers have any significant malformation (97 out of 100 babies are normal). This expected number of malformed babies is often referred to as the *background incidence* of birth defects. The concept of a background incidence of birth defects is very important to understand. It means that by chance alone a certain small number (less than 3 percent) of babies will be born with some kind of birth defect. Most of these birth defects will be insignificant, but some can be quite serious. Because of the background incidence of birth defects it is often difficult to tell whether a drug given during the first trimester was the responsible agent or merely a coincidental occurrence in a pregnancy that was destined to result in a child with a birth defect.

What causes birth defects? It is human nature to look for a cause when a baby is born with a birth defect. In fact, the cause of most birth defects is never known. Yet we do know that some birth defects can be genetic (just as we inherit other characteristics like eye color or general appearance), while others result from environmental causes such as certain viral infections, drugs, or chemicals. Drugs or other chemical agents known to cause birth defects are referred to as *teratogens.* Fortunately, most medications do not cause harm. Drug exposure accounts for fewer than 2 percent of birth defects, approximately 25 percent are genetic, but for the majority (over 70 percent) of birth defects no cause is ever found.

Whether a drug or chemical can cause a birth defect depends on several factors—the type of drug, the dosage, and the stage of pregnancy in which the exposure occurs. During certain weeks of the pregnancy the baby is extremely vulnerable to the toxic effects of a drug or chemical. On the other hand, at times the baby is relatively resistant even to known toxic substances. To understand the concept of the *vulnerable period* during pregnancy, let's examine the process of normal fetal development.

From Embryo to Newborn

Growth and development from a fertilized egg to a newborn passes through a number of stages over the nine months (40 weeks) of pregnancy. Generally, we divide pregnancy into three equal periods called *trimesters.* Each trimester is approximately three months or a little over 13 weeks long. (It's a good idea to get in the habit of knowing how many weeks pregnant you are. Most health-care professionals tend to talk about weeks rather than months. Also, physicians begin calculating dates during pregnancy from the last menstrual period even if you know the exact date you conceived.)

During the first two weeks of gestation (pregnancy), the fertilized egg has formed the beginnings of the placenta and attaches itself to the wall of the mother's uterus. Interestingly, if exposure to a harmful substance takes place during the first four weeks after the last menstrual period, there is what's called an *all or none effect*. An exposure around the time of conception or when the fertilized egg first implants into the wall of the uterus will either kill the embryo and a woman may not even know she was pregnant, or the pregnancy will progress without harm to the embryo. In other words, the embryo survives unaffected or it dies and miscarries.

The stage between five and ten weeks after the last menstrual period is very important because the limbs and organs form during this time. No major organs form after the twelfth week of pregnancy. If a birth defect is going to occur, it happens sometime during the first ten weeks of pregnancy. If the fetus is exposed to a harmful substance during the early embryo stage (about 5 weeks after the last menstrual period), the result may be a defect in the heart or central nervous system (the brain or spinal cord). Nearer the end of the embryo stage (about 10 weeks after the last menstrual period) defects in the palate or ears are more likely. If there is concern about the effects of a drug taken during pregnancy, the exact time the drug was taken and the precise date of the last menstrual period will be very important for your physician or genetic counselor.

After the embryo stage is complete, the rest of pregnancy is devoted to growth and maturation of the various organs. The vital organs have all been formed by this stage. Therefore, exposure to a harmful substance will not result in a birth defect. Yet damage can still occur in other ways. Because organs grow during this period, drugs or chemicals can potentially alter or slow that growth. One of the best examples is the risk of mental retardation caused by the effect of alcohol on the growing brain. Other drugs can cause slowing of the entire growth process, resulting in a low birth-weight baby. Nevertheless, it is important to remember that exposures during the second and third trimesters do not cause structural birth defects in any of the baby's organs.

And What About Breastfeeding?

You've given birth to a healthy baby. Do the same concerns and limitations now apply to the use of medications during breastfeeding? Do drugs and chemicals enter breast milk? What effect might they have on the newborn? During the past decade there has been a large movement by medical professionals as well as new mothers in support of breastfeeding. Breastfeeding is known to offer nutritional and immunologic (resistance to infection) properties superior to those found in infant formulas. Studies have also emphasized the significant psychologic benefits for both mother and child. Yet we also know that virtually every drug taken by a nursing mother enters breast milk. It would be easy to recommend that mothers taking medication not nurse. But not only would such advice deny the clear advantages of breastfeeding, it would very likely be ignored by many women.

From studies performed in animals we are able to provide some information about excretion of many drugs into breast milk. And from careful observation of breastfed newborns, we are able to predict the effects of many drugs. With some drugs little more than a cautionary warning about possible adverse behavioral effects in the newborn is necessary. Other drug exposures during breastfeeding pose too great a risk and require that either the drug or breastfeeding be discontinued.

In 1983 the American Academy of Pediatrics published an extensive list of medications that had been studied in breastfeeding mothers and their infants. In this publication there was an attempt to list potential adverse effects and to offer advice about the safety of many drugs during breastfeeding. Recommendations about the use of medications during breastfeeding have been primarily derived from the information published by the American Academy of Pediatrics.

Medical Problems during Pregnancy

Although few medical disorders prevent pregnancy, virtually any illness can complicate it. The various changes of pregnancy are capable of affecting the course of many diseases, and conversely, medical disorders can have a profound effect on both mother and child. In the past, many women with chronic medical disorders such as diabetes or rheumatic heart disease were warned never to become pregnant. Others were told that no medications are safe during pregnancy and sometimes suffered disastrous consequences. We now confront the occurrence of medical diseases during pregnancy with a decidedly more informed view. Today, most women with chronic medical disorders should be confident that contemporary medical and obstetric care can offer a healthy pregnancy and a happy outcome.

This section should help you understand the consequences of some of the common medical problems that complicate pregnancy. It is necessary to be cautious about taking any drug during pregnancy, but bear in mind that an untreated illness can be even more dangerous than the careful use of most medications.

Diabetes

Diabetes is a disease characterized by an excess of glucose (sugar) in the blood. There are several types of diabetes, and each can affect pregnancy. When the pancreas of a child or young adult cannot produce any insulin, we call this condition *type I* or *insulin-dependent diabetes* (formerly called *juvenile diabetes*). Individuals with type I diabetes must follow a special diet, exercise program, and they must get injections of insulin (p. 181) every day. People who develop diabetes at an older age (usually over age 40) have *type II diabetes* (formerly called *adult-onset diabetes*). In this type of diabetes insulin is still produced by the pancreas, but it does not work properly. People with type II diabetes are usually able to control their disease by following a careful diet and exercise program. Some, however, need to take pills (e.g., chlorpropamide, p. 107, glyburide, p. 160, glipizide, p. 157, tolazamide, p. 296) or inject insulin to lower the level of glucose in their blood.

A third type of diabetes, unique to pregnancy, is called *gestational diabetes*. Women with gestational diabetes produce insulin, but the effect or action of their insulin is partially blocked by other hormones (human placental lactogen, estrogen, and cortisol) made by the placenta. The inability of insulin to do its job effectively during pregnancy is referred to as *insulin resistance*, and it usually begins about midway through pregnancy (20 to 24 weeks). In most women the pancreas makes additional insulin to overcome the insulin resistance. But when the pancreas makes all the insulin it possibly can and there still isn't enough to overcome the insulin resistance, gestational diabetes results. Approximately 5 percent of pregnant women develop gestational diabetes. For most women the problem goes away immediately after delivery.

How do you know whether you have gestational diabetes? Gestational diabetes does not usually cause specific symptoms. In fact, many of the symptoms usually associated with diabetes in nonpregnant individuals (frequent urination, thirst, and fatigue) occur in almost all pregnant women whether or not they have gestational diabetes. To accurately diagnose this type of diabetes a blood test, called a glucose tolerance test, must be performed in the hospital laboratory or physician's office. Testing urine for the presence of glucose is not an accurate way to diagnose gestational diabetes. Therefore, most physicians believe that all pregnant women should undergo a blood test for the disorder between 24 and 28 weeks of pregnancy. A simple test, called the screening test for gestational diabetes, takes only one hour and is often used to see if a woman is likely to have gestational diabetes. If the screening test is abnormal, a complete three-hour glucose tolerance test must be done to confirm the diagnosis of gestational diabetes.

How Does Diabetes Affect the Baby?

Common to all types of diabetes is too much glucose in the blood. For women with type I or II diabetes before pregnancy, excessive amounts of blood glucose during the first trimester when the baby's organs are being formed can cause birth defects. Women with normal blood glucose levels during early pregnancy, however, are at no greater risk of having a baby with a birth defect than a woman without diabetes. Women with gestational diabetes do not have an increased risk of having a birth defective child, because gestational diabetes does not usually begin until at least 20 to 24 weeks of pregnancy, several weeks after the first trimester when the vital organs are formed.

Offspring of women with any type of diabetes, including gestational diabetes, may have abnormal growth during the second and third trimesters, a condition called *macrosomia*. Macrosomia literally means "large body" and refers to a baby who is considerably larger than normal. It's worth taking a moment to understand how this condition develops.

All the nutrients the fetus receives come directly from the mother's blood. If maternal blood has too much glucose, the pancreas of the fetus senses the high glucose levels and produces more of its own insulin in an attempt to use the glucose. The insulin causes the baby to grow bigger and fatter. Vaginal delivery of an unusually large baby can be very difficult. There is a chance that the baby's arms or shoulders will be injured. Occasionally, the baby is even too large to be delivered through the vagina and a cesarean delivery must be performed. Your physician can determine if the baby is macrosomic by estimating its size with a sonogram (ultrasound).

Management of Diabetes During Pregnancy

Virtually all of the potential complications of diabetes can be eliminated by careful medical and obstetric care. Most women with diabetes will be cared for by a team of health-care professionals made up of an obstetrician, internist or diabetologist, dietician, nurse-educator, and a neonatologist to care for the baby. Health-care professionals agree that certain goals should be met by all pregnant women with diabetes:

1. If you have either type I or type II diabetes, consult your physician before attempting to become pregnant. This will help ensure that your blood glucose levels are optimal during the critical early stage of pregnancy.
2. Keep blood glucose levels normal. Normal blood glucose levels vary depending on when you last ate, but they are usually in the range of 60 to 120 mg/dl. If blood glucose levels are normal during the stage of organ formation in the first trimester, the risk of a birth defect is no greater than for any other woman. By keeping

the blood glucose levels normal during the second and third trimesters the fetus will not make too much insulin and is less likely to become macrosomic.

3. Follow a well-balanced diet. You will need to follow a special diet that is designed to meet the nutritional needs of pregnancy and keep blood glucose levels normal. It is best to consult a registered dietitian to guide you in the proper diet.
4. Have blood glucose levels checked periodically. This may be done in your physician's office or at home with special glucose testing equipment. By checking blood glucose levels you and your physician can tell whether your diet is maintaining normal glucose levels.
5. For women who were taking insulin before pregnancy, it will be necessary to adjust the dosage at various times during pregnancy. Women with gestational diabetes must begin insulin if glucose levels cannot be properly controlled with diet alone. Your physician will tell you if you need insulin. Pills used by some women with type II diabetes should not be taken during pregnancy.
6. Follow up with your health-care team after delivery. You will need to adjust your diet and exercise. You should be advised about future pregnancies and contraception.
7. If you have gestational diabetes, have a repeat glucose tolerance test performed within a few months of delivery to ensure that everything has returned to normal.

Thyroid Problems

Hypothyroidism

The thyroid gland makes, stores, and secretes two hormones—thyroxine and triiodothyronine—important for normal growth and metabolism. Individuals who suffer from an underactive thyroid gland, *hypothyroidism*, often complain of fatigue, weight gain, constipation, intolerance to cold, and dry skin. Women with severe hypothyroidism may lack normal menstrual periods and find it difficult to become pregnant. The disorder is usually diagnosed by measuring the amount of thyroid hormone in a blood sample. Mild hypothyroidism presents few problems during pregnancy. Treatment includes taking a thyroid hormone pill (p. 294) daily. The pediatrician will want to check the baby's blood level of thyroid hormone, since hypothyroidism in the newborn can be a serious, but correctable, problem.

Hyperthyroidism

The thyroid gland is also capable of producing too much thyroid hormone, hyperthyroidism. When this occurs, an individual often complains of shakiness, excessive sweating, rapid heart rate, diarrhea, difficulty sleeping, intolerance to heat, and weight loss. A blood test is necessary to confirm the diagnosis.

Pregnant women with hyperthyroidism may have difficulty gaining the appropriate weight for pregnancy, but in general a mildly overactive thyroid is well tolerated during pregnancy. With one particular type of hyperthyroidism called Graves's disease, the newborn can also have an overactive thyroid. The pediatrician will check the baby shortly after delivery.

Treatment is usually accomplished by taking medicine that blocks the production of excessive hormone production in the thyroid gland. The two most commonly used medications, propylthiouracil (p. 266) and methimazole (p. 212), cross the placenta and are taken up by the baby's thyroid. Although these medications have been used safely during pregnancy, they must be given in the lowest possible dosage in order to prevent the fetal thyroid gland from growing too large, a condition called a goiter. Nonpregnant patients with hyperthyroidism are often treated with radioactive iodine to destroy overactive thyroid tissue. Radioactive iodine, however, must not be used during pregnancy because it will destroy the baby's thyroid as well.

Hypertension and Preeclampsia

Hypertension

Hypertension is the medical term for persistently elevated blood pressure. Contrary to popular belief it is not synonymous with nervous tension or anxiety, nor is it often accompanied by hyperactive behavior or a florid complexion. In most cases hypertension causes no symptoms at all.

During pregnancy women normally experience a fall in blood pressure. In the first trimester average blood pressure is about 100/70 mm Hg. Near the end of gestation average blood pressure rises only a little to about 110/70 mm Hg. Blood pressure that consistently exceeds 130/80 mm Hg is considered abnormally high any time during pregnancy.

Various medications are used to treat hypertension in nonpregnant patients. Many of these drugs have been used during pregnancy for years, but experience is lacking with some of the newer medications.

If you are being treated for hypertension and are planning pregnancy, consult your physician to see whether the medications you are taking are safe for use during pregnancy. Remember, it is often well into the first trimester before pregnancy is diagnosed in many women.

Preeclampsia

Preeclampsia, also known as *toxemia*, is a condition of unknown cause manifest by hypertension, edema (swelling) of the hands, ankles, and face, rapid weight gain, and protein in the urine (determined by urinalysis in the doctor's office). The disorder may begin with very few symptoms but progress rapidly. It is important to emphasize that women usually feel well in the early stage of preeclampsia. This sense of well-being should not minimize the seriousness of the condition. If preeclampsia is promptly recognized and treated, no harm comes to the baby or mother. Delay in treatment, however, can lead to serious complications. In the worst cases preeclampsia may advance to a severe condition called *eclampsia*, usually accompanied by convulsions.

Treatment of preeclampsia depends on the severity of high blood pressure, the condition of the baby, and the stage of pregnancy. Some obstetricians will permit women with mild preeclampsia to go home and remain at strict bedrest. For women with more severe preeclampsia or women whose home setting will not permit adequate rest, hospitalization may be necessary. While in the hospital some patients will need medications to lower their blood pressure and prevent eclampsia. The condition of the baby can be monitored by a test called the *nonstress test (NST)*. This test measures the baby's heart rate immediately after it kicks or moves. If the test indicates that the baby is in jeopardy, the obstetrician may elect to deliver the baby before the due date, sometimes even weeks ahead of schedule. The best treatment for preeclampsia is prevention. Regular visits to the obstetrician with blood pressure measured at each visit should permit early recognition of even a subtle rise in pressure.

Heart Problems

Normal pregnancy is accompanied by several changes in the heart and circulation. The volume of blood in the circulation of a pregnant woman increases by as much as 40 percent. For most women the heart has no difficulty increasing its output to accommodate for the increased blood volume. However, patients with certain heart valve abnormalities or patients whose heart muscle has been weakened by

16

disease may not be able to meet the increased demands of pregnancy. A few cardiac disorders are associated with such a high risk to both mother and child that pregnancy is not advisable. Fortunately, the majority of women with heart problems can conceive and safely carry a baby to term. A few general principles of care are worth keeping in mind.

1. If you know that you have some kind of heart problem, consult your internist or cardiologist before you plan to become pregnant. Special tests may need to be done to assess the severity of your problem. Some patients may even require surgery before pregnancy to correct an abnormal heart valve. You should also find out if your heart problem is the kind that could be genetically passed on to your baby.
2. If you take heart medications, review them with your doctor before becoming pregnant. If they can be safely taken during pregnancy, do not stop taking them. Stopping your medication may subject you and the baby to severe complications.
3. Regular visits to the doctor are essential throughout pregnancy to detect any subtle signs of heart dysfunction.
4. Call the doctor immediately if you notice any sudden shortness of breath (mild shortness of breath, however, often accompanies normal pregnancy), persistent rapid or irregular heart beats, rapid weight gain or swelling of the ankles, excessive fatigue, dizziness, or fainting. Since many of these symptoms can occur in women with normal hearts, you must be in tune with your body to recognize any changes. When in doubt, call the doctor!
5. Plan for daily rest periods. Ask your doctor whether you need to limit your usual activities, including work.
6. Find out from your obstetrician whether any special arrangements will be necessary at the time of delivery. It is safer to deliver some women with heart problems by cesarean delivery. You should know this well before your due date.
7. Many women with abnormal heart valves are treated with antibiotics before and immediately after delivery to prevent *endocarditis,* a severe heart valve infection. There are several safe choices of antibiotics.

Phlebitis

The word *phlebitis* literally means inflammation of a vein. Phlebitis is often accompanied by a thrombus (clot) in the vein, a condition called *thrombophlebitis. Superficial phlebitis,* inflammation of one of the surface veins of the leg, is relatively common during pregnancy. It results in pain and redness but is not associated with any major complications.

A clot that forms in a deep vein of the leg is called *deep vein thrombophlebitis*, a condition that can be accompanied by severe consequences. If a clot in a deep leg vein breaks loose, it has a direct path through the bloodstream to the lungs. A clot that travels to the lungs, called a *pulmonary embolus*, can be life-threatening. There is a slightly greater risk of deep vein thrombophlebitis during pregnancy. For most women the risk is so small that no special precautions are necessary. Women whose risk of this problem is high include those with a past history of deep vein thrombophlebitis or a pulmonary embolus, a known blood clotting problem (some people have an inherited tendency to form clots), an illness that requires weeks of confinement to bed, massive obesity, and certain other medical conditions like heart failure. The risk of forming a blood clot is particularly great after a cesarean delivery.

Medications called anticoagulants can be given to treat a blood clot or in some cases to prevent one from forming in patients at special risk. Unfortunately, one of the anticoagulants used in nonpregnant patients called warfarin (coumarin, p. 121) can cause birth defects if used during the first trimester. Use during the second trimester is also thought to be hazardous because the drug crosses the placenta and may cause abnormalities of the brain or spinal cord. If warfarin is used near the time of delivery, the baby is at risk of hemorrhage during delivery. Whenever possible warfarin should not be used during pregnancy.

Another medication called heparin (p. 166) can be used as an anticoagulant during pregnancy. Heparin does not cross the placenta and has no direct effect on the fetus. Unlike warfarin which can be taken as a pill, heparin must be given by subcutaneous injection two or three times each day. This is obviously uncomfortable, but heparin is the only safe anticoagulant during pregnancy.

Asthma

Asthma is a disease in which the bronchial tubes (bronchioles) constrict by overreacting to various stimuli. It is the most common respiratory disorder in women of childbearing age. Attacks of asthma are manifest by shortness of breath, wheezing, and coughing. Viral respiratory infections such as colds, sinusitis, and bronchitis are the most common triggers of asthma, but there are other triggers as well. Exercise, especially in cold weather, pollutants, allergens, and occasionally emotions can all trigger acute attacks.

The course of asthma during pregnancy is not necessarily predictable. Some women have an increase in the frequency and severity of attacks, while others actually improve. A few generalizations can be made:

1. For women with mild and infrequent asthma before pregnancy, a smooth course during pregnancy is likely.
2. The severity of asthma in a previous pregnancy is often predictive of subsequent pregnancies. This is not the case with all illnesses, but for asthma the rule is fairly reliable.
3. Most of the medications and inhalers used to successfully manage asthma in nonpregnant patients can be safely continued during pregnancy.
4. Severe attacks during labor are unlikely if asthma has been well controlled up until then.
5. If there has been a worsening of asthma during pregnancy, it is likely that things will return to the same level of difficulty experienced before pregnancy within three months of delivery.

Although asthma is not an allergy, allergy does play a significant role in approximately 10 percent of people with asthma. Many people with asthma benefit from an evaluation by an allergist to identify the dusts, molds, pollens, foods, animal danders, and other allergens capable of triggering an acute episode of wheezing. Difficult as it may be to get rid of the family pet, danders from dogs, cats, and other furry animals are common triggers that are nearly impossible to eliminate from the home without removing the animal. Allergy skin tests may be helpful before pregnancy to identify other avoidable triggers.

Not long ago allergy shots were overused in the treatment of asthma. The advent of more effective drug treatment has limited their use. Nevertheless, many patients clearly benefit from shots. If effective, this form of treatment may be continued during pregnancy. The usual maintenance dosage can be continued throughout pregnancy except during allergy season, when it should be reduced by approximately one-third. It is not considered a good idea to initiate therapy during pregnancy. Rarely, some individuals will have very strong reactions to the first shots, and this small possibility should be avoided during pregnancy.

The treatment of asthma involves taking measures to avoid substances (triggers) known to begin attacks. In some case medications can be avoided or their dosage reduced if care is taken to avoid known triggers. Mild or infrequent attacks can usually be managed by inhaled medications (bronchodilators), while women with more frequent or severe attacks of asthma may need daily doses of an oral medication. It is important not to stop your asthma medications without consulting your physician just because you are pregnant, since asthma itself can deprive the fetus of oxygen.

Inhaled bronchodilators such as albuterol (p. 66), metaproterenol (p. 208), and epinephrine (p. 142) can relieve symptoms of an acute attack within minutes, and the effect may last up to several hours. Moreover, inhaled preparations can be used preventatively to avoid constriction of the bronchioles before exercise or exposure to cold. The safety of inhaled bronchodilators has not been fully established during pregnancy. However, these drugs have been used for many years without reports of adverse effects. Inhaled medications work directly on contact with the bronchioles, and relatively little is absorbed into the bloodstream. These same medications are available in pill forms that offer little or no advantage over the inhaled preparations and may be accompanied by side effects of shakiness, rapid heart rate, and occasionally, nausea.

Another type of medication taken by inhalation is called cromolyn (p. 122). Cromolyn is a very fine powder capable of preventing cells within the bronchioles from releasing substances, like histamine, known to aggravate bronchial constriction. Cromolyn is not absorbed into the bloodstream and has no adverse effect on the baby.

Medications containing theophylline (p. 292) are often used to control wheezing in patients who have frequent attacks of asthma. They can be used alone or with inhaled bronchodilators. Like inhaled bronchodilators, they relax the muscle in the bronchioles allowing air to move freely. Theophylline may take up to several hours to begin working, but there are several sustained-release preparations capable of working up to 24 hours. Theophylline has been used during pregnancy for many years and has been shown to be safe.

Another group of medications used for the treatment of severe asthma, corticosteroids (p. 119), can be used to treat sudden, severe attacks or in small dosages may be used daily for patients who suffer from continuous wheezing. Corticosteroids should be reserved for only the most severe cases of asthma when other medications have not worked. They may be used during pregnancy when they are needed.

Digestive and Intestinal Disorders

Nausea

Nausea is one of the most common and bothersome symptoms of pregnancy. It affects as many as half of all women and is most common during the first trimester. The precise cause of nausea during early gestation remains a mystery, but most women can be reassured that it disappears after the first trimester. Rarely, some women suffer from a severe, persistent form of nausea and vomiting called *hyperemesis gravidarum*. This problem usually requires hospitalization, intravenous fluids, and medications to control vomiting.

Several years ago an important antinausea medication, doxylamine (Bendectin, p. 80), was removed from the market in the United States despite a long record of safety during pregnancy. The manufacturer, not the FDA, removed the drug from the market for economic and legal reasons. This left a major therapeutic gap in the ability to care for pregnant women. The safety of other antinausea medications (prochlorperazine, p. 262, trimethobenzamide, p. 308) is not as well established. These drugs should generally not be used to treat mild nausea during the first trimester but may be used in severe cases.

Fortunately, most women can satisfactorily control their symptoms with some simple, nonpharmacologic measures:

- Avoid foods that appear or smell offensive to you. This may seem blatantly obvious, but the role of the psyche in nausea is a very important one.
- Avoid an empty stomach. Eat several small meals throughout the day rather than two or three larger ones. If a large meal is necessary, midday is probably the best time for it.
- Avoid greasy or fatty foods. Substitute foods rich in complex carbohydrates such as whole-grain breads, cereals, and pasta. Fresh green leafy vegetables may help alleviate nausea because they are rich in vitamin B_6.
- Eat a small snack at bedtime and save two crackers at the bedside. On awakening, eat the crackers before getting out of bed and remain in bed for an additional few minutes.
- Drink plenty of fluids throughout the day to avoid dehydration.
- If nausea does occur, lie down. It helps. In fact, many women find that frequent rest periods forestall the discomfort.

Heartburn

Heartburn is a burning sensation in the chest or upper abdomen usually caused by reflux of acidic stomach contents into the esophagus. It has nothing to do with the heart. Symptoms are most common during the last trimester. There are some tips for relief:

- Avoid large meals; substitute frequent small ones.
- Do not lie down for at least one hour after a meal to allow food to empty from the stomach.

- Sleeping with your head propped up or the head of the bed elevated may help prevent regurgitation of food during the night.
- Avoid exercise or activity that involves bending.
- If physical maneuvers are not successful in alleviating symptoms, you may use small amounts of low-sodium antacids (p. 78). Do not use baking soda because it is very high in sodium and may cause fluid retention.

Constipation

Constipation is one of the most common gastrointestinal complaints during pregnancy even for women who were previously very regular. It is likely caused by the combined factors of pressure from the enlarging uterus and relaxation of intestinal muscle due to pregnancy hormones. Most women can control this problem by the following measures:

- Include some high-fiber cereal, prunes, or figs with breakfast. Do not, however, eat excessive amounts of fiber. It may be irritating to the stomach.
- Drink hot liquid with breakfast. This often has a stimulating effect on the colon.
- Allow plenty of time for appropriate bowel habits in the morning.
- Milk of magnesia (p. 199) can be used sparingly at night, but harsh laxatives should be avoided. Some laxatives can cause the uterus to contract.

Hemorrhoids

Hemorrhoids are dilated and enlarged veins in the rectum. They are extremely common during pregnancy but usually disappear within several months of delivery. Constipation, straining during bowel movements, and pressure from the enlarging uterus contribute to their formation.

Symptoms can usually be controlled with an appropriate diet to avoid constipation, a warm sitz bath (water temperature should not exceed 100° Fahrenheit), and a mild stool softener to prevent straining. Glycerin or petroleum jelly ointments may be used, but suppositories or ointments containing cortisone should be avoided.

Ulcers

Stomach or duodenal ulcers do not occur with greater frequency during pregnancy. Some studies have even suggested that they are less common among pregnant women. For those with previously diagnosed ulcers, the safest choice of treatment is the frequent use of low-sodium antacids (p. 78). Most of the newer medications (cimetidine, p. 110, ranitidine, p. 272) used to block the production of acid in the stomach have not been used extensively enough during pregnancy to ensure their safety.

Colitis

Problems related to the colon range from occasional constipation and abdominal cramping to chronic inflammatory bowel disease (Crohn's disease or ulcerative colitis). Constipation and mild abdominal cramps can usually be controlled with diet (see above). On the other hand, women with inflammatory bowel disease may suffer severe abdominal pain, diarrhea, bleeding, and malnutrition.

The vast majority of women with chronic inflammatory bowel disease are able to conceive and successfully complete pregnancy. For most patients pregnancy does not cause any worsening of their condition. Women with inflammatory bowel disease can be particularly reassured if their disease was inactive at the time they became pregnant.

The most commonly used medications for the treatment of inflammatory bowel disease are sulfasalazine (p. 283) and corticosteroids (p. 119). These medicines have been used successfully during pregnancy, but they do present some theoretical problems.

Infections and Immunizations

Common Viral Infections and Influenza

Viral respiratory infections can be epidemic in a community during the winter and frequently are transmitted to pregnant women by school-age children in the family. They are characterized by cough, general malaise, fever, and fatigue. Most viral respiratory infections are trivial and present no significant risk to the mother or fetus.

Influenza, on the other hand, is usually a more severe illness caused by influenza virus type A or B. The onset is usually abrupt, following an incubation period of one to two days. Symptoms include fatigue, fever (sometimes as high as 103°F), severe headache, muscle aches (often including the muscles of the eyes), joint aches, and cough. Most physicians believe that there is no special risk of influenza during pregnancy.

Treatment of most common viral respiratory infections and influenza involves rest, adequate fluids, and acetaminophen (p. 63) to reduce fever. Many antihistamines (p. 79) and decongestants (p. 80) have been used safely during pregnancy. The drug amantadine (p. 71) has been used in nonpregnant patients to treat influenza type A. However, this drug has been shown to cause birth defects in rats and should not be used during pregnancy.

Vaccination against influenza has been used safely during pregnancy. Vaccination is usually reserved, however, for women at risk of special complications from influenza. Such patients include those with chronic respiratory or heart conditions, diabetes, chronic kidney disease, sickle cell disease, cystic fibrosis, or other chronic debilitating illnesses. The ideal time for vaccination is before pregnancy.

Other Serious Viral Infections

Acquired Immunodeficiency Syndrome (AIDS): AIDS is one of the most important public health problems we face today, and nowhere is the disease more tragic than in a newborn. In the United States 80 percent of children with AIDS are known to have a parent who has AIDS or who is at risk of the disease and presumably infected with the human immunodeficiency virus (HIV). This virus may be transmitted from infected women to their offspring by three possible routes: (1) to the fetus while in the uterus through the maternal circulation, (2) to the infant during labor and delivery by contact with blood, and (3) to the infant shortly after birth through infected breast milk. The exact rate of transmission of the AIDS virus from mother to newborn is unknown, but it appears to be substantially less than 100 percent. A rough estimate of 40 to 50 percent is likely.

Since there is no current way to cure AIDS or prevent its transmission to the newborn, women who carry the AIDS virus (HIV) must be identified and counseled about the risks. Because many people infected with HIV have not developed AIDS, it is possible for a woman who feels perfectly well to pass the virus to her baby. Some hospitals have a policy of testing all pregnant women for HIV. Others recommend testing only women thought to be at high risk, such as

- Women with physical evidence of AIDS,
- Intravenous drug users,
- Women born in countries where heterosexual transmission is thought to play a major role in the transmission of the virus (including most countries of Central and East Africa, and Haiti),
- Women who have engaged in prostitution,
- Women who are or have been sexual partners of intravenous drug abusers, bisexual men, men with hemophilia, men with evidence of AIDS, or men who were born in countries where heterosexual transmission is thought to play a major role.

Rubella: Women infected with rubella (German measles) during the first trimester can infect the fetus and cause a syndrome of birth defects known as the congenital rubella syndrome. Some of the defects included in the syndrome are deafness, cataracts, congenital heart disease, and mental retardation. Since the introduction of the rubella vaccine in the late 1960s, rubella is much less common, and the congenital rubella syndrome has almost disappeared.

The rubella vaccine (p. 276) is made of a live virus and is theoretically capable of being transmitted to the fetus. Women who have not had rubella, have not been immunized, or have no evidence from a blood test that they are immune to rubella should be immunized at a time when they are certain they are not pregnant. Pregnancy should be postponed for at least three months following immunization.

What if a woman was inadvertently immunized against rubella during the first trimester of pregnancy? The Centers for Disease Control has followed 153 such women. None of their children suffered any of the defects associated with the congenital rubella syndrome. Thus, inadvertent rubella vaccination during the first trimester is not considered an automatic indication to terminate pregnancy.

Cytomegalovirus (CMV): CMV is a virus that exists throughout the world. Mothers who acquire the disease while pregnant can infect the fetus and cause a variety of congenital defects including hearing loss and mental retardation. Most women, however, have encountered the virus at some time during their lives prior to pregnancy and have acquired immunity to further infection. Since the majority of CMV infections cause no symptoms in adults, women are usually unaware of ever having had the disease. There is no medical treatment for CMV infection in adults or children. Prevention remains the best defense against the virus during pregnancy. Women who work in occupations where contact with CMV is known to be great (day-care personnel, nurses in kidney dialysis units, newborn nursery staff, and pediatric nurses) can be tested before pregnancy to see whether they have evidence of immunity. Those who have no indication of antibody (resistance) to the virus should consider transfer to another position during pregnancy. Regardless of prior exposure to the virus, all pregnant women who work with small children should practice meticulous hygiene, such as hand washing after each contact with urine and respiratory tract or other potentially infectious secretions, as well as careful handling and disposal of diapers.

Varicella-zoster (chicken pox and shingles): The varicella-zoster virus is responsible for the two different diseases, chicken pox and shingles. Approximately 95 percent of adults are immune to chicken pox because of contact with the virus during childhood. Many women, however, remain uncertain about past exposure and become concerned when there is contact during pregnancy with an infected child.

Because most pregnant women are immune to chicken pox, the disease is not very common during pregnancy. Nevertheless, if acquired during the first 20 weeks of pregnancy, it can infect the fetus and cause damage. Infection later in pregnancy probably does not harm the baby, but if a mother develops active chicken pox within a five-day period before delivery, the newborn may also be infected.

For women in doubt about prior exposure to chicken pox a blood test can reveal evidence of past infection and immunity. Pregnant women immune to chicken pox have nothing to fear if they are exposed to children with the disease. Women exposed to active chicken pox who are not immune can be treated with a drug called varicella-zoster immune globulin (VZIG). VZIG can be safely injected during pregnancy and is likely to suppress the disease if it is given within 72 hours of exposure. VZIG may also be given to a newborn exposed to chicken pox. A new vaccine is currently under development for prevention of chicken pox, but it is not yet available in the United States. A woman with active chicken pox at the time of delivery should not have contact with her child until all the skin sores (vesicles) have dried or disappeared.

Shingles: Shingles is a disease that usually affects older individuals. The same virus responsible for chicken pox, varicella-zoster, may remain dormant in nerve roots for many years. For unknown reasons, the virus can become reactivated and travel down the nerve to produce the painful sores of shingles. Shingles does not often complicate pregnancy and its effects on the fetus are not known.

Measles: Because of widespread vaccination in the United States, measles is uncommon in adults. There are, however, about 100 cases reported each year, usually in college students or foreign travelers. No clear link has been established between measles acquired during pregnancy and birth defects, but there are reports of an increased rate of miscarriage and premature birth. Vaccination is usually performed during childhood with a *live virus vaccine*. In general, vaccines made from live viruses should not be used during pregnancy.

Mumps: Mumps is an uncommon infectious disease in adults, and it is less contagious than measles or chicken pox. There is no conclusive evidence linking mumps to any specific birth defects. Because the vaccine used to prevent mumps is a live virus vaccine, it should not be given during pregnancy.

Parvovirus (Fifth disease): Parvovirus B19 causes an infectious disease called fifth disease or erythema infectiosum. The disease is most common in children. A child with fifth disease is typically healthy except for fever and a red rash on the face giving the appearance of slapped cheeks. A rash may also appear on the trunk and extremities. The disease goes away by itself and does not require treatment. Infection with parvovirus B19 can also occur in adults. Besides the rash and fever, disease in adults commonly includes painful swollen joints.

Recently, there has been some evidence that maternal infection during the first 20 weeks of pregnancy may lead to miscarriage. Fortunately, most adults were exposed to the virus sometime during childhood and are immune. It is currently estimated that the risk of miscarriage for women infected with the virus is less than 10 percent. If your child has a fever and rash, see your pediatrician or family physician to establish a diagnosis and determine whether the disease has any special significance during pregnancy.

Viral hepatitis: Viral hepatitis is an acute inflammation of the liver caused by one of several viruses. The most common of these are the hepatitis A virus and hepatitis B virus.

Hepatitis A usually has an abrupt onset with symptoms of fever, jaundice, diminished appetite, nausea, and abdominal pain. The disease is transmitted by contact with feces or oral secretions of an infected individual. The period of time one person can transmit the infection to another is usually confined to the two-week period before the infected person develops jaundice. Symptoms of hepatitis A typically begin approximately 30 days after exposure. Although hepatitis A can cause significant illness, it is not life-threatening and usually is not transmitted to the baby. The greatest risk of hepatitis A during pregnancy entails persistent nausea and vomiting and poor nutrition. There is no specific treatment for hepatitis A, but adequate rest, fluids, and appropriate nutrition are usually recommended.

Hepatitis A can be prevented or its severity minimized by an injection of immune globulin (p. 177) (previously called gamma globulin) before or immediately after exposure to the virus. Its preventative value is greatest (80 to 90 percent effective) when given early in the incubation period of the disease or before exposure to the virus. There is no evidence that immune globulin is harmful to the baby. It is recommended for the following individuals (including pregnant women):

- Travelers to Third World countries who will be eating in areas of poor sanitation or who will be visiting extensively with local people, especially children, who live in areas of poor sanitation,
- Household and sexual contacts of persons with hepatitis A,
- Staff of child day-care centers in which one or more cases of hepatitis A are recognized among children or employees or in which cases are recognized in two or more households of center attendees,
- Staff of a prison or facility for the developmentally disabled when an outbreak occurs.

Routine administration of immune globulin is *not* recommended for the following individuals:

- Office or factory workers who have had casual contact (not intimate) with an infected coworker,
- Pupils or teachers in elementary or secondary schools who have had contact with a single individual with hepatitis A, unless there is evidence of a school or classroom-centered outbreak,
- Hospital personnel, including nurses, who have cared for an individual with hepatitis A. Rather, sound hygienic practices should be emphasized.

Unlike hepatitis A, infection with the hepatitis B virus is a major worldwide cause of acute and chronic hepatitis, cirrhosis, and liver cancer. Transmission of hepatitis B around the time of delivery to the newborn of a woman with active hepatitis B can be as high as 90 percent. With currently available immune globulin and hepatitis B vaccine (p. 167), disease of the newborn can be prevented.

The hepatitis B virus is transmitted primarily by infected blood, saliva, and semen. Transmission by contact with feces is negligible. Blood transfusions, sexual contacts with numerous partners, and use of illicit intravenous drugs increase the risk of acquiring the disease. The incubation period for hepatitis B is longer than for hepatitis A, usually 60 to 90 days after exposure to an infected individual. Symptoms of hepatitis B include fever, jaundice, nausea, vomiting, abdominal pain, loss of appetite, rashes, and acute painful joints (arthritis).

Individuals at substantial risk of acquiring hepatitis B should be vaccinated to prevent the disease. Hepatitis B vaccine (p. 167) is safe for use during pregnancy, but the ideal time to receive hepatitis B vaccine is before pregnancy. Those at high risk who should be vaccinated include

- Health-care workers exposed to blood or blood products,
- Clients and staff of institutions for people who are mentally retarded,
- Patients with kidney failure receiving hemodialysis,
- Women with bisexual male partners (homosexually active women are not at increased risk of sexually transmitted hepatitis B),
- Patients with bleeding disorders who receive intravenous infusions of clotting factor concentrates,
- Household and sexual contacts of hepatitis B carriers,
- Inmates of long-term correctional facilities,
- International travelers who plan to reside more than six months in areas with high levels of endemic hepatitis B (the Centers for Disease Control in Atlanta, Georgia, publishes a list of countries with endemic hepatitis B),
- Families accepting orphans or unaccompanied minors from countries known to have endemic hepatitis B should have the children tested for the presence of hepatitis B (a simple blood test); if the result is positive, family members should be vaccinated;
- Individuals exposed to hepatitis B from an accidental stick by a needle contaminated with the blood of an individual with hepatitis B,
- Sexual partners of individuals known to carry the hepatitis B virus,
- Infants born to mothers with active hepatitis B or chronic carriers of the virus should be vaccinated immediately after birth; the vaccine is safe for newborns and is highly effective in preventing the disease.

Mononucleosis: The incidence of mononucleosis is low during pregnancy, since most women have had prior exposure and are immune. There has been no clear association between mononucleosis and birth defects. Treatment for the disease includes rest and good nutrition. Acetaminophen can be used during pregnancy to reduce fever.

Sexually Transmitted Diseases

Gonorrhea: Gonorrhea is one of the most frequently reported sexually transmitted diseases in the United States. Part of the explanation for the high incidence lies in the fact that women often harbor the infection without being aware of it. During the first trimester gonorrhea can cause infection of the fallopian tubes and even septic abortion. If gonorrhea is present at the time of delivery, the newborn can be infected, leading to eye damage and even blindness. Penicillin (p. 244) is the most commonly used drug for treatment, but several alternate antibiotic choices can be safely used during pregnancy for women allergic to penicillin.

Syphilis: The incidence of syphilis has steadily increased since 1977, and the disease remains a problem during pregnancy. Since most women with the disease have no symptoms, a blood test for syphilis is usually performed on all women during early pregnancy. Infants of mothers with untreated disease can be infected. Treatment of syphilis during the first and second trimesters with penicillin (p. 244), or erythromycin (p. 144) for patients allergic to penicillin, is virtually 100 percent effective. A few treatment failures have occurred in women treated during the third trimester, and careful follow-up of these patients is important.

Chlamydia: Chlamydia trachomatis is now the most common sexually transmitted disease in the United States. The organism can infect any of the pelvic organs and lead to infertility. Women infected with chlamydia can pass the infection to their baby during birth. In a newborn, chlamydia may cause eye infections, ear infections, pneumonia, intestinal infections, and poor weight gain.

Chlamydia infections in the mother may produce symptoms of burning during urination, painful intercourse and, occasionally, fever. A specimen from the urethra or cervix can be cultured for the organism. Treatment of chlamydia in nonpregnant women is usually accomplished with tetracycline (p. 291). However, tetracycline should not be used during pregnancy. Instead, erythromycin (p. 144) may be substituted. Male sexual partners of women infected with chlamydia should also be treated.

Genital Herpes: There are two types of herpes simplex virus. Herpes simplex virus, type 1, causes cold sores on the lips and in the mouth. Herpes simplex virus, type 2 (genital herpes), can cause sores on the labia, in the vagina, on the cervix, or around the rectum. In men type 2 virus can produce sores on the penis.

The initial infection with herpes simplex virus, called primary infection, has potentially the most devastating effects during pregnancy. During the first 20 weeks of gestation, primary infection is associated with an increased risk of miscarriage and congenital malformations. Primary infection at term poses a great risk of infection to the fetus, possibly as high as 50 percent with vaginal delivery.

Recurrence of herpes from a previous bout is the most common form of infection during pregnancy. The risk of infecting the baby during birth is much less than with primary herpes, approximately 5 percent. Nevertheless, neonatal herpes virus infection can be devastating. As many as 60 percent of infected newborns die, and about half of the surviving infants suffer permanent impairment.

The management of herpes during pregnancy has undergone considerable change in recent years. It is essential that any woman with a history of herpes virus infection make this information known to her obstetrician. It is also important to know whether any sexual partners have herpes even if a woman has no history of infection. Your physician will explain when, and if, cultures for the herpes virus will be necessary during pregnancy and before delivery. Women with active herpes, whether primary or recurrent, during labor will likely be delivered by cesarean section.

Bacterial Infections

Urinary Tract Infections: Infections of the urinary tract (the urethra, bladder, or kidneys) are common in young women. Most infections are confined to the lower urinary tract, the urethra and bladder. Many cause no pain or discomfort and are referred to as asymptomatic bacteriuria. Occasionally, however, bacteria can ascend from the bladder to one or both kidneys and cause a very serious infection of the kidney called pyelonephritis.

Asymptomatic bacteriuria is discovered from a routine urine culture performed at the initial prenatal visit. It should be treated with one of many safe antibiotics and followed up with a repeat urine culture. Symptomatic lower urinary tract infections also require treatment with an oral antibiotic and appropriate follow-up. Pyelonephritis, on the other hand, is a very serious infection that requires hospitalization and treatment with intravenous antibiotics.

Pneumonia: In the past pneumonia was responsible for a significant incidence of premature birth. With current antibiotics this is no longer the case. In many cases pneumonia can be diagnosed by a physician's examination. Occasionally, however, a chest X ray is necessary to confirm the diagnosis. A simple chest X ray can be safely performed during pregnancy with appropriate shielding of the fetus.

Toxoplasmosis

Toxoplasmosis is a parasitic disease sometimes contracted from eating raw meat or having contact with cat feces. The disease may produce no symptoms and go unnoticed, or it can cause high fever and a rash. The diagnosis is made from a special blood test. Infection with toxoplasmosis during pregnancy can result in miscarriage, stillbirth, or the birth of a child infected with the disease.

Most of the drugs used to treat toxoplasmosis are hazardous for use during pregnancy. Ideally, measures should be taken by all pregnant women to avoid the disease:

- Adequately cook all meat.
- Wash your hands after touching raw meat, and avoid touching your eyes while preparing meat.
- Wash all kitchen surfaces that come in contact with uncooked meats.
- Avoid contact with cat feces in litter boxes, and avoid gardening in soil contaminated with cat feces.

Immunizations

The single most effective means of infectious disease prevention is active vaccination. Ideally, all women should review the status of their immunizations with their doctor before becoming pregnant. The decision to vaccinate during pregnancy should be based on the relative risk of exposure to the disease, susceptibility to the disease, the stage of pregnancy, and the safety of the vaccine being considered. Some vaccines are made from killed viruses, while others are made from live inactivated viruses. Killed virus vaccines are generally thought to be safe for use during pregnancy. Live virus vaccines are best withheld during pregnancy unless absolutely needed. If a live virus vaccine is necessary, its use should be postponed until after the first trimester.

Blood Disorders

Anemia

Anemia refers to a deficiency in the number of red blood cells or hemoglobin (the oxygen-carrying component of red blood cells) in the blood. Anemia results when red blood cells are lost, as in bleeding; when they are destroyed prematurely because they are abnormally fragile; or when too few red cells are produced by the bone marrow, often because of iron deficiency.

Some degree of anemia is present in most pregnant women. A minimal decrease in the prepregnancy blood count occurs because more fluid in the circulation during pregnancy "dilutes" the red blood cells, but by far the most common cause of significant anemia is iron deficiency. Iron is an essential component in the oxygen-carrying material called hemoglobin. Most women begin pregnancy with some degree of iron deficiency due to monthly loss of blood during menstruation. Pregnancy places further demands on reserves. Therefore, iron needs must be met on a day-to-day basis or else red blood cell production will decline. In many cases diet alone is not enough to meet maternal and fetal needs. Iron supplements (ferrous sulfate, p. 185; ferrous gluconate, p. 185) may be necessary to prevent anemia.

Sickle cell anemia is an hereditary disorder characterized by abnormally shaped red blood cells. The disease primarily affects black people. In sickle cell anemia hemoglobin undergoes a chemical change in which it crystallizes and distorts the red cells to a rigid sickle shape. Sickling of red cells can occur when the oxygen content of the blood is low, when there is an acute infection, dehydration, or high fever. The abnormally shaped cells can obstruct small blood vessels and cause severe pain or bleeding.

Hemoglobin formation is controlled by genes inherited from both parents. When one sickle cell hemoglobin gene and one normal gene are inherited, the individual will be a carrier of the sickle cell trait but will usually not manifest any characteristics of the disease. If both sickle cell genes are inherited, the offspring will have sickle cell anemia. Approximately 0.3 percent of the black population in the United States suffers from the disease.

Sickle cell anemia can be associated with a variety of problems during pregnancy including severe worsening of the disease. These patients should be followed in a medical center with expert care. Many patients will require blood transfusions during pregnancy to correct severe anemia. Screening programs to detect abnormal genes are now available to identify couples who are both carriers. With this information couples can decide whether they want to assume the risk of having a baby with sickle cell anemia.

Bleeding Problems

Thrombocytopenia: Thrombocytopenia refers to a decreased number of platelets in the blood. Platelets are specialized cells in the blood that help form the clot that halts bleeding. Thrombocytopenia can result from a variety of causes including infections, drugs, a disease called systemic lupus erythematosus (p. 34), and preeclampsia, or it can occur without any apparent cause. In fact, in most cases the cause remains unknown and the condition is referred to by the long medical name, *idiopathic thrombocytopenic purpura* (ITP). Low platelets are suspected when there is prolonged bleeding from minor wounds, or easy bruising. The condition is confirmed by counting the actual number of platelets in a blood sample.

Because thrombocytopenia impairs the blood's ability to properly clot, prolonged bleeding after delivery is a risk. In some cases the fetus may also have a low platelet count and therefore be at risk of hemorrhage during birth. A corticosteroid drug (p. 119) is often used to increase platelets in the mother before delivery. Some women with persistently low platelets may require cesarean delivery rather than risk trauma to the baby during vaginal delivery.

Von Willebrand's Disease: Von Willebrand's disease is an inherited bleeding disorder of both men and women. Individuals with the disorder often have a history of prolonged bleeding after minor surgical procedures or even associated with minor wounds or lacerations. The diagnosis is made by measuring the blood level of factor VIII, an important substance in blood essential for normal clotting. Women known to have von Willebrand's disease can be treated with supplements of clotting factor before delivery to prevent hemorrhage.

Systemic Lupus Erythematosus

Systemic lupus erythematosus, usually called SLE or lupus, is an *autoimmune disease* caused by the abnormal formation of antibodies against some of the body's own tissues as if these normal tissues were harmful invaders. SLE affects women of reproductive age five to ten times more frequently than men. The disease can affect the skin causing a characteristic butterfly-shaped rash across the face, as well as other tissues including the joints, kidneys, heart, and nervous system. Although most women suffer only a mild form of the disease, at its worst SLE can lead to kidney failure or other severe disabling problems.

The effect of pregnancy on SLE is not completely understood. It is, however, known that pregnant women with SLE face a greater risk of miscarriage or premature birth. Rarely, children born to women with SLE can have an abnormality of the heart's electrical conduction system, called complete heart block. Offspring of women with SLE can also be born with a rash suggestive of SLE, called neonatal lupus. The rash usually disappears within six months.

SLE is usually treated with a corticosteroid drug (p. 119) or a drug that blocks the body's immune system called azathioprine (p. 85). Patients with SLE treated with these drugs before pregnancy should usually continue them during pregnancy unless advised otherwise by their physician. Women treated with a corticosteroid drug will usually have the dosage increased during labor and for several days following delivery.

Rheumatoid Arthritis

Rheumatoid arthritis is a potentially disabling form of arthritis that may affect women of reproductive age. The joints of both hands and wrists are most often involved, but other joints may also be affected. For unknown reasons up to 75 percent of women with rheumatoid arthritis demonstrate significant improvement in joint pain and swelling during pregnancy. Unfortunately, symptoms usually recur within two months after delivery.

The most commonly used drug to treat rheumatoid arthritis is aspirin (p. 82) in a dosage of six to eight tablets each day. In this disease aspirin is not just for relief of pain. It actually controls inflammation within the joints. Most physicians believe that aspirin may be safely used in women with rheumatoid arthritis throughout pregnancy. Since the disease often improves during pregnancy, it may be possible to reduce the dosage. Another group of medications used to treat rheumatoid arthritis called nonsteroidal anti-inflammatory drugs (e.g., indomethacin p. 179, ibuprofen p. 175, naproxen p. 232, sulindac p. 285, and others) are usually avoided during pregnancy. Occasionally the disease is so severe that treatment with corticosteroids (p. 119) is necessary. In all cases adequate rest and physical therapy should be maximized in order to avoid or reduce the dosage of medications during pregnancy.

Skin Problems

The interaction of pregnancy and the skin is conveniently categorized into normal changes associated with pregnancy, abnormal conditions unique to pregnancy, and preexisting conditions that may be affected by pregnancy. Several normal skin changes occur during pregnancy:

- Chloasma or "mask of pregnancy" refers to areas of increased skin pigment involving the forehead, bridge of the nose, and cheeks.

This usually disappears after pregnancy. A strong sun block should be used during the summer to prevent further darkening.

- Palmar erythema or red palms is commonly associated with pregnancy and is due to the increased levels of estrogen in the blood. It goes away after pregnancy and does not require treatment.
- Linea nigra refers to a dark line that occurs from the pubic bone to the umbilicus and remains throughout pregnancy. Similar darkening occurs of the areola, the area around the nipple.
- Striae or stretch marks develop in about 90 percent of pregnant women. They usually fade after delivery but may never go away completely.
- Hair and nail changes occur in virtually all pregnancies. During pregnancy hair growth may increase and hair may be unusually thick. Soon after pregnancy, however, there may be extensive hair loss lasting up to a year. Hair loss is not permanent. It will return to normal within a year or sooner. Nails may become brittle or grooved during pregnancy, but will return to normal following delivery.

A variety of skin rashes occur only during pregnancy. Some of these conditions can be very significant and should be brought to the attention of a dermatologist. Other common conditions such as acne require a change in the medications used before pregnancy. Neither topical medications nor pills containing tetracycline (p. 291) should be used to treat acne during pregnancy. Furthermore, it is essential that the drug isotretinoin (brand name Accutane p. 187) not be used during pregnancy. It causes birth defects. This drug should not be used to treat acne in any young woman capable of becoming pregnant. Topical medications that contain corticosteroids should be used only under a physician's care.

Neurologic Problems

Headaches

The most common type of headaches—tension or muscular contraction headaches—are no more or less frequent during pregnancy. They can usually be managed effectively with rest, massage, stress reduction, or acetaminophen (p. 63). It is best to avoid tranquilizers.

Migraine, or vascular, headaches often diminish in severity and frequency during pregnancy. For those who continue to suffer migraines during pregnancy, treatment with some medications must be altered. Ergotamine drugs (p. 143) should generally be avoided because they can stimulate contractions of the uterus. Most infrequent migraines may be safely treated with acetaminophen (p. 63) or codeine (p. 118).

Epilepsy

Epilepsy is a general term for at least 30 chronic disorders of the brain characterized by periods of impaired consciousness or convulsions. The most common types of epilepsy are grand mal seizures and petit mal seizures. The grand mal variety involve loss of consciousness, spasms of the muscles, and rapid jerking of various body parts. The beginning of a grand mal seizure is often heralded by a so-called aura, a peculiar feeling in the stomach, flashes of light, noises in the ear, or vertigo. Petit mal seizures are brief attacks of impaired consciousness. They may be little more than a subtle "tuning out" of the environment.

Most forms of epilepsy can be effectively managed with currently available medications (phenytoin, p. 252, phenobarbital, p. 247, carbamazepine, p. 98, primidone, p. 260, ethosuximide, p. 146, valproic acid, p. 313). Many of these, however, have been associated with birth defects when taken during pregnancy. All women with a history of epilepsy should consult a neurologist before pregnancy to discuss their current medication program and its potential effect on pregnancy. If a woman has been free of seizures for several years, her physician may want to consider discontinuing medications for a period of time before she attempts to conceive. Some patients who remain free of seizures can complete pregnancy without medications. Women who continue to have seizures, however, should not stop their medications. Grand mal seizures may be associated with birth defects even if no drug was taken. If medications must be taken, they should be given in a sufficient, but not excessive, dosage. Ideally, the least number of drugs necessary to control seizures should be taken. It is necessary to change the dosage of many of these medications as pregnancy progresses. The exact dosage can best be determined by measuring the level of medication in the blood. Never stop taking your medications without medical advice.

Multiple Sclerosis

Multiple sclerosis (MS) is a chronic disease of the central nervous system characterized by the degeneration and loss of myelin, an insulating substance that covers nerves and is necessary for normal transmission of electrical impulses. Symptoms of MS range from mild, transient loss of sensation to severe weakness or paralysis, impaired sensation, and visual problems. The disease is particularly common in young adults between the ages of 20 and 40.

MS can have a variable course during pregnancy. Some patients notice an improvement in symptoms, particularly during the third trimester. A return of symptoms, however, is common following delivery. In the past it was thought that the disease becomes worse after pregnancy, but more recent studies have not confirmed this observation. Birth defects do not occur more frequently in the offspring of women with MS. There is no specific treatment for MS. Acute attacks are traditionally managed with rest and a brief course of corticosteroids (p. 119).

Cancer

Of all the complications of pregnancy, none can be more devastating to the expectant mother, her family, and her physician than cancer. The very word conjures up visions of a wasted, pain-ridden, dying mother, a motherless child, and a grieving family. Fortunately, this image is often wrong. With the advent of successful anticancer drugs, many malignancies can be cured or at least put in remission. One of the most frequently asked questions, and one of the most difficult to answer is, "What are the effects of chemotherapy on the developing fetus?" Some answers are currently available.

Most anticancer drugs act on dividing cells. Since the fetus contains a high proportion of dividing cells, one would expect significant effects of such drugs on the developing fetus. The fetus is particularly vulnerable during the first trimester during the period of organ formation when birth defects are most likely to occur. What is also clear, however, is that the DNA repair mechanisms in the fetus have a remarkable capacity to repair chromosomal injuries after the first trimester. In recent years experience has mounted suggesting that some anticancer drugs can be administered during the second and third trimesters without apparent harm to the baby. Yet it must be remembered that the long-term effects of anticancer medications on offspring of mothers treated during pregnancy have not been determined. Absolutely no assurance can as yet be given that a child exposed to chemotherapy in the uterus will have continued normal growth and development. In general, the risk of birth defects in children exposed to anticancer drugs during the first trimester should be considered high. All patients should have expert counseling regarding these risks before deciding to continue pregnancy.

Psychiatric Disorders

Many psychiatric problems can be effectively managed with counseling, but many psychotic disorders cannot be properly controlled without medications. Virtually all drugs used to treat psychotic disorders cross the placenta and are taken up by the fetus. The nature of these drugs is that they affect the brain of the mother and the developing fetus. Since the brain develops throughout pregnancy, drugs that directly affect the central nervous system have potential for harm during each trimester. If discontinuation of a psychiatric drug predisposes a woman to severe psychotic symptoms, the physician must carefully weigh the dangers of the psychotic process against the potential harm to the baby. Antipsychotic medications are excreted into breast milk and are capable of causing profound behavioral and neurologic side effects in the newborn. Mothers who must take these medications are usually discouraged from breastfeeding their newborns.

Environmental and Occupational Hazards during Pregnancy

Potential hazards to reproductive health may be found virtually anywhere—in the home, the environment, and the workplace. Among them are chemicals, drugs, infectious agents, ionizing radiation, and physical factors such as heat, cold, noise, and injury. Workers, both men and women, have two principal concerns related to their reproductive health—exposure to substances that can increase the difficulty of conception and exposure to substances that can endanger the health and development of their offspring. Concerns may be further complicated by fear for job security and loss of income.

If you are planning a pregnancy, carefully evaluate your home and workplace for possible chemical hazards. Initially, any substance should be suspected, even though most will turn out to be safe. If you have been unable to become pregnant, if your partner suspects he may be infertile, if you've had several miscarriages, or if you've had a child with a birth defect, be particularly suspicious. If you have concerns about your workplace, you and your physician should discuss with your employer the best way to avoid hazardous substances while allowing you to remain on the job without compromising productivity.

You have a right to know and your employer has an obligation to inform you of any substance that might be harmful to reproduction. If you've been exposed to chemicals at work or at home and later find out you are pregnant, don't panic. Risk depends on the amount and time of exposure, and potentially harmful substances may well have no effect on you or your baby. Discuss this exposure with your physician, and provide as much information as you possibly can. Try to obtain the exact name of any chemical, and if possible bring in actual container labels or product information. Attempt to quantify the amount of exposure, the duration of exposure, and what safety precautions were used (gloves, special clothing, hoods, ventilation, etc.). The date of your last menstrual period will be very important in helping your physician determine the stage of pregnancy during which the exposure took place. (If you are not certain of the date of your last menstrual period, an ultrasound test done during the first trimester can accurately determine the age of pregnancy.) Although no physician can guarantee with 100 percent certainty that no harm has occurred, in most cases you will be reassured to discover that the risk, if any, is very slight. In addition, there are tests and procedures that can be performed to see whether the baby is all right.

Far too often occupational reproductive hazards have been viewed as a "woman's problem" and "corrected" by removing the worker from her job. You cannot legally be fired from your job merely because of pregnancy. The 1978 Pregnancy Discrimination Act, an amendment to Title VII of the 1964 Civil Rights Act, requires that pregnant women must be treated the same as other employees and applicants for employment when an employer determines their probable ability or inability to perform a job. This law protects a woman from being fired or refused a job or promotion merely because she is pregnant. A woman unable to work for pregnancy-related reasons is entitled to disability benefits, sick leave, and health insurance (except for abortions) just like employees disabled for other medical reasons. Pregnant workers temporarily unable to perform their jobs must be treated in the same manner as other disabled workers, such as modifying the task, changing the work assignment, granting disability leave or leave without pay.

Work is not the only place you might encounter potentially hazardous substances, though. There are chemicals right at home that should be used with care. No scientific studies have proven that the occasional inhalation of ordinary household cleansers has any harmful effects during pregnancy, but common sense should tell you to avoid using oven cleaners and dry-cleaning solvents whose labels warn of their danger during pregnancy. Wear gloves when using any strong cleaner. If a household product has a strong odor or fumes, don't breathe it in directly. Use it in a well-ventilated area, or don't use it at all. Most important, never mix ammonia with chlorine-based products: You can create a very toxic chlorine gas.

This chapter presents some, but by no means all, of the common hazards pregnant women encounter in the environment, workplace, and home. In most cases little more is needed than awareness of the potential hazards and some simple avoidance measures. Common sense will take you a long way.

Despite the deluge of warnings in the media about everything from the air we breathe to water from the tap, there has never been a safer time to have a baby. Rather than quit your job because there are chemicals around, discuss the risks openly with your physician and employer. In most cases simple adjustments can be made to keep your employer happy while you remain on the job throughout most of your pregnancy.

Rather than avoid fresh fruits and vegetables for fear of insecticides, wash them carefully with detergent and water before eating. And rather than risking your health and your baby's by refusing an X-ray examination, understand the minimal risk of diagnostic X rays and ultrasound as well as their potential benefit for diagnosing serious medical illnesses. In short, never expose yourself or your baby to any unnecessary drug or chemical, yet understand that the vast majority of common substances in our homes and workplaces have been used by generations of pregnant women without harm.

Type of Exposure: Air Pollution

POTENTIAL HAZARDS: Carbon monoxide, ozone

COMMON SOURCES OF EXPOSURE: Residents of urban areas with high pollution; bus, taxi, and other vehicle drivers; some airline workers; workers in poorly ventilated buildings; chronic cigarette smokers

SPECIAL CONCERNS DURING PREGNANCY: Carbon monoxide can rapidly enter the bloodstream, firmly attach to red blood cells, and prevent the uptake of oxygen by red blood cells. Carbon monoxide also diffuses across the placenta reaching levels in the fetus that may actually exceed its mother's by 10 to 15 percent. In very high concentrations carbon monoxide has clearly been associated with fetal harm. Reproductive studies in rats exposed to high concentrations of carbon monoxide have demonstrated decreased birth weight, increased risk of miscarriage and stillbirth, and in some instances, birth defects and brain damage. However, even in our most polluted cities you are not likely to be exposed to such high concentrations. Since the amount of exposure necessary to cause harm during human pregnancy is not known, prudence dictates avoiding those settings where carbon monoxide levels are likely to be very high.

Ozone is both a normal constituent of the earth's upper atmosphere and potentially a hazardous substance in the air we breathe. In cities prone to high pollution, such as Los Angeles, ozone levels on high-pollution days may reach 0.1 parts per million (ppm). Fortunately, research has shown that exposure of laboratory rats to ozone in concentrations as high as 2 ppm (20 times the amount in the air on a very polluted day) does not cause birth defects. Although the exact risk to human fetuses remains unknown, the usual urban levels of ozone do not appear to place the fetus at special risk.

Other less common gases can pollute the air of factories, plants, and even hospitals. In most situations ensuring adequate ventilation will prevent any harm to mother and baby.

PRECAUTIONS:

- Avoid cigarette smoke. If you smoke, stop! Encourage other smokers in the family to stop, or at least to refrain from smoking in your presence. Avoid smoke-filled rooms for extended, repeated periods. Although "passive" exposure to cigarette smoke has not been shown to cause harm, it can't be good.
- If a high-pollution alert is called in your city, stay indoors as much as possible, and certainly avoid vigorous outdoor exercise.
- Be sure your car is in good repair, especially the exhaust system. Never run the car in a closed garage.
- If there is any concern about the possibility of a faulty home heating system, ask your local utility company to check the level of carbon monoxide in your home.
- Insist that your work area is well ventilated, especially if you suspect potentially toxic vapors may enter the air.

Type of Exposure: Food Additives and Contaminants

POTENTIAL HAZARDS: Food dyes; artificial sweeteners; preservatives; contaminants; naturally occurring toxic foods

COMMON SOURCES OF EXPOSURE: There are basically two ways by which chemicals that are not a natural part of food enter what we eat: (1) by deliberate addition for the purpose of color, preservation, or taste enhancement; or (2) by accidental contamination with substances such as diethylstilbestrol (DES) and polychlorinated biphenyls (PCBs).

SPECIAL CONCERNS DURING PREGNANCY: Food dyes have long been the source of considerable controversy. No food dye has come under closer scrutiny or criticism than Red Dye Number 2, a dye formerly used in soft drinks, gelatins, cereals, candy, lipsticks, and pill coatings. Before the dye was removed from the market, it was accused of causing birth defects and cancer in laboratory animals. More recent studies have not been able to confirm the alleged toxicity of Red Dye Number 2. Similarly, none of the dyes currently used to color food have been shown to cause birth defects in humans.

The most commonly used artificial sweeteners in the United States are aspartame (p. 81) and saccharin. Questions are commonly raised about their safety during pregnancy. Saccharin has been shown to cross the placenta, but it is not known if this poses any special risk for the baby. Still, most physicians and dieticians recommend avoiding saccharin during pregnancy.

The artificial sweetener aspartame is composed of two chemicals, aspartate and phenylalanine. Aspartate seems to be of little concern during pregnancy because it does not cross the placenta. Phenylalanine does cross the placenta, but it is unlikely that eating or drinking a moderate amount (such as one can of diet soda or one serving of aspartame sweetened dessert per day) would be harmful. New artificial sweeteners are now being introduced into the U.S. market. Acesulfame potassium (Sunette brand) is a new calorie-free sweetener that reportedly has no adverse reproductive effects in laboratory animals. Its safety during human pregnancy has not been established.

Sodium nitrite, a food preservative, has come under fire because it is converted by bacteria in the intestine to nitrosamines. Nitrosamines are of concern because they can cause mutations and cancer in rats, chicks, and hamsters. As is the case with many chemicals, however, the dosage necessary to produce harm in laboratory animals is considerably greater than any imaginable human ingestion. One of the highest dietary sources of nitrosamines is beer, which should be avoided during pregnancy for many reasons (see alcohol, p. 67). Other foods preserved with nitrites include frankfurters, salami, bacon, luncheon meats, and smoked meats and fish.

Another possible food contaminant is diethylstilbestrol (DES). This hormone was once used to fatten beef and poultry, but no longer. Today, we are aware of the potential harm of DES during pregnancy because for a time it was given to pregnant women to prevent threatened miscarriage (see p. 132). Later it was discovered that the drug not only failed to prevent miscarriage but caused birth defects, cancer and reproductive problems in the offspring.

A potentially serious source of food contamination comes from a group of compounds called polychlorinated biphenyls (PCBs). Careless disposal of these industrial toxins has contaminated soil and water systems throughout the country. Over the past few decades these substances have entered the food chain primarily through fish and other animals fed fish meal (e,g,, chickens). In humans, the most extensive information on the effects of PCB exposure during pregnancy comes from two episodes of PCB poisonings in rice oil in Japan in 1968 and in Taiwan in 1979. In both cases, cooking oil was accidentally contaminated with large amounts of PCBs. Abnormalities associated with these poisonings included cola-colored discoloration of the skin and nails, and lower than expected birth weight. Nearly all the exposed mothers exhibited evidence of poisoning as well. After delivery the babies demonstrated "catch-up" growth, and skin discoloration slowly disappeared.

PCBs are difficult to avoid entirely, but a few simple rules will help limit exposure. Since PCBs are stored in animal fat, carefully trim fat and skin. As a general rule ocean fish such as tuna, sea bass, flounder, sole, and snapper are relatively free of PCBs, but many freshwater fish from contaminated waterways, such as Lake Michigan and the St. Lawrence Seaway, can have significant concentrations of PCBs.

Pesticides (see p. 52) remain a source of significant concern when they enter our grains, drinking water, and even the tissues of animals. However, with the exception of only a few herbicides (agents used to kill unwanted plants), studies have not been able to link most pesticides to fetal harm. This is the kind of reassurance that tends to comfort manufacturers and even some scientists, but offers little solace to pregnant women. Whenever possible, it is still best to avoid these substances by carefully washing fresh fruits and vegetables.

PRECAUTIONS: Is any food safe to eat during pregnancy? Clearly, the answer is yes, but some thoughtful selection should reduce even the small risk of harm from food contamination:

- Whenever possible, use fresh fruits and vegetables, and wash them thoroughly in a detergent bath before cooking or eating. Fresh foods not only help avoid questionable ingredients but also provide better nutritional value.
- Choose products free of artificial coloring and flavoring.
- Limit your intake of artificial sweeteners.

- Avoid foods preserved with nitrates and nitrites such as hot dogs, salami, smoked meats and fish, and luncheon meats.
- Avoid alcohol.
- Eat only the lean cuts of meats. Chemicals given to livestock are primarily stored in fat and organ meats.
- Avoid freshwater game fish, or at least check with the local Environmental Protection Agency (EPA) to find out if local fish are contaminated with PCBs.
- Do not assume that products labeled "natural" or "organic" are guaranteed safe. Such labels are often little more than a marketing gimmick.
- Many potentially toxic substances from food can enter breast milk. Be just as careful about your diet during breastfeeding as you were during pregnancy.

Type of Exposure: Hyperthermia (Excessive Heat)

COMMON SOURCES OF EXPOSURE: Hot tubs, saunas, prolonged high fever, possibly some work environments, and possibly extreme, prolonged exercise

SPECIAL CONCERNS DURING PREGNANCY: Hyperthermia has been suspected of causing birth defects when the temperature of the uterus exceeds 104° F for at least one day during weeks three to seven of gestation. In the absence of a severe infection, such high fever is very rare and in most cases fever above 102° F can be reduced with regular use of acetaminophen (p. 63) or a cool bath. Normal, nonpregnant women have been tested in hot tubs and saunas to see how much exposure was necessary to raise their body temperature to 102° F. None of the 20 women in this study was able to remain in the sauna long enough to raise her body temperature to 102° F. It is unlikely then, that pregnant workers would remain in a work environment sufficiently hot to raise their temperatures high enough to cause harm to their babies. Prolonged, intense exercise can also raise body temperature. Consequently, exercise should be kept moderate during pregnancy.

Hyperthermia has long been known to have adverse effects on sperm production in men. Infertile couples should consider this possibility when undergoing a medical evaluation for the source of their problem.

PRECAUTIONS:

- Although hot tubs, saunas, or steam baths are unlikely to raise your body temperature to dangerous levels, it is best to avoid them during the first trimester. If you sat in a hot tub before you found out you were pregnant, there is very little chance of any harm to the baby.
- Be sure to have a thermometer at home and report any temperature over 100° F to your physician. Both the fever and the cause of the fever are important. Temperatures less than 104° F are unlikely to cause any harm. In most cases acetaminophen (p. 63) can be safely taken throughout pregnancy to reduce the temperature. A cool bath may also be helpful.
- Exercise moderately. Pregnancy is not the time to participate in extremely vigorous or competitive sports. Try to exercise during the coolest part of the day and always be sure to drink sufficient fluids to prevent dehydration.
- Although it is very unlikely that your workplace will be hot enough to raise your temperature to dangerous levels, make every attempt to ensure a comfortable environment.

Type of Exposure: Hospital and Health-care Hazards

POTENTIAL HAZARDS:: Infections, drugs and chemicals, anesthetic gases, X rays, physical injury, emotional stress

SPECIAL CONCERNS DURING PREGNANCY: More than 2.3 million women work in hospitals and another 4.5 million in other health-care services. Pregnant health-care workers face several unusual risks as a direct result of their occupation. Health-care providers are frequently exposed to infectious diseases of all types. Exposure may come in the form of direct patient contact, accidental laboratory contamination, direct contact with patients' blood and other body fluids, and respiratory transmission of bacteria due to poor ventilation. Infections of particular concern to pregnant workers include hepatitis A and B (p. 27), rubella (p. 25), influenza (p. 23), cytomegalovirus (CMV, p. 25), parvovirus B19 (p. 27), chicken pox (p. 25), tuberculosis (p. 311), and AIDS (p. 24). Although it may be true that many healthcare workers have immunity to certain infectious agents that protects them from some diseases, nothing less than the strictest sterile technique should be used whenever caring for patients with communicable diseases.

Hospital workers also are exposed to a wide variety of drugs, and chemicals used for cleaning, sterilizing, and lab analysis. Of particular concern is the risk of preparing and administering chemotherapy to patients with cancer. Many such drugs are known to cause infertility, birth defects, and fetal loss.

Anesthetic gases, such as nitrous oxide, have been implicated in the cause of miscarriage and birth defects. Measures must be taken to ensure appropriate ventilation in operating rooms to minimize exposure of pregnant operating room personnel to these vapors.

Exposure to X rays (see p. 55) has long been a concern to pregnant women. In most cases the risk of Xray exposure to hospital personnel is minimal and unlikely to adversely affect the baby.

Nurses and other health-care workers also are known to have a high rate of injury. Hazards contributing to this high accident rate include electrical hazards from the extensive use of monitoring equipment, needle sticks, falls suffered on slippery floors, and injury due to moving heavy equipment. Pregnancy may increase this risk even further as the growing uterus makes it more difficult to get close enough to equipment and patients for proper lifting.

PRECAUTIONS:

- Hospitals must assess the effectiveness of control measures for handling toxic medications and chemicals. For example, exposure to ethylene oxide and other toxic gases can be minimized by complete evacuation of sterilizer units before opening, use of aeration cabinets and catalytic converters, and careful equipment maintenance.
- Infection control procedures should be developed to ensure appropriate gown and glove technique and careful handling of potentially infectious body fluids.
- Hospitals must provide adequate ventilation in infectious disease units and operating rooms.
- X-ray equipment must be regularly maintained to ensure minimal emission of scattered radiation and appropriate shielding for all employees should be used.
- Work shifts should be of reasonable length and punctuated by sufficient rest to minimize stress and maintain the highest standards of patient care.
- Dangerous drugs and chemicals should be clearly labeled. Direct contact with chemotherapeutic drugs should be avoided during pregnancy or at least during the first trimester.
- In the vast majority of cases it is not reasonable to arbitrarily

exclude women of childbearing potential from potentially hazardous health-care jobs. Hospital administrators, physicians, nurses, and worker groups should be able to develop and implement safe policies and procedures for pregnant workers.

Type of Exposure: Solvents and Cleaners

POTENTIAL HAZARDS: Acetone, benzene, carbon tetrachloride, chloroform, dimethyl sulfoxide (DMSO), gasoline, methyl ethyl ketone, tetrachloroethylene, toluene, vinyl chloride, xylene

COMMON SOURCES OF EXPOSURE: Domestic workers and janitors (homes, hotels, motels, office buildings), professional launderers and dry cleaners, painters, hairdressers and cosmetologists, hospital personnel

SPECIAL CONCERNS DURING PREGNANCY: Concerns about exposure during pregnancy to organic solvents and cleaners are common, whether these substances come from industrial sources or household cleaners, paints, thinners, or a multitude of other products. Many of these chemicals have proven harmful in laboratory animals, but their effects during human pregnancy are not fully understood. Much of the information known about the hazards of organic solvents comes from the outcome of pregnancies where women deliberately abused solvents in the form of sniffing gasoline, glue, fingernail polish remover, paint thinner, lighter fluid, and others. Such abusive behavior has been reported to cause birth defects, miscarriages, and growth retardation of the fetus. The effects of chronic lower-level exposures to organic solvents is only now beginning to be investigated. Since many cleaning products have been in common use for decades and no link has ever been established between normal use of household cleaners and birth defects, it is unlikely that disinfecting your toilet or polishing your furniture will in any way harm your baby. Even occasional inadvertent inhalation of solvent vapors is not likely to be harmful.

PRECAUTIONS:

- Pay attention to your nose. If something has a strong, caustic odor, avoid directly inhaling it.
- Clean and paint in a well-ventilated area large enough to let fumes dissipate. Use latex rather than oil-based paints.

- Paint strippers can emit toxic fumes and should be avoided or used only in a well-ventilated area.
- Wear gloves when you're cleaning.
- If your clothing becomes contaminated with chemicals, wash them before wearing them again.
- Use pump sprays instead of aerosols.
- If possible, avoid strong oven cleaners and dry-cleaning agents during pregnancy.
- Heat a small bowl of ammonia in the oven overnight, then wip with a damp cloth and baking soda.
- Never mix ammonia with chlorine-based products. The combination produces abundant toxic chlorine gas fumes.

Type of Exposure: Heavy Metals

POTENTIAL HAZARDS: Lead, methyl mercury, lithium, selenium, arsenic, cadmium, and copper

COMMON SOURCES OF EXPOSURE:

Lead: Makers of batteries, ceramics, enamels, glass, lubricants, paints, pigments, and enamels; brass founders; painters; insecticide workers; plumbers; solderers

Methyl mercury: Makers of disinfectants and fungicides; seed handlers; wood preservers

SPECIAL CONCERNS DURING PREGNANCY: Of all classes of chemical compounds, the heavy metals are said to have the greatest potential for causing birth defects, miscarriage, and mental retardation. Heavy metal compounds that are definitely harmful to the human fetus include lead and methyl mercury. Other metals suspected of causing harm include lithium, selenium, arsenic, cadmium, and copper.

Lead has clearly been shown to cause an increased rate of miscarriages, birth defects, low birth weight, brain damage, mental retardation, and convulsions. At the turn of the century, the ability of lead to induce abortions was well known and was used illegally to terminate unwanted pregnancies. The abortion rate was high, but so was maternal toxicity, including brain damage and blindness. Lead is also capable of impairing sperm production.

Methyl mercury is used to prevent the growth of fungi on grain seed, and many accidental poisonings have occurred when contaminated grain was inadvertently consumed. In 1953 mercury compounds used as catalysts in a plastics plant in Japan at Minimata Bay were dumped into the bay. About 700 cases of human poisonings were recorded including many pregnant women. Many of the infants of exposed pregnant women suffered brain damage, convulsions, mental retardation, and blindness. This constellation of abnormalities has since become known as Minimata disease. Clearly, methyl mercury is one of the most potent of all fetal toxins.

PRECAUTIONS:

- Use only latex paints and paint in an open, well-ventilated area.
- Although lead- and arsenic-based paints are seldom used any longer, such paints are still on walls painted many years ago. Be very careful when removing old paint. It may contain significant amounts of lead.
- Many ceramic dishes and cups are made with significant amounts of lead, especially some European ceramic dishes. Simple kits are available to test dishes for lead content.
- If you're concerned that your drinking water is contaminated by lead from the pipes, have the lead content of your water tested.
- Methyl mercury is not a common contaminant of food or water. Nevertheless, if mercury contamination is suspected in grain seed or in the water supply, avoid exposure until a responsible agency can ensure there is no danger.

Type of Exposure: Pesticides (Includes Insecticides, Herbicides, Fungicides)

POTENTIAL HAZARDS:

Insecticides: Aldrin, DDT, DDE, dieldrin, heptachlorepoxide, lindane (the most popular insecticide for indoor use), malathion, parathion, toxaphene (the most heavily applied outdoor insecticide in the United States), zectran

Herbicides: 2,4-D (the most widely used herbicide), "agent orange" (used as a defoliant in Vietnam), 2,3,7,8-tetrachlorodibenzo-p-dioxin (TCDD)

Fungicides: Captan, cycloheximide, ethylene oxide, folpet

COMMON SOURCES OF EXPOSURE: Contaminated vegetables, grains, and water, and some animal meat (particularly fat and skin), direct contact through farming and gardening, and exposure during manufacturing and distribution

SPECIAL CONCERNS DURING PREGNANCY: In few other areas do economic issues and concern for the unborn come into such direct conflict. The importance of pesticides in American agriculture is vast. Use of chemical pesticides in the United States has increased tenfold during the past 30 years. The pesticide industry uses approximately 1,400 active ingredients in an estimated 60,000 products available worldwide.

Animal studies using very intense exposure to pesticides have demonstrated abnormal growth and some birth defects in the offspring of exposed mothers. Similarly, observations of human populations accidentally exposed to pesticides (e.g., lindane exposure in Love Canal, New York; dioxin exposure in Times Beach, Missouri; agent orange exposure in Vietnam; and TCDD exposure in Alsea, Oregon, and in New Zealand) have suggested, but not proven, that these chemicals can increase the risk of miscarriage, stillbirth, birth defects, and growth retardation when pregnant women (or in some cases their husbands) are exposed to extraordinarily high concentrations. At present no conclusive studies have demonstrated a significant risk during pregnancy associated with the usual levels of pesticides to which we are exposed in foods and by direct contact. On the other hand, their safety is far from assured, and avoidance should be the rule. Also, remember that some pesticides can interfere with normal sperm production, resulting in infertility.

PRECAUTIONS:

- Wash all fruits and vegetables thoroughly in a bath of liquid detergent.
- Although some moths and insects may offend your aesthetic sense, it may be safer to live with them for a few months than to eliminate them with insecticide sprays. Insect traps such as roach "motels" appear to be safe. Also cockroaches and ants can be effectively killed with boric acid (safe unless ingested) sprinkled in troublesome areas.
- If tree spraying is in progress in your neighbor's yard, stay inside with the windows closed until the smell of chemicals has disappeared.
- Pull weeds or use soapy water rather than weed-killing sprays.

- If your work places you in constant contact with pesticides, consider a change of duties and location during pregnancy.

Type of Exposure: Physical Exertion

SPECIAL CONCERNS DURING PREGNANCY: Studies suggest that a woman's aerobic capacity does not change during pregnancy, except during the last few months. However, the ability to lift heavy objects will be altered during later pregnancy as the center of gravity shifts and as the expanding abdomen prevents objects from being lifted close to the body. In addition, ligaments and joints become more relaxed during pregnancy, making lifting potentially more hazardous. Low back injury appears to be particularly common among pregnant workers who lift heavy loads or stand for prolonged periods.

Recently, researchers have studied the effect of heavy lifting and strenuous exercise on pregnancy outcome. Some studies have suggested that prolonged standing and strenuous activity during the last half of gestation increase the risk of premature birth and may result in newborns that are smaller than average.

PRECAUTIONS:

- For at least the first half of pregnancy women can continue activities to which they are accustomed, but pregnancy is not the time to begin strenuous activities.
- Whether or not it is safe to continue strenuous activities until the time you deliver should be determined by you and your physician, taking into account the requirements of your job, your general health status, any complications of pregnancy such as high blood pressure, premature uterine contractions, excessive weight gain or fluid retention, and other health problems.
- The American Medical Association has issued guidelines that suggest women who work at jobs requiring more than four hours a day on their feet should quit by the twenty-fourth week, and that those who must stand for 30 minutes out of each hour should quit by the thirty-second week. It has also been recommended that women not remain at jobs that require lifting, climbing stairs or ladders, or bending below waist level past the twentieth week if this work is intensive, and past the twenty-eighth week if it is moderate. Nevertheless, many physicians will permit women in good health with uncomplicated pregnancies to work longer.
- As long as you remain on the job, take frequent breaks. Stand up

and walk around if you've been sitting; sit down with your feet elevated if you've been standing.

- Listen to your body. Stop work and rest if you become fatigued.
- If you must stand for prolonged periods, resting one foot on a stool or box with the knee slightly bent will help prevent back pain.
- Avoid strenuous recreation when you are not working. Enlist the family or hire domestic help to assist with household chores ("It's doctor's orders.").
- Whenever possible lie on your left side during breaks. Resting in this position aids blood flow from the legs to the heart.
- If possible, reduce your hours or your workload during the last trimester.
- Despite your plans to work until the day you deliver, be realistic. Develop contingency plans for the possibility that complications may force you to quit working earlier than you'd like.

Type of Exposure: Radiation, Microwaves, and Ultrasound

COMMON SOURCES OF EXPOSURE:

Radiation: Patients exposed to diagnostic or therapeutic radiation; X-ray technicians; nurses; physicians; video display terminal (VDT) users

Microwaves: Individuals working near FM radio stations, radar, and microwave ovens

Ultrasound: Patients exposed to diagnostic ultrasound; ultrasound technicians; nurses; physicians

SPECIAL CONCERNS DURING PREGNANCY: Few words strike more fear into the hearts of pregnant women than *radiation*. Confusion about the effects and hazards of radiation begin with misunderstanding of the word itself. Too often the term *radiation* is incorrectly applied equally to X rays, microwaves, and ultrasound. Actually, these three forms of energy have quite different biologic effects and risks.

Ionizing Radiation: Radiation, or more correctly, ionizing radiation is a powerful natural force that relates to the release of energy from atoms. Its power has been harnessed by scientists for such diverse purposes as medical diagnosis and treatment, power plants, and nuclear warheads. Much of our fear of radiation comes from its association with bombs and nuclear waste. To be sure, ionizing radiation can cause harm to the fetus. The good news is that radiation has probably been studied more extensively than any other environmental hazard. Information about reproductive hazards comes from animal studies, pregnant women exposed to low levels of diagnostic radiation, and those Japanese women and their offspring exposed to massive radiation following the bombings during World War II. Years of study and research have determined that there is no harm to the fetus if levels of radiation remain below 5 rads (rads are the units used to measure radiation). Even if your physician or dentist orders several X-ray examinations, you and your baby will be exposed to far less than 1 rad. In fact, there is virtually no radiation exposure to the baby when it is properly shielded with a lead apron placed over your abdomen. Certainly, no X-ray studies should be performed during pregnancy (or even if you might be pregnant) unless they are absolutely necessary. Nevertheless, the Committee on Radiology of the American Academy of Pediatrics says that because the possibility of birth defects resulting from X-ray exposure during pregnancy is extremely low, even abdominal X-ray examination need not be postponed if it is genuinely needed. If you had an X ray at a time when you didn't know you were pregnant, don't spend time worrying. There is no significant risk to the baby.

On the other hand, large dosages of radiation used for the purpose of treating cancer often exceed several thousand rads and may harm the baby. Pregnant women who must undergo therapeutic radiation for cancer should discuss the risks with their physician and consider either postponing therapy until after pregnancy or terminating pregnancy.

Microwaves: Microwaves are another source of concern during pregnancy. For busy mothers a microwave oven can be one of the most valuable pieces of equipment in the house. But what about exposure to the fetus? Theoretically, if a microwave oven had a significant door leak, you could expose yourself and the baby by placing a part of your body in direct contact with the oven. In this way it is conceivable that after several hours you might receive a measurable exposure. Yet, short of such irrational behavior there is virtually no way to obtain enough exposure to microwaves to harm the baby.

To date there are no published studies linking ordinary use of microwave ovens and harm to the baby. If you're concerned about the safety of your microwave oven, have it checked with a meter to detect any significant leaks and don't stand near the oven while it's in operation. Studies have shown that women who work near FM radio transmitters or radar are not exposed to significant levels of microwaves.

Ultrasound: Few diagnostic techniques have contributed more to the improved outcome of pregnancy than ultrasonography. Diagnostic ultrasonography is often performed at various times during pregnancy to determine the rate of growth of the fetus and to estimate its size before delivery. It is also used to look for birth defects, but due to the limitations of the technology, it cannot identify all possible birth defects. The technique works by bouncing high-frequency sound waves (ultrasound) off internal structures, including the baby, and back to a screen forming an image. This procedure has been used for about 20 years in obstetrics and has been shown to be safe. The ultrasound machine does not emit X rays.

Ultrasound can also be used in higher dosages as physical therapy for back and muscle injuries. Therapeutic ultrasound uses much higher dosages than standard diagnostic ultrasonography. Since the effects of high-dosage ultrasound on the fetus are not known, it is best avoided during pregnancy.

Video Display Terminals: In recent years considerable media attention has been devoted to "clusters" of pregnancy complications (such as miscarriage, premature delivery, and birth defects) from exposure to video display terminals (VDTs). The hazards are alleged to be ionizing radiation. In fact, the Food and Drug Administration (FDA), the National Institute for Occupational Safety and Health, as well as a number of private organizations have measured the radiation emissions from VDTs and have found that under normal conditions they emit essentially no ionizing radiation. Even under the worst possible conditions, the dose of ionizing radiation to the fetus from a VDT would be extremely low, roughly 1,000 times below that known to possibly cause any harm to the baby. The National Academy of Sciences says that the fetus is exposed to more ionizing radiation from natural sources in the environment than from its mother's work with a VDT. The reported "clusters" of adverse pregnancy outcomes are most likely chance occurrences among the millions of women who work with VDTs. Remember that approximately 3 percent of normal, healthy pregnant women have a child with a significant birth defect. When a birth defect occurs, it is always tempting to look for a cause, and often VDTs have gotten the blame.

PRECAUTIONS:

- If you are pregnant or think you might be pregnant, always inform the doctor ordering the X ray or the technician performing the X ray so your abdomen can be properly shielded with a lead apron. In many cases your doctor may decide that the X ray will not be helpful enough to warrant even slight exposure.

- Ask whether another diagnostic test will provide the same information as an X ray. In some cases ultrasonography can be substituted.
- Have X rays performed only at licensed, regularly inspected facilities with certified X-ray technicians.
- Carefully follow the technician's directions about preparation for an X-ray examination so there will be no need for repeat studies.
- If you are concerned about the safety of your microwave oven, have it checked with a meter to determine whether there is any significant leak.
- Follow the manufacturer's directions for the use of your microwave oven, and don't stand right next to it when it's in operation.
- Relax about the use of ultrasound. Ultrasonography can safely provide valuable information about the condition of your baby.
- With currently available scientific information you can be confident that neither you nor your baby is at any risk from radiation emitted by video display terminals. Nevertheless, extended work at a VDT can be associated with other problems such as glare, fatigue, tendonitis, and back pain. Be sure your working environment is comfortable and well lighted and that your chair is comfortable and positioned properly for data entry.

❧ The Safe Use of Medications during Pregnancy and Breastfeeding

T his section profiles many of the most common prescription and over-the-counter (nonprescription) medications used in the United States. Like medications themselves, this information should be used with caution. It is not intended to be a self-treatment manual. Read this information with the goal of supplementing what your physician has already told you, and use it to ask additional questions about why medication is being prescribed, what the possible side effects are, how safe the medication is during pregnancy and breastfeeding, and whether there is an appropriate alternative to taking a drug. It would be unthinkable for me or anyone else unfamiliar with your care to suggest specific medical therapy. Yet I believe that understanding your medications will allow you to participate more actively and confidently in medical decisions affecting you and your unborn child. Knowing more about medications and asking thoughtful questions may even prevent potentially disastrous consequences of a drug misused during pregnancy.

Each drug profile contains the following information:

GENERIC NAME: The generic name of a medication refers to the scientific or chemical name given to all drugs. Although each drug has only one generic name, it may have different brand names given by different manufacturers. Most generic names are long and difficult to pronounce. They are not the way you usually talk about your medications. Nevertheless, generic names are necessary to categorize drugs and prevent needless repetition of the many different brands of the same drug. Today, there are also manufacturers making less expensive medications sold as "generic drugs" and labeled with only the generic name. Learn to read the label of any medication you intend to take and make a list of each active ingredient. You can easily look up any brand name or generic name in the index to find the information you desire. Don't be overwhelmed by the generic name.

COMMON BRANDS: The name the manufacturer gives to a drug is called the brand name or trade name. These names usually bear no resemblance to the generic name. For example, the pain reliever acetaminophen is marketed under the brand names Tylenol, Datril, Tempra, Anacin-3, and many others. Many drugs are also available in a "generic form" and will be labeled with only the appropriate generic name. Finally, many drugs combine two or more active ingredients in one preparation. For example, the prescription cough suppressant Robitussin A-C contains guaifenesin, codeine, and alcohol. You can find information about Robitussin A-C by identifying its active ingredients on the product label and looking them up in the index of generic drugs or you can look up the brand name in the index of brand names. New products are constantly being developed and marketed. It is impossible to list all the brand name products currently available. However, most of these products are not really new. They are different combinations or a new dosage of existing drugs. If you can't find a particular drug by its brand name, look up its generic name in the index.

TYPE OF DRUG: This section indicates whether a drug is available over-the-counter without a prescription or from a pharmacist only with a physician's prescription. In this section there is also a brief indication of the major pharmacologic use of the drug—e.g., antihistamine, anticonvulsant, antidiarrheal, antibiotic, and so forth. Some medications will have more than one use, and many medications are prescribed for purposes that have not been specifically approved by the FDA. Only your physician can explain why a particular medication has been chosen to treat your medical problem.

FDA RISK CATEGORY FOR PREGNANCY: In 1980 the FDA defined levels of risk (A, B, C, D, X) that a prescription drug poses to the fetus. The definitions used for these risk categories are listed below. (The categories do not pertain to the risk of medications during breastfeeding.)

- A Controlled studies of these drugs in pregnant women have shown no risk to the fetus. Therefore, the possibility of harm to the fetus appears remote.
- B There has been no evidence of risk in animals, but insufficient information is available about use in humans. This category also includes those drugs that have shown an adverse effect in animals that could not be confirmed in humans.
- C For drugs in this category risk cannot be ruled out. Human studies are lacking, or animal studies have either demonstrated fetal risk or are lacking as well. However, potential benefits of medications in this category may justify the risk.
- D Drugs in this category have demonstrated evidence of human fetal risk. Nevertheless, the benefits from use of these drugs during pregnancy may be acceptable despite the risk—for example, if the drug is needed in a life-threatening situation or for a serious disease for which safer drugs are not available.
- X Drugs in this category should be avoided throughout pregnancy. Studies in animals or humans have shown fetal risk that clearly outweighs any possible benefit to the patient.

In many ways this classification tends to oversimplify a very complex problem. Most drugs fall in categories B or C where complete safety cannot be certain. Your physician will help you understand whether the need to treat your particular problem with a medication justifies any risk to the baby. *Will It Hurt the Baby?* will give you some of the basic information about the risk of medications during pregnancy and should help you formulate questions to ask your doctor.

GENERAL INFORMATION: This section describes in more detail the type of drug and its usual indication for use. Because this information is general, it applies to all patients and not just pregnant women. The fact that general advice about a drug is presented in this section does not imply that the drug is safe for use during pregnancy. It is not intended to replace specific instructions or warnings given to you by your physician.

POSSIBLE MATERNAL SIDE EFFECTS: Few drugs, if any, are completely free of side effects. This section contains some of the more common mild side effects, as well as uncommon serious ones. This is by no means a complete list of potential adverse effects, nor have possible adverse interactions with other medications or foods been included. If you are not sure whether you are experiencing a side effect of a medication, always call your doctor.

Any drug can cause an allergic reaction ranging from a mild rash to severe difficulty breathing or even shock. Many drug reference guides give a standard warning for each drug entry that the medication should not be taken if there is any history of allergy to that medication. Since this advice is appropriate for every drug in this book, I have chosen not to restate that warning with each discussion. Nevertheless, the warning about allergy is important. Always be sure your physician has a complete and up-to-date list of any medication allergies or intolerances.

USE DURING PREGNANCY: You probably bought the book because of the information in this section. It would be easy to recommend that no drugs be taken during pregnancy. Certainly everyone would agree that no drug should be taken during pregnancy unless the potential benefit outweighs any risk. Nevertheless, a blanket warning against the use of all drugs during pregnancy denies a woman relief from troublesome symptoms such as nausea and vomiting, or subjects her and the baby to potentially dangerous consequences of curable illnesses like infections.

There is now considerable information available to guide physicians in the rational and safe use of medications during pregnancy. I have drawn from many sources (see references) in order to provide useful and current information about the special considerations and risks of each medication taken during pregnancy. One important source of information is a large study called the Collaborative Perinatal Project, in which more than 50,000 pregnancies were studied very carefully to ascertain any birth defects that may have occurred as a result of a drug taken during the first four months of pregnancy. No single study to date is as large as this one. In the discussion of several drugs you will find the statement that the Collaborative Perinatal Project could not establish a link between the drug and any birth defects or fetal malformations. This does not guarantee that no harm is possible, but it does offer the reassurance that no harm could be found in the pregnancies monitored. Unfortunately, there is too little experience with many drugs to ensure their safety during pregnancy. Most medications fall into the category where safety is likely, but even a small risk must be considered when choosing a particular medication.

USE DURING BREASTFEEDING: Most drugs are excreted in breast milk to some extent. The mere presence of a drug in breast milk, however, does not imply that the newborn is at any risk of adverse effects from the drug. Some drugs are present in breast milk in such small quantities that they have very little, if any, effect on the newborn. Other drugs, however, may have significant effects in the breast-fed newborn even in small amounts. In 1983 the American Academy of Pediatrics published an extensive list of medications that had been studied in breastfeeding mothers and their infants. In this publication there was an attempt to list potential adverse effects and to offer advice about the safety of many drugs during breastfeeding. I have drawn heavily from the information published by the American Academy of Pediatrics for the recommendations in this section. Unfortunately, information is not always available about every drug.

ALTERNATIVES TO MEDICATIONS: Whenever possible I have recommended alternatives to the use of medications during pregnancy. Some of these recommendations may suffice for relief of troublesome symptoms without medications during the critical first trimester, and some may allow you to abstain from medications throughout pregnancy. On the other hand, certain medical conditions must be treated with medications since failure to treat might place both you and your baby at jeopardy. At no time should you stop taking medication without consulting your physician!

GENERIC NAME: Acetaminophen

COMMON BRANDS: Anacin-3, Bromo Seltzer, Datril, Liquiprin, Panadol, Phenaphen, Tempra, Tylenol, Valorin

TYPE OF DRUG: (Over-the-counter) Analgesic, antipyretic

FDA PREGNANCY CATEGORY: B

GENERAL INFORMATION: Acetaminophen has been routinely used during pregnancy to reduce pain and to lower fever. Its mechanism of action is not completely understood.

POSSIBLE MATERNAL SIDE EFFECTS: In the usual dosage it has no side effects.

USE DURING PREGNANCY: Although the drug crosses the placenta, there have been no reports of fetal harm. Massive overdose of acetaminophen can cause liver damage in the mother and presumably in the fetus.

USE DURING BREASTFEEDING: The drug is excreted into breast milk in small amounts. There have been no reports of adverse effects in the newborn. The American Academy of Pediatrics considers acetaminophen compatible with breastfeeding.

ALTERNATIVES TO MEDICATIONS: Musculoskeletal pain can often be relieved with warm baths and massage. In some patients chronic pain can be controlled with relaxation techniques and biofeedback. Nevertheless, acetaminophen is probably the safest medication to take during pregnancy for relief of minor pain.

GENERIC NAME: Acetazolamide

COMMON BRANDS: Diamox

TYPE OF DRUG: (Prescription) Carbonic anhydrase inhibitor, diuretic

FDA RISK CATEGORY FOR PREGNANCY: C

GENERAL INFORMATION: Acetazolamide is a form of diuretic. It can be used to decrease excess fluid and pressure in the eye in patients with glaucoma. It has also been used for prevention of high-altitude (mountain) sickness in individuals going from sea level to high altitude.

POSSIBLE MATERNAL SIDE EFFECTS: Side effects are rare, but changes in blood concentration of sodium and potassium can occur.

USE DURING PREGNANCY: When the drug was given to pregnant rats in a dosage 10 times the usual human dosage, abnormalities of the limbs were noted. There have been no reports, however, linking acetazolamide to birth defects in humans. The Collaborative Perinatal Project monitored over 50,000 pregnant women; 1,024 exposures to acetazolamide were noted, and there was no evidence the drug causes birth defects.

USE DURING BREASTFEEDING: No information is available.

ALTERNATIVES TO MEDICATIONS: The use of diuretics during pregnancy is usually reserved for women with heart problems or kidney disease. Mild edema (fluid retention) is a common occurrence during pregnancy and does not require treatment. If edema becomes uncomfortable, it can usually be relieved by lying on your side for periods of 30 to 60 minutes. In some cases mild restriction of dietary salt intake may be necessary. Severe salt restriction, however, is not appropriate and may even be harmful. There is no evidence that so-called natural diuretics found in health food stores are effective, and their safety during pregnancy cannot be assured.

GENERIC NAME: Acyclovir

COMMON BRANDS: Zovirax

TYPE OF DRUG: (Prescription) Antiviral, antiherpes

FDA RISK CATEGORY FOR PREGNANCY: C

GENERAL INFORMATION: Acyclovir capsules are indicated for the treatment of primary (initial) and recurrent genital herpes. The drug is also available as an ointment for topical treatment of herpes, but the ointment is not as effective as the pills.

POSSIBLE MATERNAL SIDE EFFECTS: Acyclovir usually has very few side effects. The oral form can cause nausea, vomiting, and headaches. The ointment can occasionally cause a rash.

USE DURING PREGNANCY: Acyclovir has been studied in animals and has not been shown to cause birth defects. There have been a few reports of the use of acyclovir in humans during pregnancy and no evidence of birth defects. A man with a history of recurrent herpes can be treated with acyclovir capsules throughout gestation to limit viral shedding and reduce the possibility of infecting his pregnant partner.

USE DURING BREASTFEEDING: No information is available.

ALTERNATIVES TO MEDICATIONS: There is no other medication or topical preparation available to kill the herpes virus. The oral form of the drug may be particularly helpful for treatment of primary herpes virus infection during pregnancy, and therefore its use may outweigh any theoretical risk. Acyclovir may also be helpful in preventing genital herpes infection in a woman by treating her partner with the drug and hastening recovery of his infection. The disease may also be prevented by abstinence from sex when your partner has an active herpes lesion. At other times use condoms if your partner has a history of herpes.

GENERIC NAME: Albuterol

COMMON BRANDS: Proventil, Ventolin

TYPE OF DRUG: (Prescription) Bronchodilator

FDA RISK CATEGORY FOR PREGNANCY: C

GENERAL INFORMATION: Albuterol is available as a pill or inhaler. It is used for the prevention or relief of bronchial spasm in patients with asthma. The pill form begins to work in approximately 30 minutes, and its effect lasts about 4 hours. The inhaler begins to work in less than 15 minutes and lasts 3 to 4 hours.

POSSIBLE MATERNAL SIDE EFFECTS: Possible side effects include palpitations, rapid heart rate, dizziness, anxiety, tremor, nausea, loss of appetite, and insomnia. Side effects are generally fewer with the inhaled form.

USE DURING PREGNANCY: There have been no reports linking albuterol to birth defects. Very little of the inhaled form is absorbed into the blood; therefore, there is little effect on the fetus. Blood levels can be significant when the drug is taken by pill. Rapid heart rate can occur in both mother and fetus. Albuterol can also increase maternal blood glucose levels, possibly worsening gestational diabetes. For the treatment of asthma there is little to be gained by taking albuterol by pill. The inhaled form works more rapidly and has fewer side effects.

Because it inhibits contractions of the uterus, albuterol has also been used to prevent premature labor.

USE DURING BREASTFEEDING: Albuterol enters breast milk and can cause rapid heart rate in the baby when it is taken by pill. Nevertheless, it appears to be safe for use during breastfeeding.

ALTERNATIVES TO MEDICATIONS: In some cases asthma can be prevented by avoidance of known allergens, particularly animals. If you smoke, stop. It is generally a good rule, however, to use a bronchodilating inhaler at the earliest indication of wheezing. Often prompt effective relief of asthma can prevent minor episodes from becoming more severe and prolonged.

GENERIC NAME: Alcohol (Ethanol)

COMMON BRANDS: Variety of cough syrups, liquor, wine, and beer

TYPE OF DRUG: (Over-the-counter)

FDA RISK CATEGORY FOR PREGNANCY: X

GENERAL INFORMATION: In the past alcohol was used during pregnancy to halt premature labor. It is no longer used for this purpose and has no medical use during pregnancy.

POSSIBLE MATERNAL SIDE EFFECTS: Side effects include intoxication, loss of judgment, difficulty with balance and gait, impaired ability to drive, and psychological dependency.

USE DURING PREGNANCY: Clinical studies have shown that heavy use of alcohol by pregnant women often results in a pattern of severe and irreversible abnormalities in their offspring called the fetal alcohol syndrome. Babies born with fetal alcohol syndrome are abnormally small at birth and usually do not catch up as they get older. They may suffer from various facial malformations and major organ defects, particularly of the heart. Most babies with fetal alcohol syndrome have small brains, some degree of mental retardation, and behavioral problems. Women who drink the equivalent of three ounces of pure alcohol each day (six average mixed drinks or six cans of beer) frequently give birth to babies who have the complete fetal alcohol syndrome. Moderate amounts of alcohol during pregnancy (two to five drinks daily) also can damage the fetus. At this time it is not known how little alcohol must be consumed to produce the syndrome. In the past many women were advised to have a drink each day "to relax." We now know it is best to avoid all alcohol during pregnancy, particularly during the first trimester. On the other hand if you had a few drinks before you found out you were pregnant, don't despair. There's no evidence that a few drinks on a couple of occasions early in pregnancy will prove harmful to your baby.

USE DURING BREASTFEEDING: Alcohol enters breast milk and can cause sedation in the newborn. Furthermore, a recent study of women who had at least one drink of alcohol daily demonstrated a significant detrimental effect on motor development of their infants at one year of age.

ALTERNATIVES TO MEDICATIONS: There is no reason to consume alcohol during pregnancy. Be careful to read the labels of over-the-counter cough syrups and cold preparations. Many of them contain significant quantities of alcohol.

GENERIC NAME: Allopurinol

COMMON BRANDS: Lopurin, Zyloprim

TYPE OF DRUG: (Prescription) Antigout (lowers uric acid in the blood)

FDA RISK CATEGORY FOR PREGNANCY: C

GENERAL INFORMATION: Allopurinol is used to lower the blood concentration of uric acid in individuals with gout or certain kinds of kidney stones. It acts by reducing the production of uric acid in the body. The drug is not commonly used by young women since problems due to an elevated uric acid level are far more common in men.

POSSIBLE MATERNAL SIDE EFFECTS: Possible side effects include nausea, skin rash, low white blood cell count, and elevated liver function tests.

USE DURING PREGNANCY: Studies have been performed with allopurinol in pregnant mice and rabbits with dosages 20 times the usual human dosage. It was concluded that there was no impairment of fertility or harm to the fetus. Studies have not been performed, however, in humans.

USE DURING BREASTFEEDING: Allopurinol enters breast milk, but there is no information about its effect on breastfed infants.

ALTERNATIVES TO MEDICATIONS: Although there is an increased risk of gout and kidney stones in individuals with an elevated uric acid level, these are uncommon problems in young women. In most cases allopurinol can be withheld during at least the first trimester, if not throughout pregnancy. Diet therapy to reduce uric acid levels is generally not effective.

GENERIC NAME: Aloe

COMMON BRANDS: Nature's Remedy, and many other "natural" laxatives and creams available at health food stores.

TYPE OF DRUG: (Over-the-counter) Laxative (oral), skin cream

FDA RISK CATEGORY FOR PREGNANCY: D (oral)

GENERAL INFORMATION: Aloe is derived from the aloe vera plant. It is used in a variety of skin creams and in oral laxative preparations. The drug is widely available in pharmacies, health food stores, and vitamin stores.

POSSIBLE MATERNAL SIDE EFFECTS: Side effects are minimal, but diarrhea can occur.

USE DURING PREGNANCY: Aloe should not be used as a laxative during pregnancy. It can cross the placenta and stimulate the fetal intestine, leading to contamination of the amniotic fluid with meconium. Meconium is the greenish-brown residue that fills the fetal intestine and is usually not passed until after birth.

USE DURING BREASTFEEDING: No information is available.

ALTERNATIVES TO MEDICATIONS: Aloe-containing laxatives should not be used during pregnancy. High-fiber foods and fruits along with plenty of fluids should help avoid constipation in most cases. However, large quantities of bran should be avoided, especially if diarrhea results. Too much bran can interfere with absorption of minerals from food.

GENERIC NAME: Alprazolam

COMMON BRANDS: Xanax

TYPE OF DRUG: (Prescription) Antianxiety, sedative

FDA RISK CATEGORY FOR PREGNANCY: D

GENERAL INFORMATION: Alprazolam is a member of a group of antianxiety medications called benzodiazepines. These drugs are used for the treatment of anxiety and insomnia. Alprazolam is used primarily as a sedative or for insomnia. Benzodiazepines work by relaxing skeletal muscles and by a direct action on the brain. Any of these drugs can be abused if taken indiscriminately or for a long period of time. Withdrawal symptoms including tremor, agitation, insomnia, muscle cramps, nausea, and seizures can occur if these drugs are discontinued abruptly after chronic use. Benzodiazepines should not be taken without careful medical supervision.

POSSIBLE MATERNAL SIDE EFFECTS: Common side effects with all benzodiazepines include sedation, depression, mental confusion, dizziness, unsteady gait, nightmares, fatigue, dry mouth, and low blood pressure. These drugs can interfere with the ability to safely drive a car or operate dangerous equipment. Physical and psychological dependence can occur with chronic use.

USE DURING PREGNANCY: All benzodiazepines rapidly cross the placenta and enter the fetal circulation. Blood levels in the fetus equal that of the mother's within one hour of taking a pill. Several studies have demonstrated a link between first-trimester use of benzodiazepines and birth defects. The most commonly reported malformations are cleft lip and cleft palate. Used near term benzodiazepines have been associated with lethargy, respiratory problems, and withdrawal symptoms in the newborn. Most authorities believe that it is best to avoid these medications during the first trimester and if possible throughout pregnancy.

USE DURING BREASTFEEDING: Benzodiazepines are excreted into breast milk in significant quantities. They can cause sedation in the newborn and should be avoided during breastfeeding.

ALTERNATIVES TO MEDICATIONS: Before using medications to control anxiety or stress consider the following strategy:

1. Identify the source of your anxiety. Worry often persists because of an inability to identify a problem and take action to solve it. Visualization can begin the process. Close your eyes and take a few deep breaths. Allow an image of the problem to arise.
2. Once you've defined the source of your anxiety, gather information. For example, if you are worried about the outcome of your pregnancy because of a possible hereditary problem or a medication you took before you knew you were pregnant, get information from your physician or a genetic counselor. In most cases what you discover will be very comforting.

3. After obtaining information, decide on a plan of action. Do what you can to deal with the problem, but once you've done all you can, change your focus and move on to other parts of life. Instead of worrying, concentrate on your life beyond the worry. Exercise or take walks. Plan how you will spend the evening or the weekend. Treat yourself to something pleasant, or think up a surprise for someone you care about. As your mind gets busy with other thoughts, you'll find that stress will begin to fade.
4. If anxiety persists despite your best efforts, see a therapist. Often only a few counseling sessions can effectively reduce anxiety and stress and eliminate the need for medication.

GENERIC NAME: Amantadine

COMMON BRANDS: Symmetrel

TYPE OF DRUG: (Prescription) Anti-Parkinson's disease, antiviral

FDA RISK CATEGORY FOR PREGNANCY: C

GENERAL INFORMATION: In older individuals amantadine is used to control the tremors of Parkinson's disease, but this disease is extremely rare in women of reproductive age. For unknown reasons the drug also has an antiviral action against the influenza A virus. In some instances amantadine is given to prevent influenza in healthy individuals exposed to known cases. It may also be given to reduce symptoms even after the onset of the disease.

POSSIBLE MATERNAL SIDE EFFECTS: Side effects include light-headedness, dizziness, confusion, hallucinations, anxiety, dry mouth, nausea, and diminished appetite.

USE DURING PREGNANCY: Amantadine has been shown to cause birth defects in laboratory animals. There are no large-scale studies of the drug in human pregnancies, but there is one report of a baby born with a heart defect whose mother took amantadine during the first trimester. The drug should not be used for the treatment of routine viral infections or uncomplicated influenza during pregnancy. Women at risk of severe complications from influenza should be vaccinated against the disease before pregnancy or, in some cases, even during pregnancy rather than take amantadine.

USE DURING BREASTFEEDING: Amantadine is excreted into breast milk in low concentrations. The drug can cause skin rash, vomiting, or difficulty emptying the bladder in infants and should therefore be avoided during breastfeeding.

ALTERNATIVES TO MEDICATIONS: Women with chronic medical disorders such as diabetes, heart disease, or kidney disease should be immunized against influenza before pregnancy. Most pregnant women are not at any unusual risk from influenza and do not need to take amantadine.

GENERIC NAME: Aminoglycosides

COMMON BRANDS: Amikacin (Amikin), Gentamicin (Garamycin), Kanamycin (Kantrex), Streptomycin, Tobramycin (Nebcin)

TYPE OF DRUG: (Prescription) Antibiotics

FDA RISK CATEGORY FOR PREGNANCY: C

GENERAL INFORMATION: Aminoglycoside antibiotics are usually given only to hospital patients with severe infections. They are administered by intramuscular or intravenous injection.

POSSIBLE MATERNAL SIDE EFFECTS: In excessive dosages aminoglycoside antibiotics can cause hearing loss and damage to the kidneys.

USE DURING PREGNANCY: During pregnancy an aminoglycoside antibiotic might be given for serious infections of the kidneys, amniotic fluid, or perforation of the intestine. A single dose may be given immediately before delivery to any woman with a known abnormal heart valve in order to prevent infection of the valve (endocarditis). Kanamycin and streptomycin have been shown to cause deafness in some infants exposed to the drug for prolonged periods during pregnancy. Ideally, these antibiotics should be avoided during the first trimester, but they should not be withheld when a serious infection threatens the health of the mother. There is no evidence that these drugs are harmful when given during the third trimester.

USE DURING BREASTFEEDING: Aminoglycosides are excreted into breast milk in low concentrations. All of these drugs are poorly absorbed when taken by mouth. Therefore, the nursing infant is not likely to receive a significant amount. These antibiotics may be used during breastfeeding to treat serious infections with minimal risk to the infant.

ALTERNATIVES TO MEDICATIONS: Because aminoglycosides are reserved for the treatment of serious infections, there is no non-pharmacologic alternative to their use. Their safety can be enhanced by measuring blood levels to ensure that the dosage is not toxic.

GENERIC NAME: Amitriptyline

COMMON BRANDS: Elavil, Endep, Etraton, Limbitrol, Triavil

TYPE OF DRUG: (Prescription) Antidepressant

FDA RISK CATEGORY FOR PREGNANCY: D

GENERAL INFORMATION: Amitriptyline is used in nonpregnant patients to treat chronic, severe depression.

POSSIBLE MATERNAL SIDE EFFECTS: The drug has several side effects including drowsiness, confusion, dry mouth, nausea, difficulty passing urine, and abnormal heart rhythms.

USE DURING PREGNANCY: Abnormal development of the legs or arms has been noted in some infants exposed to amitriptyline in the first trimester. It should be avoided during pregnancy.

USE DURING BREASTFEEDING: The drug is excreted into breast milk in low concentrations. The effect of even small amounts on the infant remains unknown.

ALTERNATIVES TO MEDICATIONS: Depression often gives rise to hopelessness, negativity toward oneself, and at times an inability to carry out normal activities of daily living. Some individuals may become intensely sad or grief-stricken over the loss of someone or something close to them. Others may suffer from chronic depression unrelated to a specific event. In many cases counseling is necessary to truly understand the cause and extent of depression. There are, however, a number of things you can do to deal with depression on your own.

1. Try to identify the specific situation or personal interaction that has caused your sense of hopelessness and negativity.

2. Make a fresh start at correcting the problem. Talk it through. If necessary, repair relationships with previously available support systems. Often family or close friends can serve to reduce your distress.
3. Realize that there are options for most situations. Seldom is there truly "no choice."
4. Understand some of the warning signs that indicate you have severe depression requiring professional counseling. Such signs include
   - Intense sadness, frequent bouts of crying, or depressed mood most of the day,
   - Uncharacteristically negative thoughts about yourself,
   - Markedly diminished interest or pleasure in most activities,
   - Diminished appetite and weight loss,
   - Chronic insomnia or sleeping excessively,
   - Feelings of worthlessness or guilt,
   - Persistent fatigue or lack of energy,
   - Inability to think or concentrate,
   - Thoughts or plans for suicide.
5. Patients with severe depression should not stop taking antidepressant medications without careful psychiatric supervision.

GENERIC NAME: Amoxicillin

COMMON BRANDS: Amoxil, Augmentin, Larotid, Polymox, Trimox, Wymox

TYPE OF DRUG: (Prescription) Antibiotic

FDA RISK CATEGORY FOR PREGNANCY: B

GENERAL INFORMATION: Amoxicillin is a penicillin-type antibiotic used to treat common respiratory, sinus, and urinary tract infections.

POSSIBLE MATERNAL SIDE EFFECTS: Side effects are uncommon, but diarrhea may result from treatment with any antibiotic and should be reported to your physician if it lasts longer than 48 hours. Amoxicillin should not be taken if you have a history of allergy to penicillin or any other penicillin-type antibiotic.

USE DURING PREGNANCY: Amoxicillin has been used extensively in pregnant women. No evidence has been reported linking the drug to birth defects or abnormal fetal growth.

USE DURING BREASTFEEDING: Amoxicillin is excreted into breast milk in low concentrations. No adverse effects have been reported in nursing infants. Theoretically, however, an infant could be sensitized to amoxicillin causing an allergic reaction to subsequent treatment with any penicillin-type antibiotic.

ALTERNATIVES TO MEDICATIONS: Antibiotic treatment of bacterial infections such as urinary tract infections should not be withheld because of pregnancy. Most common colds and viral infections, however, do not require antibiotic therapy. Mild decongestants and acetaminophen may be used to control persistent symptoms.

GENERIC NAME: Amphetamines

COMMON BRANDS: Benzedrine, Dexedrine, Obetrol

TYPE OF DRUG: (Prescription) Appetite-suppressant

FDA RISK CATEGORY FOR PREGNANCY: X

GENERAL INFORMATION: Amphetamines have a high potential for abuse. Their use as appetite-suppressants may lead to drug dependency. They are occasionally used to treat a rare disorder of excessive sleeping called narcolepsy.

POSSIBLE MATERNAL SIDE EFFECTS: Side effects of amphetamines are common and may be severe or life-threatening including sudden, severe high blood pressure, rapid, irregular heart rate, hallucinations, psychosis, and sudden death. Chronic use can lead to dependency.

USE DURING PREGNANCY: These drugs clearly cause birth defects in mice. In addition, there are reports of heart defects and cleft palate in infants exposed to amphetamines during the first trimester. Infants born to mothers dependent on amphetamines manifest symptoms of drug withdrawal agitation and poor feeding. Amphetamines should not be used during pregnancy.

USE DURING BREASTFEEDING: Amphetamines are excreted into breast milk and can cause irritability, poor feeding, and sleep disturbance in infants. They should not be taken during breastfeeding.

ALTERNATIVES TO MEDICATIONS: These drugs should not be taken during pregnancy. Women who take amphetamines should seek psychiatric counseling to assist with a plan for withdrawal.

GENERIC NAME: Amphotericin B

COMMON BRANDS: Fungizone

TYPE OF DRUG: (Prescription) Antifungal

FDA RISK CATEGORY FOR PREGNANCY: B

GENERAL INFORMATION: Amphotericin B should be administered only in the hospital to patients with potentially fatal or progressive fungus infections. It should not be used to treat most common forms of skin or nail fungus infections.

POSSIBLE MATERNAL SIDE EFFECTS: When the drug is given intravenously, a variety of side effects are common, including headache, nerve pain, loss of appetite, nausea, and weight loss. The most serious side effect is severe kidney damage.

USE DURING PREGNANCY: There are several reports of treatment with amphotericin B during various stages of pregnancy. No link has been established between the drug and any specific birth defects or fetal harm. Nevertheless, its use during pregnancy should be restricted to treatment of severe fungus infections.

USE DURING BREASTFEEDING: No information is available about the use of amphotericin B during breastfeeding.

ALTERNATIVES TO MEDICATIONS: Minor chronic fungus infection of skin or nails does not require treatment with amphotericin B. The drug should be reserved only for severe infections.

GENERIC NAME: Ampicillin

COMMON BRANDS: Amcap, Amcill, Omnipen, Polycillin, Principen, Suspen, Unasyn

TYPE OF DRUG: (Prescription) Antibiotic

FDA RISK CATEGORY FOR PREGNANCY: B

GENERAL INFORMATION: Ampicillin is a penicillin-type antibiotic used to treat common respiratory, sinus, and urinary tract infections.

POSSIBLE MATERNAL SIDE EFFECTS: Side effects are uncommon, but diarrhea may result from treatment with any antibiotic and should be reported to your physician if it lasts longer than 48 hours. Ampicillin should not be taken if you have a history of allergy to penicillin or any other penicillin-type antibiotic.

USE DURING PREGNANCY: Ampicillin has been used extensively in pregnant women. No evidence has been reported linking the drug to birth defects or abnormal fetal growth.

USE DURING BREASTFEEDING: Ampicillin is excreted into breast milk in low concentrations. No adverse effects have been reported in nursing infants. Theoretically, however, an infant could be sensitized to ampicillin causing an allergic reaction to subsequent treatment with any penicillin-type antibiotic.

ALTERNATIVES TO MEDICATIONS: Antibiotic treatment of bacterial infections such as urinary tract infections should not be withheld because of pregnancy. Most common colds and viral infections, however, do not require antibiotic therapy. Mild decongestants and acetaminophen may be used to control persistent symptoms.

GENERIC NAME: **Anabolic steroids**

COMMON BRANDS: Anadrol-50, Anavar, Deca-Durabolin, Durabolin

TYPE OF DRUG: (Prescription and illicit) Anabolic steroids

FDA RISK CATEGORY FOR PREGNANCY: X

GENERAL INFORMATION: Anabolic steroids are closely related to the naturally occurring male hormone, testosterone. They are legitimately used to stimulate the production of red blood cells in certain types of anemia and to treat some patients with severe weight loss from chronic debilitating disease. Unfortunately, they are also used by male and female athletes to enhance muscle building.

POSSIBLE MATERNAL SIDE EFFECTS: Because these drugs are chemically similar to male hormones, they can cause masculinization in women including excessive hair growth, deepening of the voice, clitoral enlargement, oily skin, and acne. Very important, they can also interfere with normal menses resulting in infertility. Other risks include liver cell tumors and an increased chance of developing coronary heart disease.

USE DURING PREGNANCY: Anabolic steroids should not be taken during pregnancy, nor should they be taken by women who are not using adequate contraception. These drugs have been shown to cause birth defects, fetal death, and masculinization of female offspring.

USE DURING BREASTFEEDING: It is not known whether anabolic steroids enter breast milk. Nevertheless, because of the potential of adverse effects to the nursing infant, they should not be taken during breastfeeding.

ALTERNATIVES TO MEDICATIONS: Anabolic steroids should not be used during pregnancy. There is no need for alternatives.

GENERIC NAME: Antacids

COMMON BRANDS:

Aluminum antacids: Amphojel, Basaljel, Phosphaljel, Rolaids
Calcium antacids: calcium carbonate, Chooz, Titralac, Tums
Magnesium antacids: Camalox, Di-Gel, Haley's M-O, Gaviscon, Maalox, Mylanta, Phillips' Milk of Magnesia, Rolaids
Sodium bicarbonate antacids: Alka-Seltzer, Arm & Hammer pure baking soda
Aluminum plus magnesium antacids: Delcid, Gaviscon, Maalox, Riopan, Triconsil, WinGel
Calcium plus magnesium antacids: Bisodol, Lo-Sol
Aluminum plus calcium plus magnesium antacids: Camalox
Aluminum plus magnesium plus simethicone antacids: Di-Gel, Gelusil, Maalox Plus, Mylanta, Riopan Plus
Aluminum plus magnesium plus calcium plus simethicone antacids: Tempo

TYPE OF DRUG: (Over-the-counter) Stomach acid neutralizer

FDA RISK CATEGORY FOR PREGNANCY: Not classified

GENERAL INFORMATION: Antacids are used to treat heartburn, acid reflux, gastritis, and ulcers. Although there are dozens of antacids on the market, there are only a few basic types: aluminum, calcium, magnesium, simethicone (an antigas ingredient), and sodium. Each works by chemically neutralizing acid produced in the stomach. To be effective, antacids must be taken in a sufficient dosage (1 to 2 tablespoons) at least one hour to three hours after meals and at bedtime.

POSSIBLE MATERNAL SIDE EFFECTS: Side effects depend on the ingredients in each preparation. Aluminum- and calcium-containing antacids frequently cause constipation. Magnesium-containing products often cause diarrhea. Combination preparations may offset these side effects. Sodium-containing antacids can cause fluid retention and edema (swelling). Antacids can affect the absorption of other drugs. Most drugs should not be taken for at least one to two hours after taking antacids.

USE DURING PREGNANCY: Most antacids are considered safe for use in small quantities during pregnancy. No link between first trimester use and birth defects has been established. Each antacid has its particular side effects, which can adversely affect pregnancy. Sodium-containing antacids such as sodium bicarbonate can cause fluid retention, aluminum- and calcium-containing products can cause constipation, and magnesium-containing antacids may lead to diarrhea.

USE DURING BREASTFEEDING: There are no reported adverse effects of antacid treatment during breastfeeding.

ALTERNATIVES TO MEDICATIONS: As an alternative to the use of antacids for nausea and morning sickness, try the following:
- Avoid large meals; substitute frequent small ones.
- Do not lie down for at least one hour after a meal to allow food to empty from the stomach.
- Sleeping with your head propped up or the head of the bed elevated may help prevent regurgitation of food or stomach acid during the night.
- Avoid exercise or activity that involves bending.
- If physical maneuvers are not successful, you may use small amounts of low-sodium antacids such as Gelusil or Maalox. Do not use baking soda (sodium bicarbonate) because it is very high in sodium and may cause fluid retention.

GENERIC NAME: Antihistamines

COMMON BRANDS:

Astemizole: Hismanal

Azatadine: Optimine

Brompheniramine: Dimetane, Dimetapp, Drixoral

Chlorpheniramine: A.R.M. Allergy Relief Medicine, Alka-Seltzer Plus, Allerest, Chlor-Trimeton, Comtrex, Contac, Coricidin, Co-Tylenol, Fedahist, Novahistine, Sine-Off, Teldrin, Triaminic, Vicks Formula 44 Cough Mixture

Clemastine: Tavist

Cyclizine: Marezine

Cyproheptadine: Periactin

Dexchlorpheniramine: Polaramine

Dimenhydrinate: Dramamine

Diphenhydramine: Benadryl, Benylin, Nytol, Sinutab, Sominex

Doxylamine: Bendectin (No longer available), Unisom

Meclizine: Antivert, Bonine

Terfenadine: Seldane

Tripelennamine: PBZ

TYPE OF DRUG: (Over-the-counter and prescription) Antihistamine

FDA RISK CATEGORY FOR PREGNANCY: C (Risk category B for clemastine)

GENERAL INFORMATION: Antihistamines are frequently used alone or in combination with decongestants, expectorants, and analgesics to relieve the symptoms of runny nose, itching eyes, and sore throat caused by viruses or hay fever. They also can be used to treat rashes, hives, and itching from allergic reactions. Unlike antibiotics, they are not capable of curing infections.

POSSIBLE MATERNAL SIDE EFFECTS: The most common side effects include drowsiness, dry mouth, blurred vision, dizziness, and nervousness.

USE DURING PREGNANCY: Most antihistamines are not associated with birth defects. In the Collaborative Perinatal Study there were 1,070 exposures to the common antihistamine chlorpheniramine and there was no link to birth defects. However, brompheniramine (in Dimetane, Dimetapp, and Drixoral) was associated with a three-fold risk of birth defects when used during the first trimester and therefore should be avoided. One of the commonly prescribed new antihistamines, terfenadine, has not been studied extensively enough during pregnancy to assure its safety.

Many over-the-counter antihistamine preparations also contain decongestants. In the Collaborative Perinatal Project an association was found between the first-trimester use of the decongestants epinephrine (p. 142) and phenylpropanolamine (p. 251) and an increased risk of birth defects. Preparations containing these drugs should be avoided. If a decongestant alone is necessary, pseudoephedrine (p. 267) is recommended. For combinations with an antihistamine, pseudoephedrine plus triprolidine (Actifed), or pseudoephedrine plus chlorpheniramine (Chlortrimeton or Sudafed Plus) are recommended.

Antihistamines are also used frequently during pregnancy for relief of first-trimester nausea. One of the most widely used and well-studied antihistamines for the control of nausea is meclizine. In 1,014 patients who took meclizine in the Collaborative Perinatal Study there was no increased risk of birth defects. The antihistamine (antinausea) drug Bendectin, which contained doxylamine and vitamin B_6, was removed from the market by the manufacturer in 1984. Despite extensive use of this drug during pregnancy and no scientific evidence that it caused birth defects, the cost of defending several lawsuits forced removal of the drug from the market. The active ingredient of Bendectin, doxylamine, is still available over-the-counter as Unisom. One Unisom 25 mg and one vitamin B_6 25 mg is similar to two Bendectin.

USE DURING BREASTFEEDING: Antihistamines can inhibit milk production. In addition, small amounts are excreted into breast milk and can cause sedation in nursing infants. Antihistamines should be avoided during breastfeeding if they cause sedation or poor feeding in the newborn.

ALTERNATIVES TO MEDICATIONS: As an alternative to antihistamines or decongestants for the relief of nasal congestion, saline (salt water) nose drops may be helpful. As an alternative to the use of antihistamines for nausea and morning sickness, try the following:

- Avoid large meals; substitute frequent small ones.
- Do not lie down for at least one hour after a meal to allow food to empty from the stomach.
- Sleeping with your head propped up or the head of the bed elevated may help prevent regurgitation of food during the night.
- Avoid exercise or activity that involves bending.

GENERIC NAME: Aspartame

COMMON BRANDS: Equal, Nutrasweet

TYPE OF DRUG: (Over-the-counter) Artificial sweetener

FDA RISK CATEGORY FOR PREGNANCY: Not classified

GENERAL INFORMATION: Aspartame is a nonnutritive artificial sweetener found in many low-calorie, dietetic foods and beverages. It is available in tablet form, with one tablet containing 19 mg aspartame, the sweetening equivalent of 1 teaspoon of sugar. Low-calorie carbonated beverages contain about 230 mg aspartame per 12-ounce can.

POSSIBLE MATERNAL SIDE EFFECTS: Aspartame has no significant side effects. It should, however, not be used by individuals with phenylketonuria.

USE DURING PREGNANCY: The FDA has approved the use of aspartame by pregnant and lactating women. There have been no reports of birth defects from first-trimester use of the drug. The major theoretical concern about the use of aspartame during pregnancy is that it is composed of aspartic acid and phenylalanine, and that high maternal levels of phenylalanine have been associated with mental retardation in infants of mothers with the disorder *phenylketonuria* who did not limit their intake of phenylalanine during pregnancy. The FDA considers a toxic level of phenylalanine to be above 100 μmol/dl in adults. To reach that level an average-sized adult would have to consume 600 aspartame tablets or approximately 75 12-ounce cans of aspartame-sweetened beverage at a single sitting. Nevertheless, women with known phenylketonuria should not consume aspartame during pregnancy.

USE DURING BREASTFEEDING: In studies of lactating laboratory animals, barely detectable increases in phenylalanine and aspartate levels were found in the milk of mothers fed very large amounts of aspartame.

ALTERNATIVES TO MEDICATIONS: In place of aspartame or sugar-containing beverages, try seltzer, which contains no calories, sugar, or salt. (In contrast, tonic water contains sugar, and club soda contains salt.) For flavor, add a squeeze of lemon or a little fruit juice.

GENERIC NAME: Aspirin

COMMON BRANDS: Alka-Seltzer, Anacin, Arthritis Pain Formula, Ascriptin, Bayer, Bufferin, Ecotrin, Empirin, Equagesic, 4-Way Cold Tablets, Fiorinal, Norgesic, Percodan, Robaxisal, Soma, Synalgos-DC, Excedrin, Vanquish

82

TYPE OF DRUG: (Over-the-counter and prescription) Analgesic, anti-inflammatory, antifever

FDA RISK CATEGORY FOR PREGNANCY: C

GENERAL INFORMATION: Aspirin is found in literally hundreds of over-the-counter products. Its uses are varied, including relief of mild pain and inflammation, lowering of body temperature, and inhibition of clotting in patients prone to stroke or heart attack.

POSSIBLE MATERNAL SIDE EFFECTS: Side effects of aspirin include nausea, stomach irritation, bleeding from the stomach, easy bruising, and possibly asthma in individuals allergic to aspirin.

USE DURING PREGNANCY: It is likely that no other drug has been used as extensively during pregnancy as aspirin. Nevertheless, its safety remains controversial. In the past, two studies that included only a small number of women suggested that taking aspirin during the first trimester slightly increased the risk of cardiac birth defects. A recent study, however, of more than 1800 women who took aspirin during the first trimester demonstrated that the risk of cardiac birth defects was no greater in the women who took aspirin than in those who did not.

Aspirin, even as little as one or two tablets, can prolong maternal bleeding time. Theoretically, during the third trimester, this could worsen the bleeding that follows vaginal or cesarean delivery. However, there is new information that low doses of aspirin (one baby aspirin per day) may help prevent preeclampsia in women with chronic hypertension. It may also reduce the risk of miscarriage in some patients known to be at high risk. To be on the safe side, *always* consult your physician before taking aspirin during any trimester of pregnancy. For relief of pain or fever, acetaminophen appears to be the safest choice. Nevertheless, most physicians believe that if you took aspirin before you knew you were pregnant, there is very little chance that your baby will be harmed in any way.

USE DURING BREASTFEEDING: Aspirin is excreted into breast milk in low concentrations. Theoretically, it could cause prolonged bleeding or easy bruising in infants.

ALTERNATIVES TO MEDICATIONS: Musculoskeletal pain can often be relieved with warm baths and massage. In some patients chronic pain can be controlled with relaxation techniques and biofeedback. If an analgesic is needed or fever needs to be reduced, acetaminophen should generally be used instead of aspirin.

GENERIC NAME: Atenolol

COMMON BRANDS: Tenoretic, Tenormin

TYPE OF DRUG: (Prescription) Antihypertensives

FDA RISK CATEGORY FOR PREGNANCY: C

GENERAL INFORMATION: Atenolol is a member of a group of drugs called beta blockers. Beta blockers act by inhibiting a major chemical reaction in the nervous system. Each of these drugs is capable of slowing the heart rate and lowering blood pressure. Their uses in the general population include treatment of high blood pressure, control of abnormal rhythms of the heart, control of acute hyperthyroidism (overactive thyroid gland), relief of angina (heart pain), prevention of migraine headaches, and prevention of performance anxiety (stage fright).

POSSIBLE MATERNAL SIDE EFFECTS: Possible side effects include slow heart rate, fatigue, wheezing (in patients with asthma), and depression.

USE DURING PREGNANCY: Beta blockers cross the placenta, but they have not been linked to congenital malformations. A large study of beta blockers during pregnancy revealed no evidence of abnormal fetal growth or development. They are now being used more frequently for the treatment of high blood pressure during pregnancy. Newborn infants of women who took atenolol near delivery should be checked closely in the newborn nursery for slow heart rate and low blood sugar.

USE DURING BREASTFEEDING: Beta blockers are excreted into breast milk and theoretically could slow the baby's heart rate. Nevertheless, the American Academy of Pediatrics considers atenolol and other beta blockers compatible with breastfeeding.

ALTERNATIVES TO MEDICATIONS: With a program of weight loss, mild salt restriction, exercise, and cessation of smoking many women can successfully decrease their blood pressure before pregnancy and remain off medications throughout at least the first trimester. However, if antihypertensive medication is necessary, another drug with a proven record of safety during pregnancy (such as methyldopa, p. 215) should be considered.

GENERIC NAME: Azathioprine

COMMON BRANDS: Imuran

TYPE OF DRUG: (Prescription) Antitransplant rejection, immunosuppressant

FDA RISK CATEGORY FOR PREGNANCY: D

GENERAL INFORMATION: In patients who have undergone kidney or liver transplantation azathioprine is given to prevent rejection of the transplanted organ. Its use has substantially improved the success of organ transplantation. The drug is also used to control joint pain and swelling in patients with rheumatoid arthritis and systemic lupus erythematosus. Azathioprine is frequently given in combination with prednisone (p. 119).

POSSIBLE MATERNAL SIDE EFFECTS: Possible side effects include an increased risk of infections, liver damage, anemia, low white blood cell count, and low platelet count.

USE DURING PREGNANCY: Azathioprine is a potent and potentially toxic drug. Use during pregnancy should be limited to severe or life-threatening conditions. Nevertheless, there are now many cases of transplant recipients treated with azathioprine throughout pregnancy who delivered normal, healthy infants. There have been a few case reports in the medical literature of infants with birth defects or chromosomal damage who were exposed to the drug during pregnancy. There is, however, no clear pattern of fetal harm, and isolated reports cannot establish a definite link between azathioprine and birth defects.

Women who must take the drug during pregnancy should be checked often for signs of infection. Even minor respiratory, urinary, or skin infections must be reported immediately to a physician. It is necessary to check blood counts and liver tests every one to three weeks throughout gestation. In addition, the newborn must be checked for abnormal blood tests and signs of infection. Despite these warnings, pregnant women who have received a kidney or liver transplant face greater danger from organ rejection than from the careful use of azathioprine.

USE DURING BREASTFEEDING: There is very little experience with the use of azathioprine during breastfeeding. Theoretically, the drug could diminish the newborn's immunity against infections and lower its blood counts. Breastfed infants must be followed carefully by the pediatrician.

ALTERNATIVES TO MEDICATIONS: There is no nonpharmacologic alternative to azathioprine for prevention of organ transplant rejection.

GENERIC NAME: **Barbiturates**

COMMON BRANDS:

Amobarbital: Amytal
Pentobarbital: Nembutal
Phenobarbital: Eskabarb, Sedadrops, SK-Phenobarbital, or generic
Secobarbital: Seconal
Secobarbital plus amobarbital: Tuinal

TYPE OF DRUG: (Prescription) Anticonvulsant, sedative

FDA RISK CATEGORY FOR PREGNANCY: D

GENERAL INFORMATION: Barbiturates are used to prevent epileptic seizures and as tranquilizers or sleeping pills. Abrupt discontinuation of these drugs in patients with epilepsy may cause seizures. Most patients should have barbiturate blood levels checked at various intervals during pregnancy to ensure the dosage is within a safe and effective range. Barbiturates are included in several combination medications in order to reduce side effects of anxiety.

POSSIBLE MATERNAL SIDE EFFECTS: Common side effects include sedation, confusion, fatigue, dizziness, and unsteadiness. Stopping barbiturates abruptly after chronic therapy may result in withdrawal symptoms of agitation and insomnia.

USE DURING PREGNANCY: Barbiturates should be used with great caution during pregnancy. Phenobarbital, and presumably other members of this class of drugs, have been linked to various birth defects including cleft lip, congenital heart disease, and microcephaly.

Ideally, any woman taking a barbiturate for prevention of seizures should consult her physician before pregnancy to see whether she still needs to take the drug. These medications should not, however, be discontinued without careful consultation. An epileptic seizure caused by stopping medication can be more harmful to both mother and fetus than taking the drug.

Blood levels of the medication should be checked often throughout pregnancy. The dosage of phenobarbital may need to be increased as pregnancy progresses to maintain the blood level in the effective range. If an increased dosage is necessary during the third trimester, the dosage will need to be reduced immediately following delivery.

Infants of women who take barbiturates must be examined for signs of withdrawal (restlessness and poor feeding). These newborns may also have a tendency to bleed excessively, a problem that can be prevented by giving the baby an injection of vitamin K shortly after birth.

USE DURING BREASTFEEDING: The American Academy of Pediatrics considers barbiturates compatible with breastfeeding. However, they do enter breast milk and can cause sedation in the newborn.

ALTERNATIVES TO MEDICATIONS: When barbiturates are being given to prevent seizures, they should not be discontinued without consulting a physician. If they are being taken for anxiety or sedation, strong consideration should be given to discontinuing their use during or ideally before pregnancy.

Insomnia may be relieved by some of the following techniques:

- Generally, try to avoid daytime naps. However, for some women sleeping patterns change during pregnancy, and a nap may be necessary to supplement abbreviated nighttime sleep.
- Go to bed only when tired. Instead of lying in bed when you are wide awake, get up, do something, and then return to bed when you feel tired.
- Try to establish a regular sleep pattern. Recognize when you *are* able to sleep and build on that.
- Exercise daily. Even a 30-minute walk will aid relaxation.
- Learn techniques of progressive relaxation. These techniques are simple to learn and effective.

- Avoid stimulant drinks such as coffee, tea, and caffeine-containing colas. On the other hand, warm milk may help make you sleepy.
- Never use alcohol to induce sleep.
- If you awaken during the night, recall the dream just before you awoke. Reentering the dream can return you to sleep.
- Make love. Sex is relaxing and often ends with sleep.
- If you are lying awake because a problem is on your mind, talk it through with someone until it's resolved.

GENERIC NAME: Beclomethasone

COMMON BRANDS: Beclovent, Beconase, Vancenase, Vanceril

TYPE OF DRUG: (Prescription) Corticosteroid inhaler (oral and nasal)

FDA RISK CATEGORY FOR PREGNANCY: C

GENERAL INFORMATION: Beclomethasone oral inhaler is used for the treatment of chronic asthma. The drug is a form of corticosteroid (p. 119) effective for prevention of wheezing when used in a regular dosage twice each day. It is not effective for relief of acute wheezing. The nasal inhaler is used for the prevention of allergic rhinitis (nasal congestion).

POSSIBLE MATERNAL SIDE EFFECTS: Possible side effects include hoarseness, thrush (yeast infection of the mouth), and a dry, irritated throat.

USE DURING PREGNANCY: In recommended dosages beclomethasone has not been shown to cause malformations in humans. However, when given in extremely high dosages corticosteroids have been associated with an increased risk of cleft palate in laboratory rabbits and rats.

USE DURING BREASTFEEDING: It is not known whether beclomethasone is excreted into breast milk.

ALTERNATIVES TO MEDICATIONS: In some cases asthma can be prevented by avoidance of known allergens, particularly animals. If you smoke, stop. It is generally a good rule, however, to use a bronchodilating inhaler such as albuterol (p. 66) at the earliest indication of wheezing. Often prompt effective relief of asthma can prevent minor episodes from becoming more severe and prolonged.

GENERIC NAME: Belladonna

COMMON BRANDS: Belladenal, Bellaspaz, Bellergal, Kinesed

TYPE OF DRUG: (Prescription) Antidiarrheal, gastrointestinal anti-spasmodic

FDA RISK CATEGORY FOR PREGNANCY: C

GENERAL INFORMATION: By decreasing spasms of the colon (large intestine), belladonna is effective in the treatment of irritable bowel syndrome, often called spastic colon or functional bowel syndrome. Several combination prescription products also include barbiturates such as phenobarbital (p. 247).

POSSIBLE MATERNAL SIDE EFFECTS: The most common side effects include dry mouth, blurred vision, drowsiness (especially when combined with an antihistamine or barbiturate), difficulty urinating, and palpitations.

USE DURING PREGNANCY: The Collaborative Perinatal Project found a slight increase in the number of birth defects following first-trimester exposure to belladonna. Belladonna should be avoided during the first trimester, but use during the second and third trimesters appears to be safe.

USE DURING BREASTFEEDING: Belladonna enters breast milk and could cause lethargy or poor feeding in the newborn.

ALTERNATIVES TO MEDICATIONS: Alternatives to taking belladonna for treatment of irritable bowel syndrome include additional dietary fiber, regular exercise, and avoidance of gas-forming foods such as beans, onions, cabbage, dried fruits (apricots, dates, raisins), apple juice, and foods made with all-purpose refined white flour.

GENERIC NAME: Birth control pills (Oral contraceptives)

COMMON BRANDS: Brevicon, Demulen, Levelen, Loestrin, Lo/Ovral, Micronor, Modicon, Nordette, Norethin, Norinyl, Ortho-Novum, Ovcon, Ovral, Ovrette, Tri-Levlen, Triphasil

TYPE OF DRUG: (Prescription) Estrogen/Progestin hormones

FDA RISK CATEGORY FOR PREGNANCY: X

GENERAL INFORMATION: Birth control pills (oral contraceptives) are synthetic hormones consisting of a combination of estrogen and progestin, or progestin alone. Their use is to prevent pregnancy.

POSSIBLE MATERNAL SIDE EFFECTS: The most common side effects include nausea, abdominal bloating, and headaches. The most serious adverse effects include worsening of migraine headaches, phlebitis (blood clot in a major vein of the leg), pulmonary embolism (blood clot in the lung), high blood pressure, stroke, and heart attack. Fortunately, these serious adverse effects are rare.

USE DURING PREGNANCY: Ideally, oral contraceptives should be stopped three months, or at least two normal menstrual cycles, before attempting to conceive. Rarely, pregnancy can occur while taking the pill. Statistically, there appears to be no reason for alarm. Most studies have shown little, if any, risk to the fetus if birth control pills were inadvertently taken during the first weeks of pregnancy. Becoming pregnant while taking the pill does not warrant terminating the pregnancy.

USE DURING BREASTFEEDING: Use of oral contraceptives during breastfeeding may decrease milk production and interfere with normal infant weight gain. If birth control pills must be used during breastfeeding, the preparation with the lowest effective dosage of estrogen should be chosen, and the baby should be monitored for appropriate weight gain. Nutritional supplements may be required.

ALTERNATIVES TO MEDICATIONS: Alternatives to birth control pills include the condom, diaphragm, contraceptive sponge, IUD, and cervical cap.

GENERIC NAME: Bisacodyl

COMMON BRANDS: Biscolax, Carter's Pills, Dulcolax Pills and Suppositories, Fleet Prepkits, Theralax Suppositories

TYPE OF DRUG: (Over-the-counter) Laxative

FDA RISK CATEGORY FOR PREGNANCY: B

GENERAL INFORMATION: Bisacodyl is the active ingredient found in several over-the-counter pills and suppositories used for relief of acute constipation. The drug has a direct stimulant effect on the colon. Bisacodyl should not be used chronically. If constipation persists, medical evaluation is necessary.

POSSIBLE MATERNAL SIDE EFFECTS: The most common side effect of bisacodyl pills is nausea. Swallowing tablets whole rather than chewing or crushing them minimizes stomach irritation. Chronic use of any laxative can lead to loss of important minerals, such as potassium, and laxative dependence.

USE DURING PREGNANCY: There are no special warnings about the use of bisacodyl during pregnancy. Chronic use, however, can lead to laxative dependence. In most cases the addition of fiber in the diet and appropriate exercise will alleviate constipation during pregnancy.

USE DURING BREASTFEEDING: Bisacodyl may be used safely during breastfeeding.

ALTERNATIVES TO MEDICATIONS: Constipation is one of the most common gastrointestinal complaints during pregnancy even for women who were previously very regular. It is likely caused by the combined factors of pressure from the enlarging uterus and relaxation of intestinal muscle due to pregnancy hormones. Most women can control this problem by the following measures:

- Include some high-fiber cereal, prunes, or figs with breakfast. Do not, however, eat excessive amounts of fiber. It may be irritating to the stomach.
- Drink hot liquid with breakfast. This often has a stimulating effect on the colon.
- Allow plenty of time for appropriate bowel habits in the morning.
- With your doctor's consent milk of magnesia (p. 78) can be used sparingly at night but harsh laxatives should be avoided. Some laxatives can cause the uterus to contract.

GENERIC NAME: Bismuth subsalicylate

COMMON BRANDS: Pepto-Bismol

TYPE OF DRUG: (Over-the-counter) Antidiarrheal, antacid, antinausea

FDA RISK CATEGORY FOR PREGNANCY: B

GENERAL INFORMATION: Bismuth subsalicylate is an over-the-counter preparation most often used for the treatment of acute diarrhea. It usually controls diarrhea within 24 hours and can also relieve associated cramps and nausea. The product also contains salicylates (see aspirin, p. 82).

POSSIBLE MATERNAL SIDE EFFECTS: Bismuth may cause temporary and harmless darkening (even blackening) of the tongue and stools. Stool darkening should not be confused with bleeding in the intestinal tract. Salicylates can cause irritation of the stomach and ringing in the ears, especially if Pepto-Bismol is taken in combination with aspirin.

USE DURING PREGNANCY: In general bismuth subsalicylate is considered safe for occasional use during pregnancy. However, prolonged diarrhea or diarrhea associated with fever over 100°F should be reported to your physician.

USE DURING BREASTFEEDING: Bismuth subsalicylate is safe for use during breastfeeding.

ALTERNATIVES TO MEDICATIONS: With acute diarrhea solid foods may be discontinued for 12 to 24 hours. When diarrhea abates, start eating again with dry bread or toast and small amounts of vegetables. Since it is essential to avoid dehydration, be sure to drink plenty of liquids that contain sugar. Soup can also provide some nutrition and hydration without aggravating diarrhea. Symptoms of dehydration include thirst, dry mouth, fast breathing, and sometimes fever. An early sign of dehydration is reduction in the amount and frequency of urination. Drink enough to keep up normal urine output. If adequate hydration cannot be maintained, call the doctor.

During pregnancy consideration should be given to avoiding trips to countries where traveler's diarrhea is known to be common.

GENERIC NAME: **Bromocriptine**

COMMON BRANDS: Parlodel

TYPE OF DRUG: (Prescription) Infertility

FDA RISK CATEGORY FOR PREGNANCY: C

GENERAL INFORMATION: Bromocriptine is used to promote normal ovulation and regular menstrual periods in women with tumors of the pituitary gland. Women with these tumors are often unable to become pregnant unless they are first treated with the drug. Bromocriptine is also given to shrink the size of large pituitary tumors (greater than one-half inch).

POSSIBLE MATERNAL SIDE EFFECTS: The most common side effect of bromocriptine is nausea, which occurs in almost half the patients treated with the drug. Other side effects include dizziness, headache, fatigue, dry mouth, and difficulty urinating.

USE DURING PREGNANCY: Bromocriptine is generally discontinued once pregnancy is diagnosed. However, since pregnancy is often not confirmed until several weeks after conception, use of bromocriptine during the first trimester is common. Several studies have shown that the drug can be safely taken during any stage of pregnancy. Its use during the first trimester has not been linked to birth defects.

USE DURING BREASTFEEDING: Bromocriptine is often given to suppress milk production in women who choose not to breastfeed. Therefore, breastfeeding is usually not possible in women taking this medication.

ALTERNATIVES TO MEDICATIONS: There is no nonpharmacologic alternative to bromocriptine for induction of ovulation in women with tumors of the pituitary gland.

GENERIC NAME: Bumetanide

COMMON BRANDS: Bumex

TYPE OF DRUG: (Prescription) Diuretic

FDA RISK CATEGORY FOR PREGNANCY: C

GENERAL INFORMATION: Bumetanide is a potent diuretic used for the treatment of high blood pressure and heart failure. It is not usually used for the treatment of simple fluid retention.

POSSIBLE MATERNAL SIDE EFFECTS: Possible side effects include loss of potassium and sodium. Patients known to be allergic to sulfa medications may also be allergic to bumetanide.

USE DURING PREGNANCY: All diuretics should be used with caution during pregnancy. Bumetanide is generally reserved for women with chronic heart disorders and should not be used to treat the water retention that occurs during most normal pregnancies. The drug has not been shown to cause birth defects when given in large dosages to mice. However, there have been no careful studies in women during the first trimester.

USE DURING BREASTFEEDING: No data are available.

ALTERNATIVES TO MEDICATIONS: The use of diuretics during pregnancy is usually reserved for women with heart problems or kidney disease. Mild edema (fluid retention) is a common occurrence during pregnancy and does not require treatment. If edema becomes uncomfortable, it can usually be relieved by lying on your side for periods of 30 to 60 minutes. In some cases mild restriction of dietary salt intake may be necessary. Severe salt restriction, however, is not appropriate and may even be harmful. There is no evidence that so-called natural diuretics found in health food stores are effective and their safety during pregnancy cannot be assured.

GENERIC NAME: Buspirone

COMMON BRANDS: BuSpar

TYPE OF DRUG: (Prescription) Antianxiety, sedative

FDA RISK CATEGORY FOR PREGNANCY: B

GENERAL INFORMATION: Buspirone is a tranquilizer that is not chemically related to benzodiazepines (p. 69) or barbiturates (p. 86). It is reported to be less sedating than either benzodiazepines or barbiturates.

POSSIBLE MATERNAL SIDE EFFECTS: Common side effects include dizziness, confusion, depression, blurred vision, rapid heart rate, and dry mouth.

USE DURING PREGNANCY: Buspirone is a relatively new drug. Therefore, there is too little experience with its use during pregnancy to ensure its safety. Animal studies, however, have not revealed any link with birth defects.

USE DURING BREASTFEEDING: The extent to which buspirone is excreted into breast milk is not known.

ALTERNATIVES TO MEDICATIONS: Before using medications to control anxiety or stress consider the following strategy:

1. Identify the source of your anxiety. Worry often persists because of an inability to identify a problem and take action to solve it. Visualization can begin the process. Close your eyes and take a few deep breaths. Allow an image of the problem to arise.
2. Once you've defined the source of your anxiety, gather information. For example, if you are worried about the outcome of your pregnancy because of a possible hereditary problem or a medication you took before you knew you were pregnant, get information from your physician or a genetic counselor. In most cases what you discover will be very comforting.
3. After obtaining information, decide on a plan of action. Do what you can to deal with the problem, but once you've done all you can, change your focus and move on to other parts of life. Instead of worrying, concentrate on your life beyond the worry. Exercise or take walks. Plan how you will spend the evening or the weekend. Treat yourself to something pleasant, or think up a surprise for someone you care about. As your mind gets busy with other thoughts, you'll find that stress will begin to fade.
4. If anxiety persists despite your best efforts, see a therapist. Often only a few counseling sessions can effectively reduce anxiety and stress and eliminate the need for medication.

GENERIC NAME: ## Butoconazole

COMMON BRANDS: Femstat

TYPE OF DRUG: (Prescription) Antifungal

FDA RISK CATEGORY FOR PREGNANCY: C

GENERAL INFORMATION: Butoconazole is available in a cream for the treatment of yeast (candida) infections of the vagina and vulva. Often a vaginal discharge is mistakenly assumed to be caused by yeast infection. Since there are many other causes of acute vaginitis, treatment should not be begun without appropriate medical examination and laboratory confirmation.

POSSIBLE MATERNAL SIDE EFFECTS: Side effects are usually minimal, but vaginal burning and itching can occur.

USE DURING PREGNANCY: There has not been extensive experience with butoconazole during pregnancy. However, in studies where rats were given the drug intravaginally, there was no evidence of birth defects. Clinical studies of over 200 women treated with butoconazole during the second and third trimesters demonstrated no adverse effect on the fetus. In many cases treatment of vaginitis can be postponed until after pregnancy or at least until after the first trimester.

USE DURING BREASTFEEDING: It is not known whether butoconazole is excreted into breast milk.

ALTERNATIVES TO MEDICATIONS: To help avoid vaginal yeast infections do not take antibiotics unnecessarily, wear loose cotton underwear, avoid harsh soaps and irritants, and be sure your partner does not have a chronic yeast infection. During pregnancy it is not always necessary to treat mild yeast infections.

GENERIC NAME: Caffeine

COMMON BRANDS: Anacin, chocolate, coffee, cola, Dexatrim, Excedrin, Midol, No Doz, tea, Vanquish, Vivarin

TYPE OF DRUG: (Over-the-counter) Stimulant

FDA RISK CATEGORY FOR PREGNANCY: B

GENERAL INFORMATION: Caffeine is found in a variety of over-the-counter cold tablets, pain pills, and appetite suppressants as well as many foods and beverages. Amounts of caffeine in common products include: coffee, 15 to 150 mg per 8-ounce cup; cola beverages, 30 to 65 mg per 12 ounce can; cocoa, 5 to 10 mg per 8-ounce cup; tea, 40 to 60 mg per 8-ounce cup; allergy and pain pills, 15 to 65 mg per pill; appetite suppressants, 50 to 200 mg per pill; stimulants, 100 to 200 mg per pill.

POSSIBLE MATERNAL SIDE EFFECTS: Habitual consumption of 500 to 750 mg per day of caffeine can cause restlessness, anxiety, irritability, palpitations, and sleeplessness.

USE DURING PREGNANCY: The use of caffeine during pregnancy remains controversial. Most studies have not been able to establish a link between caffeine and birth defects. Several authors, however, have associated high caffeine consumption (6 to 8 cups of coffee per day) with decreased fertility, increased incidence of miscarriage, and low birth weights. A recent review of the published medical data suggests that until more information is available, it would be prudent to limit caffeine intake to no more than 300 mg per day during pregnancy.

USE DURING BREASTFEEDING: Caffeine enters breast milk and can cause irritability and poor sleeping patterns in the newborn. Daily intake should be limited to no more that 300 mg.

ALTERNATIVES TO MEDICATIONS: Today, most caffeine-containing beverages are available in decaffeinated alternatives.

GENERIC NAME: Calcitonin

COMMON BRANDS: Calcimar

TYPE OF DRUG: (Prescription) Hormone

FDA RISK CATEGORY FOR PREGNANCY: C

GENERAL INFORMATION: Calcitonin is a synthetic hormone used for the treatment of two chronic bone diseases—Paget's disease and osteoporosis. The drug works by blocking the normal reabsorption of calcium from bones. Both Paget's disease and osteoporosis are rare in young women.

POSSIBLE MATERNAL SIDE EFFECTS: Common side effects include facial flushing, nausea, and headaches. Since the drug affects calcium levels in the blood, it is necessary to measure blood levels at regular intervals.

USE DURING PREGNANCY: Calcitonin does not cross the placenta. However, the drug has not been sufficiently used during human pregnancy to ensure its safety.

USE DURING BREASTFEEDING: Calcitonin has been shown to interfere with breast milk production in animals. No data are available in humans.

ALTERNATIVES TO MEDICATIONS: It would be unusual for calcitonin to be necessary during pregnancy. There are no nonpharm-acologic alternatives.

GENERIC NAME: **Captopril**

> **COMMON BRANDS:** Capoten, Capozide
>
> **TYPE OF DRUG:** (Prescription) Antihypertensive
>
> **FDA RISK CATEGORY FOR PREGNANCY:** C
>
> **GENERAL INFORMATION:** Captopril is a member of a new class of powerful antihypertensive drugs called angiotensin-I converting en-zyme (ACE) inhibitors. It works by blocking the formation of a chem-ical that causes constriction of arteries.
>
> **POSSIBLE MATERNAL SIDE EFFECTS:** Side effects are usually mini-mal, but the drug should be used cautiously in patients with kidney disease.
>
> **USE DURING PREGNANCY:** Studies of captopril in animals indicate an increased risk of birth defects when the drug is given during the first trimester. There have also been isolated reports of birth defects in humans. In addition, the drug can damage the baby's kidneys. Since there are safer medications for the treatment of hypertension, captopril should not be used during pregnancy.
>
> **USE DURING BREASTFEEDING:** The drug enters breast milk, but its effects in the newborn are not known. If possible, other antihyperten-sive medications should be used in place of captopril.
>
> **ALTERNATIVES TO MEDICATIONS:** With a program of weight loss, mild salt restriction, exercise, and cessation of smoking many women can successfully decrease their blood pressure before preg-nancy and remain off medications throughout at least the first tri-mester. However, if antihypertensive medication is necessary, another drug with a proven record of safety during pregnancy (such as methyldopa, p. 215) should be substituted for captopril.

GENERIC NAME: **Carbamazepine**

> **COMMON BRANDS:** Tegretol
>
> **TYPE OF DRUG:** (Prescription) Anticonvulsant

FDA RISK CATEGORY FOR PREGNANCY: D

GENERAL INFORMATION: Carbamazepine is used for the treatment of epilepsy in adults and children. It is effective for prevention of grand mal (major motor) seizures, petit mal (minor seizures or absence attacks) seizures, and temporal lobe epilepsy. The precise mechanism of action is not known.

POSSIBLE MATERNAL SIDE EFFECTS: The most common side effects include drowsiness, unsteadiness, nausea, and fatigue. If the drug is used during pregnancy, blood concentrations should be measured at regular intervals to insure the dosage is safe and effective.

USE DURING PREGNANCY: The drug crosses the placenta and reaches levels in the blood of the fetus equal to the mother's. A recent medical study has clearly linked the first trimester use of carbamazepine with several major birth defects including cleft lip and cleft palate. With regard to the use of anticonvulsant medications during pregnancy most authorities and the American College of Obstetricians and Gynecologists recommend the following:

1. All women with epilepsy whether or not they are taking anticonvulsant medication should consult their physician before attempting pregnancy or just as soon as pregnancy is suspected.
2. Women who have been free of seizures for several years should consult their physician to see whether medication can be discontinued before pregnancy. Some anticonvulsant medications are considered safer than others and at least a change in medications may be appropriate.
3. Women with recurrent seizures should not stop taking their medications when they find out they are pregnant without first consulting a physician. The risk to both mother and baby is greater from a major epileptic seizure than from taking medication. Even if a medication must be taken during the first trimester, the chance of having a normal baby is approximately 90 percent.
4. The use of anticonvulsant medications during pregnancy requires careful medical follow-up. Blood levels of the drugs should be checked frequently, generally monthly, to ensure that the dosage is safe and effective.
5. The pediatrician should be notified before delivery if anticonvulsants were prescribed during pregnancy so the baby can be checked immediately for any problems.

USE DURING BREASTFEEDING: Cambamazepine is excreted into breast milk, but no adverse effects have been reported. The American Academy of Pediatrics considers the drug compatible with breastfeeding.

ALTERNATIVES TO MEDICATIONS: When anticonvulsant medication is needed for prevention of seizures, there is no non-pharmacologic alternative. Nevertheless, the risk of seizures can be reduced by obtaining adequate rest, avoiding alcohol, and not taking any other drug or medication without consulting a physician.

GENERIC NAME: Carbenicillin

COMMON BRANDS: Geocillin

TYPE OF DRUG: (Prescription) Antibiotic

FDA RISK CATEGORY FOR PREGNANCY: B

GENERAL INFORMATION: Carbenicillin is a penicillin-type antibiotic. It should not be used by people allergic to penicillin.

POSSIBLE MATERNAL SIDE EFFECTS: Side effects are uncommon, but diarrhea may result from treatment with any antibiotic and should be reported to your physician if it lasts longer than 48 hours. A rash can occur at any time in individuals allergic to penicillin.

USE DURING PREGNANCY: The drug is considered safe for use during any stage of pregnancy.

USE DURING BREASTFEEDING: Carbenicillin is safe for use during breastfeeding.

ALTERNATIVES TO MEDICATIONS: Carbenicillin is usually reserved for severe infections. Although there is no nonpharmacologic alternative for treatment of serious infections, occasionally other less expensive penicillin antibiotics can be used in place of carbenicillin.

GENERIC NAME: Cephalosporins

COMMON BRANDS:

Cefaclor: Ceclor
Cefazolin: Ancef
Cefadroxil: Duricef, Ultracef

Ceforanide: Precef
Cefoperazone: Cefobid
Cefotaxime: Claforan
Cefotetan: Cefotan
Ceftazidime: Fortaz
Ceftizoxime: Cefizox
Ceftriaxone: Rocephin
Cefuroxime: Ceftin, Zinacef
Cephalexin: Keflex, Keftabs
Cephapirin: Cefadyl
Cephalothin: Keflin
Cephradine: Anspor, Velosef
Moxalactam: Moxam

TYPE OF DRUG: (Prescription) Antibiotics

FDA RISK CATEGORY FOR PREGNANCY: B

GENERAL INFORMATION: Cephalosporins are broad-spectrum antibiotics used to treat a variety of infections including urinary tract infections, sinus and respiratory infections, pneumonia, and some severe systemic infections. A small number of individuals who are allergic to penicillin can also be allergic to cephalosporins.

POSSIBLE MATERNAL SIDE EFFECTS: Side effects are uncommon, but diarrhea may result from treatment with any antibiotic and should be reported to your physician if it lasts longer than 48 hours. A rash can occur at any time in individuals allergic to cephalosporins and in about 10 percent of people allergic to penicillin.

USE DURING PREGNANCY: Older cephalosporins such as cefadroxil, cefazolin, cephalexin, cephalothin, cephapirin, cephradine (first-generation cephalosporins) and cefaclor, cefamandole, cefonicid, ceforanide, cefotetan, cefoxitin, cefuroxime (second-generation cephalosporins) have been used extensively during pregnancy and have been determined to be safe. The newer cephalosporins such as cefoperazone, cefotaxime, ceftazidime, ceftizoxime, and ceftriaxone (third-generation cephalosporins) have not been used long enough to ensure their safety. Newer cephalosporins are usually reserved for severe infections when other antibiotics have been shown to be less effective.

USE DURING BREASTFEEDING: Cephalosporins enter breast milk, but appear to be safe for use during breastfeeding.

ALTERNATIVES TO MEDICATIONS: For serious bacterial infections there is no nonpharmacologic alternative to antibiotics. Most common viral infections do not require antibiotic treatment.

GENERIC NAME: Chloral hydrate

COMMON BRANDS: Noctec, Oradrate

TYPE OF DRUG: (Prescription) Sedative

FDA RISK CATEGORY FOR PREGNANCY: C

GENERAL INFORMATION: Chloral hydrate is a sedative most often used as a sleeping pill. With chronic use it can become habit-forming or addictive.

POSSIBLE MATERNAL SIDE EFFECTS: Common side effects include sedation, hangover, confusion, dizziness, nightmares, nausea, and an abnormal taste.

USE DURING PREGNANCY: All sedatives cross the placenta and should be used with caution during pregnancy. However, chloral hydrate has not been linked to birth defects or other fetal harm.

USE DURING BREASTFEEDING: The drug is excreted into breast milk and can cause sedation in the nursing infant. Sedatives should be used only if necessary during breastfeeding.

ALTERNATIVES TO MEDICATIONS: Insomnia may be relieved by some of the following techniques:

- Generally, try to avoid daytime naps. However, for some women sleeping patterns change during pregnancy, and a nap may be necessary to supplement abbreviated nighttime sleep.
- Go to bed only when tired. Instead of lying in bed when you are wide awake, get up, do something, and then return to bed when you feel tired.
- Try to establish a regular sleep pattern. Recognize when you are able to sleep and build on that.
- Exercise daily. Even a 30-minute walk will aid relaxation.
- Learn techniques of progressive relaxation. These techniques are simple to learn and effective.

- Avoid stimulant drinks such as coffee, tea, and caffeine-containing colas. On the other hand, warm milk may help make you sleepy.
- Never use alcohol to induce sleep.
- If you awaken during the night, recall the dream just before you awoke. Reentering the dream can return you to sleep.
- Make love. Sex is relaxing and often ends with sleep.
- If you are lying awake because a problem is on your mind, talk it through with someone until it's resolved.

GENERIC NAME: Chloramphenicol

COMMON BRANDS: Chloromycetin

TYPE OF DRUG: (Prescription) Antibiotic

FDA RISK CATEGORY FOR PREGNANCY: C

GENERAL INFORMATION: Chloramphenicol is an older antibiotic, which has generally been replaced by newer, safer drugs. In a few cases it has caused severe anemia by interfering with red blood cell production in the bone marrow.

POSSIBLE MATERNAL SIDE EFFECTS: The most serious adverse effect of chloramphenicol is a severe suppression of the bone marrow called aplastic anemia.

USE DURING PREGNANCY: Chloramphenicol has not been shown to cause birth defects. Used near term, however, it can cause a severe reaction in the newborn called the "gray syndrome," resulting in collapse of the cardiovascular system and death. Chloramphenicol should not be used during pregnancy unless there is no safer antibiotic available to treat a severe infection.

USE DURING BREASTFEEDING: Use of chloramphenicol during breastfeeding is controversial. Theoretically, it could suppress production of red and white blood cells in the bone marrow of the newborn. It should generally be avoided.

ALTERNATIVES TO MEDICATIONS: For the treatment of serious bacterial infections there is no nonpharmacologic alternative to antibiotics. In most cases, however, there are safer antibiotic alternatives to chloramphenicol.

GENERIC NAME: Chlordiazepoxide

COMMON BRANDS: Librax, Librium

TYPE OF DRUG: (Prescription) Antianxiety, sedative

FDA RISK CATEGORY FOR PREGNANCY: D

GENERAL INFORMATION: Chlordiazepoxide is a member of a group of antianxiety medications called benzodiazepines. These drugs are used for the treatment of anxiety, insomnia. They work by relaxing skeletal muscles and by a direct action on the brain. Benzodiazepines can be abused if taken indiscriminately or for a long period of time. Withdrawal symptoms including tremor, agitation, insomnia, muscle cramps, nausea, and seizures can occur if these drugs are discontinued abruptly after chronic use. Benzodiazepines should not be taken without careful medical supervision.

POSSIBLE MATERNAL SIDE EFFECTS: Common side effects of all benzodiazepines include sedation, depression, mental confusion, dizziness, unsteady gait, nightmares, fatigue, dry mouth, and low blood pressure. These drugs can interfere with the ability to safely drive a car or operate dangerous equipment. Physical and psychological dependence can occur with chronic use.

USE DURING PREGNANCY: All benzodiazepines rapidly cross the placenta and enter the fetal circulation. Blood levels in the fetus equal that of the mother's within one hour of taking a pill. Several studies have demonstrated a link between first-trimester use of benzodiazepines and birth defects. The most commonly reported malformations are cleft lip and cleft palate.

Used near term benzodiazepines have been associated with lethargy, respiratory problems, and withdrawal symptoms in the newborn. Most authorities believe that it is best to avoid these medications during the first trimester, and if possible, throughout pregnancy.

USE DURING BREASTFEEDING: Benzodiazepines are excreted into breast milk in significant quantities. They can cause sedation in the newborn and should be avoided during breastfeeding.

ALTERNATIVES TO MEDICATIONS: Before using medications to control anxiety or stress consider the following strategy:

1. Identify the source of your anxiety. Worry often persists because

of an inability to identify a problem and take action to solve it. Visualization can begin the process. Close your eyes and take a few deep breaths. Allow an image of the problem to arise.

2. Once you've defined the source of your anxiety, gather information. For example, if you are worried about the outcome of your pregnancy because of a possible hereditary problem or a medication you took before you knew you were pregnant, get information from your physician or a genetic counselor. In most cases what you discover will be very comforting.

3. After obtaining information, decide on a plan of action. Do what you can to deal with the problem, but once you've done all you can, change your focus and move on to other parts of life. Instead of worrying, concentrate on your life beyond the worry. Exercise or take walks. Plan how you will spend the evening or the weekend. Treat yourself to something pleasant or think up a surprise for someone you care about. As your mind gets busy with other thoughts, you'll find that stress will begin to fade.

4. If anxiety persists despite your best efforts, see a therapist. Often only a few counseling sessions can effectively reduce anxiety and stress and eliminate the need for medication.

GENERIC NAME: Chloroquine

COMMON BRANDS: Aralen

TYPE OF DRUG: (Prescription) Antimalarial

FDA RISK CATEGORY FOR PREGNANCY: C

GENERAL INFORMATION: Chloroquine is the drug of choice for prevention and treatment of malaria. The drug is usually given once each week to travelers going to countries known to have a high rate of malaria infections. It should be continued for six weeks following departure from a high-risk area. Certain areas of the world are now known to have malaria parasites resistant to chloroquine. Infections due to chloroquine-resistant strains will require additional drugs.

POSSIBLE MATERNAL SIDE EFFECTS: Possible side effects include headache, blurred vision, and nausea.

USE DURING PREGNANCY: There have been a few reports of birth defects in infants of women who took chloroquine during the first trimester. However, there have been no large studies that confirmed these isolated reports. If possible, travel to areas known to have a high incidence of malaria should be avoided during pregnancy. Nevertheless, the risk of malaria during pregnancy is probably greater than the theoretical risk of chloroquine. Chloroquine should not be withheld because of pregnancy in women who must travel to high-risk areas of the world.

USE DURING BREASTFEEDING: Chloroquine does not appear to be excreted in measurable amounts in breast milk. The American Academy of Pediatrics considers chloroquine compatible with breastfeeding.

ALTERNATIVES TO MEDICATIONS: If possible, travel to areas of the world where the risk of malaria is high should be avoided during pregnancy (or at least during the first trimester). If travel to these areas cannot be avoided, chloroquine should be taken to prevent malaria. Additional protection is available by using insect repellents containing 100 percent DEET, nets, and screens for personal protection against mosquitoes.

GENERIC NAME: Chlorpromazine

COMMON BRANDS: Thorazine

TYPE OF DRUG: (Prescription) Major tranquilizer, antipsychotic

FDA RISK CATEGORY FOR PREGNANCY: C

GENERAL INFORMATION: Chlorpromazine is a member of a class of medications called phenothiazines. It is used to treat major psychotic disorders such as schizophrenia. The drug can also be used to treat persistent nausea and vomiting.

POSSIBLE MATERNAL SIDE EFFECTS: The most common side effects include drowsiness, jaundice, and an unusual group of side effects, called extrapyramidal effects, characterized by spasm of the neck muscles and difficulty swallowing.

USE DURING PREGNANCY: Chlorpromazine has been used during pregnancy to treat persistent nausea and vomiting (hyperemesis gravidarum) during the first trimester. The Collaborative Perinatal Project found no link between the drug and birth defects. There have been a few reports of tremors and muscle spasticity in newborns when the drug was used near term. Chlorpromazine should therefore be avoided near the time of delivery.

USE DURING BREASTFEEDING: The drug enters breast milk and could cause sedation in the newborn. Nevertheless, the American Academy of Pediatrics considers chlorpromazine compatible with breastfeeding.

ALTERNATIVES TO MEDICATIONS: For patients with serious psychotic disorders such as schizophrenia, chlorpromazine should not be discontinued without careful consultation from a psychiatrist. In some cases it is possible to stop the drug or reduce the dosage by increasing the frequency of counseling sessions and by living in a controlled, well-supervised home or hospital setting.

GENERIC NAME: Chlorpropamide

COMMON BRANDS: Diabinese

TYPE OF DRUG: (Prescription) Oral diabetes medication

FDA RISK CATEGORY FOR PREGNANCY: D

GENERAL INFORMATION: Chlorpropamide is used for treatment of adult-onset (type II) diabetes. It is not appropriate for individuals with insulin-dependent (type I) diabetes. Patients with type I diabetes require daily injections of insulin.

POSSIBLE MATERNAL SIDE EFFECTS: The most significant side effect is low blood sugar (hypoglycemia). Patients allergic to sulfa drugs are likely to be allergic to chlorpropamide.

USE DURING PREGNANCY: Chlorpropamide should not be used during pregnancy. Women taking the drug before pregnancy should be switched to insulin before conception and throughout pregnancy. First-trimester use of chlorpropamide has been associated with an increased risk of birth defects. When used near term it can cause severe, prolonged hypoglycemia in the newborn.

USE DURING BREASTFEEDING: Chlorpropamide is excreted into breast milk and can theoretically cause hypoglycemia in the nursing infant.

ALTERNATIVES TO MEDICATIONS: Some women with type II diabetes treated with chlorpropamide before pregnancy can satisfactorily control their blood sugars by following a strict diet. Most pregnant women, however, will have to take injections of insulin to maintain their blood sugar levels in the range appropriate for pregnancy.

GENERIC NAME: Chlorthalidone

COMMON BRANDS: Combipres, Hygroton, Tenoretic, Thalitone

TYPE OF DRUG: (Prescription) Diuretic

FDA RISK CATEGORY FOR PREGNANCY: B

GENERAL INFORMATION: Chlorthalidone is a diuretic used for the treatment of chronic hypertension, heart failure, and edema due to certain types of kidney disorders. It works by increasing the urinary excretion of sodium and water. For treatment of high blood pressure the drug may be used alone or in combination with other antihypertensive medications. Several combination antihypertensive preparations contain chlorthalidone plus another drug.

POSSIBLE MATERNAL SIDE EFFECTS: The most significant side effect is urinary loss of potassium, which may require taking potassium supplements. Other side effects are generally mild, including nausea and loss of appetite.

USE DURING PREGNANCY: The use of chlorthalidone during pregnancy is controversial. Some physicians feel that women treated with this diuretic before pregnancy may safely continue taking the drug throughout gestation. Others are concerned about reports of a slight increase in the risk of malformations when the drug is used during the first trimester. Treatment of hypertension should be re-evaluated before attempting pregnancy, and if possible, other medications considered safer for use during pregnancy should be substituted for chlorthalidone. If, however, treatment of heart disease, kidney disease, or hypertension necessitates the use of this drug during pregnancy, most authorities believe it is relatively safe. It should not be given to alleviate the normal water retention experienced by most women during the third trimester.

USE DURING BREASTFEEDING: Use of chlorthalidone during breastfeeding is controversial. The drug enters breast milk but probably has little effect on the newborn. On the other hand, the medication can theoretically interfere with the production of breast milk.

ALTERNATIVES TO MEDICATIONS: The use of diuretics during pregnancy is usually reserved for women with chronic hypertension, heart problems, or kidney disease. Mild edema (fluid retention) is a common occurrence during pregnancy and does not require treatment. If edema becomes uncomfortable, it can usually be relieved by lying on your side for periods of 30 to 60 minutes. In some cases mild restriction of dietary salt intake may be necessary. Severe salt restriction, however, is not appropriate and may even be harmful. There is no evidence that so-called natural diuretics found in health food stores are effective and their safety during pregnancy cannot be assured.

GENERIC NAME: # Cholestyramine

COMMON BRANDS: Questran

TYPE OF DRUG: (Prescription) Lowers cholesterol

FDA RISK CATEGORY FOR PREGNANCY: C

GENERAL INFORMATION: Cholestyramine is a resin that binds bile acids in the intestine. Its action results in a lowering of serum cholesterol and can therefore be used to treat patients with an elevated serum cholesterol level. The drug is not absorbed into the blood.

POSSIBLE MATERNAL SIDE EFFECTS: Side effects are confined to the intestinal tract. Some patients complain of increased gas, bloating, and constipation. Absorption of fat-soluble vitamins can be impaired.

USE DURING PREGNANCY: Cholestyramine has been used during pregnancy to treat the itching due to a disorder called cholestasis of pregnancy. Its ability to bind bile acids in the intestine is thought to reduce the itching associated with this condition. Although large studies of cholestyramine use during pregnancy are lacking, the drug is considered safe because it is not absorbed into the blood. Since the drug can interfere with the absorption of fat-soluble vitamins, additional supplements may be required.

USE DURING BREASTFEEDING: It is unlikely that the drug enters breast milk. However, certain vitamins may be missing from breast milk because cholestyramine can interfere with their absorption from your diet.

ALTERNATIVES TO MEDICATIONS: Treatment of elevated serum cholesterol can usually be achieved with dietary restriction of cholesterol and saturated fat. The addition of dietary fiber such as oat bran may also be helpful.

GENERIC NAME: Cimetidine

COMMON BRANDS: Tagamet

TYPE OF DRUG: (Prescription) Blocks gastric acid production

FDA RISK CATEGORY FOR PREGNANCY: B

GENERAL INFORMATION: Cimetidine blocks the production of acid in the stomach. It is used for the treatment of ulcers in the stomach or duodenum (small intestine).

POSSIBLE MATERNAL SIDE EFFECTS: Cimetidine is generally well tolerated.

USE DURING PREGNANCY: The drug has not been studied extensively during human gestation, but birth defects have not been reported. When given in very high dosages to laboratory animals cimetidine has not been linked to birth defects.

USE DURING BREASTFEEDING: Cimetidine enters breast milk in high concentrations and is capable of interfering with acid production in the newborn. Although it is not clear if there is any risk to the infant, the drug should generally be avoided during breastfeeding.

ALTERNATIVES TO MEDICATIONS: A program of dietary restriction, alone, is generally not adequate for treatment of stomach or intestinal ulcers. However, an alternative to cimetidine during pregnancy is the regular use of antacids (p. 78) between meals.

GENERIC NAME: Ciprofloxacin

COMMON BRANDS: Cipro

TYPE OF DRUG: (Prescription) Antibiotic

FDA RISK CATEGORY FOR PREGNANCY: C

GENERAL INFORMATION: Ciprofloxacin is a relatively new antibiotic used for the treatment of urinary tract and respiratory infections.

POSSIBLE MATERNAL SIDE EFFECTS: Ciprofloxacin is generally well tolerated. The most frequently reported side effect is mild nausea.

USE DURING PREGNANCY: There is very little experience with ciprofloxacin during human pregnancy. Reproductive studies have been performed in mice and rats and have not demonstrated any link between the drug and birth defects. However, ciprofloxacin and chemically similar antibiotics (nalidixic acid, p. 230, and norfloxacin, p. 237) have been shown to cause abnormalities of bones and joints in immature animals. Because of this theoretical risk and the availability of safer antibiotics, ciprofloxacin should generally be avoided during pregnancy.

USE DURING BREASTFEEDING: It is not known if ciprofloxacin is excreted into breast milk. Because other safe antibiotics are available, it should generally be avoided during breastfeeding.

ALTERNATIVES TO MEDICATIONS: For the treatment of serious bacterial infections there are no nonpharmacologic alternatives. There are, however, several antibiotics with a longer record of safety during pregnancy that can be substituted for ciprofloxacin.

GENERIC NAME: Clindamycin

COMMON BRANDS: Cleocin

TYPE OF DRUG: (Prescription) Antibiotic

FDA RISK CATEGORY FOR PREGNANCY: B

GENERAL INFORMATION: Clindamycin is an antibiotic that can be administered by pill, topical cream, or intravenous solution.

POSSIBLE MATERNAL SIDE EFFECTS: Side effects are unusual unless an individual is allergic to the drug. A severe diarrheal illness called pseudomembranous colitis can result during or shortly after treatment with clindamycin. If diarrhea occurs, contact your physician immediately.

USE DURING PREGNANCY: There have been no reports linking the use of clindamycin during pregnancy with birth defects. Nevertheless, the drug is usually reserved for severe infections.

USE DURING BREASTFEEDING: The American Academy of Pediatrics considers clindamycin compatible with breastfeeding. If, however, the newborn develops diarrhea, stop taking the drug and contact your physician.

GENERIC NAME: Clomiphene

COMMON BRANDS: Clomid

TYPE OF DRUG: (Prescription) Fertility drug

FDA RISK CATEGORY FOR PREGNANCY: X

GENERAL INFORMATION: Clomiphene is used to induce ovulation in infertile women. The drug should be discontinued as soon as pregnancy is diagnosed.

POSSIBLE MATERNAL SIDE EFFECTS: Side effects include headache, blurred vision, dizziness, insomnia, nausea, abdominal pain, and ovarian enlargement.

USE DURING PREGNANCY: There is no indication for the use of clomiphene during pregnancy. There have been several case reports of birth defects associated with the use of this medication during the first trimester. These reports, however, have not been confirmed by any large-scale study. Although clomiphene should not be taken during pregnancy, it may be safely taken before pregnancy to help induce ovulation in certain infertile women.

USE DURING BREASTFEEDING: No information is available, but there is no indication for the use of this drug during breastfeeding.

ALTERNATIVES TO MEDICATIONS: Ovulation may be spontaneous at any time even in women who are thought to be infertile. However, there is no nonpharmacologic alternative for induction of ovulation.

GENERIC NAME: Clonazepam

COMMON BRANDS: Klonopin

TYPE OF DRUG: (Prescription) Antianxiety, anticonvulsant, sedative

FDA RISK CATEGORY FOR PREGNANCY: D

GENERAL INFORMATION: Clonazepam is a member of a group of antianxiety medications called benzodiazepines. These drugs are used for the treatment of anxiety and insomnia and as anticonvulsants for control of certain kinds of seizures. They work by relaxing skeletal muscles and by a direct action on the brain. Benzodiazepines can be abused if taken indiscriminately or for a long period of time. Withdrawal symptoms including tremor, agitation, insomnia, muscle cramps, nausea, and seizures can occur if these drugs are discontinued abruptly after chronic use. Benzodiazepines should not be taken without careful medical supervision.

POSSIBLE MATERNAL SIDE EFFECTS: Common side effects with all benzodiazepines include sedation, depression, mental confusion, dizziness, unsteady gait, nightmares, fatigue, dry mouth, and low blood pressure. These drugs can interfere with the ability to safely drive a car or operate dangerous equipment. Physical and psychological dependence can occur with chronic use.

USE DURING PREGNANCY: All benzodiazepines rapidly cross the placenta and enter the fetal circulation. Blood levels in the fetus equal that of the mother's within one hour of taking a pill. Several studies have demonstrated a link between first-trimester use of benzodiazepines and birth defects. The most commonly reported malformations are cleft lip and cleft palate. Used near term benzodiazepines have been associated with lethargy, respiratory problems, and withdrawal symptoms in the newborn. Most authorities believe that it is best to avoid these medications during the first trimester and if possible throughout pregnancy.

USE DURING BREASTFEEDING: Benzodiazepines are excreted into breast milk in significant quantities. They can cause sedation in the newborn and should be avoided during breastfeeding.

ALTERNATIVES TO MEDICATIONS: For treatment of seizures there is no effective nonpharmacologic alternative. There are, however, several anticonvulsant medications that may be substituted for clonazepam.

Before using medications to control anxiety or stress consider the following strategy:

1. Identify the source of your anxiety. Worry often persists because of an inability to identify a problem and take action to solve it. Visualization can begin the process. Close your eyes and take a few deep breaths. Allow an image of the problem to arise.
2. Once you've defined the source of your anxiety, gather information. For example, if you are worried about the outcome of your pregnancy because of a possible hereditary problem or a medication you took before you knew you were pregnant, get information from your physician or a genetic counselor. In most cases what you discover will be very comforting.
3. After obtaining information, decide on a plan of action. Do what you can to deal with the problem, but once you've done all you can, change your focus and move on to other parts of life. Instead of worrying, concentrate on your life beyond the worry. Exercise or take walks. Plan how you will spend the evening or the weekend. Treat yourself to something pleasant, or think up a surprise for someone you care about. As your mind gets busy with other thoughts, you'll find that stress will begin to fade.
4. If anxiety persists despite your best efforts, see a therapist. Often only a few counseling sessions can effectively reduce anxiety and stress and eliminate the need for medication.

GENERIC NAME: Clonidine

COMMON BRANDS: Catapres, Combipres

TYPE OF DRUG: (Prescription) Antihypertensive

FDA RISK CATEGORY FOR PREGNANCY: C

GENERAL INFORMATION: Clonidine is capable of lowering blood pressure within 30 minutes of the first dose. The drug can be administered by pill or absorbed through the skin from a patch. It has recently been discovered that clonidine administered by skin patch may be helpful in reducing the withdrawal symptoms associated with cessation of cigarette smoking.

POSSIBLE MATERNAL SIDE EFFECTS: Common side effects include drowsiness, fatigue, dizziness when changing position from lying to standing, dry mouth, and constipation.

USE DURING PREGNANCY: Clonidine has not been used extensively enough during pregnancy to ensure its safety. Antihypertensives with a longer record of safety during pregnancy should be substituted.

USE DURING BREASTFEEDING: The drug enters breast milk in amounts equal to or greater than that in maternal blood. The effect on the newborn is not known. Other antihypertensives should be used if possible.

ALTERNATIVES TO MEDICATIONS: With a program of weight loss, mild salt restriction, exercise, and cessation of smoking many women can successfully decrease their blood pressure before pregnancy and remain off medications throughout at least the first trimester. However, if antihypertensive medication is necessary, another drug with a proven record of safety during pregnancy (such as methyldopa, p. 215) should be substituted for clonidine.

GENERIC NAME: # Clorazepate

COMMON BRANDS: Tranxene

TYPE OF DRUG: (Prescription) Antianxiety, sedative

FDA RISK CATEGORY FOR PREGNANCY: D

GENERAL INFORMATION: Clorazepate is a member of a group of antianxiety medications called benzodiazepines. These drugs are used for the treatment of anxiety and insomnia. They work by relaxing skeletal muscles and by a direct action on the brain.

Benzodiazepines can be abused if taken indiscriminately or for a long period of time. Withdrawal symptoms including tremor, agitation, insomnia, muscle cramps, nausea, and seizures can occur if these drugs are discontinued abruptly after chronic use. Benzodiazepines should not be taken without careful medical supervision.

POSSIBLE MATERNAL SIDE EFFECTS: Common side effects with all benzodiazepines include sedation, depression, mental confusion, dizziness, unsteady gait, nightmares, fatigue, dry mouth, and low blood pressure. These drugs can interfere with the ability to safely drive a car or operate dangerous equipment. Physical and psychological dependence can occur with chronic use.

USE DURING PREGNANCY: All benzodiazepines rapidly cross the placenta and enter the fetal circulation. Blood levels in the fetus equal that of the mother's within one hour of taking a pill. Several studies have demonstrated a link between first-trimester use of benzodiazepines and birth defects. The most commonly reported malformations are cleft lip and cleft palate. Used near term benzodiazepines have been associated with lethargy, respiratory problems, and withdrawal symptoms in the newborn. Most authorities believe that it is best to avoid these medications during the first trimester and if possible throughout pregnancy.

USE DURING BREASTFEEDING: Benzodiazepines are excreted into breast milk in significant quantities. They can cause sedation in the newborn and should be avoided during breastfeeding.

ALTERNATIVES TO MEDICATIONS: Before using medications to control anxiety or stress consider the following strategy:

1. Identify the source of your anxiety. Worry often persists because of an inability to identify a problem and take action to solve it. Visualization can begin the process. Close your eyes and take a few deep breaths. Allow an image of the problem to arise.
2. Once you've defined the source of your anxiety, gather information. For example, if you are worried about the outcome of your pregnancy because of a possible hereditary problem or a medication you took before you knew you were pregnant, get information from your physician or a genetic counselor. In most cases what you discover will be very comforting.
3. After obtaining information, decide on a plan of action. Do what you can to deal with the problem, but once you've done all you can, change your focus and move on to other parts of life. Instead of worrying, concentrate on your life beyond the worry. Exercise or take walks. Plan how you will spend the evening or the weekend. Treat yourself to something pleasant, or think up a surprise for someone you care about. As your mind gets busy with other thoughts, you'll find that stress will begin to fade.
4. If anxiety persists despite your best efforts, see a therapist. Often only a few counseling sessions can effectively reduce anxiety and stress and eliminate the need for medication.

GENERIC NAME: Clotrimazole

COMMON BRANDS: Gyne-Lotrimin, Lotrimin, Mycelex

TYPE OF DRUG: (Prescription) Antifungal antibiotic

FDA RISK CATEGORY FOR PREGNANCY: B

GENERAL INFORMATION: Clotrimazole can be applied as a cream or lotion to areas of fungal skin infections. It is often used topically or by vaginal tablet for the treatment of vaginal yeast infection (candida infection).

POSSIBLE MATERNAL SIDE EFFECTS: Occasionally, vaginal irritation may occur during treatment with clotrimazole.

USE DURING PREGNANCY: The drug has been used extensively during pregnancy and has not been linked to birth defects or fetal harm.

USE DURING BREASTFEEDING: Clotrimazole is safe for use during breastfeeding.

ALTERNATIVES TO MEDICATIONS: Although there is no non-pharmacologic treatment of vaginal yeast infections, it is not necessary to treat mild vaginitis until after delivery. Use of cotton undergarments and skirts rather than nonventilating clothing might minimize moisture, thus preventing circumstances that are known to predispose to yeast infections.

Uncircumcised men may harbor yeast under the foreskin, thus continuing to infect their sexual partner. For women with recurrent infections, sexual partners should be examined and treated if there is any evidence of infection.

GENERIC NAME: Cocaine

COMMON BRANDS: none

TYPE OF DRUG: Illicit

FDA RISK CATEGORY FOR PREGNANCY: X

GENERAL INFORMATION: Cocaine is one of the most commonly abused substances in the United States. The only legitimate use of the drug is for topical anesthesia during nasal or dental surgical procedures.

POSSIBLE MATERNAL SIDE EFFECTS: Side effects of cocaine include disorientation, hallucinations, loss of appetite, and addiction.

117

USE DURING PREGNANCY: Cocaine is among the most dangerous drugs to unborn babies. Women who use cocaine during pregnancy are at least three times more likely to have a premature baby, and even if the baby is not premature, it is more likely to be much smaller than it would otherwise be. The risk of miscarriage is also considerably higher.

Babies exposed to cocaine before birth may also have neurologic and respiratory problems. Newborns experience something similar to "withdrawal" from the drug. They are very jittery and irritable, and they startle and cry at the gentlest touch or sound. Consequently, these babies are very difficult to comfort and often are described as withdrawn or unresponsive. The drug should not be used at any time during pregnancy.

USE DURING BREASTFEEDING: Cocaine should not be used during breastfeeding.

ALTERNATIVES TO MEDICATIONS: There is no legitimate use for cocaine during pregnancy. Women addicted to the drug should seek competent psychiatric care to begin a supervised withdrawal program before pregnancy.

GENERIC NAME: Codeine

COMMON BRANDS: Aspirin with Codeine, Dimetane-DC Cough Syrup, Empirin #3, Esgic with Codeine, Fiorinal with Codeine, Naldecon CX, Phenaphen with Codeine, Phenergan VC with Codeine, Robitussin AC, Robitussin DAC, Soma Compound with Codeine, Triaminic with Codeine, Tussar, Tylenol with Codeine

TYPE OF DRUG: (Prescription) Analgesic, cough suppressant

FDA RISK CATEGORY FOR PREGNANCY: C

GENERAL INFORMATION: Codeine is a narcotic pain reliever (analgesic), also effective as a cough suppressant. As an analgesic codeine is capable of relieving mild to moderate pain and is frequently combined with aspirin (p. 82) or acetaminophen (p. 63).

POSSIBLE MATERNAL SIDE EFFECTS: Possible side effects include drowsiness, nausea, loss of appetite, and constipation. As is the case with any narcotic, habituation to the drug is possible.

USE DURING PREGNANCY: The effect of codeine on the fetus remains uncertain. The Collaborative Perinatal Project could demonstrate no association between the use of codeine during the first trimester and birth defects. Other studies, however, reported a slight increased risk of cleft lip and palate when the drug was used during the first trimester. Chronic use of codeine near term can result in an infant born with respiratory depression and signs of narcotic withdrawal. In spite of these theoretical risks, codeine has been used extensively during pregnancy for suppression of persistent coughing and relief of severe pain.

USE DURING BREASTFEEDING: Codeine enters breast milk in small amounts and could theoretically cause sedation and poor feeding in nursing infants. Nevertheless, the American Academy of Pediatrics considers codeine compatible with breastfeeding.

ALTERNATIVES TO MEDICATIONS: In some patients chronic pain can be controlled with relaxation techniques and biofeedback. Musculoskeletal pain can often be relieved with warm baths and massage. Acetaminophen is probably the safest medication to take during pregnancy for relief of minor pain and if possible should be substituted for codeine.

GENERIC NAME: ## Corticosteroids

COMMON BRANDS: Celestone (Betamethasone), Decadron (Dexamethasone), Deltasone (Prednisone), Medrol or Solu-Medrol (Methylprednisolone), Prednisone, Solu-Cortef (Hydrocortisone)

TYPE OF DRUG: (Prescription) Corticosteroid

FDA RISK CATEGORY FOR PREGNANCY: C

GENERAL INFORMATION: Corticosteroids (often called steroids) are potent drugs used to treat a variety of serious medical conditions including rheumatoid arthritis, systemic lupus erythematosus, certain kidney disorders, inflammatory bowel disease, severe asthma, and insufficiency of the adrenal gland (Addison's disease). They should be given in the lowest effective dosage and never discontinued abruptly.

Patients currently taking corticosteroids should be treated with an increased dosage for several days before and after any acute stressful event such as infection, surgery, or labor and delivery. This is because taking these substances by pill suppresses the adrenal gland's natural ability to manufacture corticosteroids during times of stress. The adrenal gland's ability to produce needed amounts of corticosteroids usually returns within six months of discontinuing these medications.

POSSIBLE MATERNAL SIDE EFFECTS: Common side effects include euphoria, insomnia, restlessness, edema, stomach irritation, increased appetite, weight gain, and an increase in blood glucose concentration (and possibly gestational diabetes). When these drugs are used for long periods (usually longer than several months), additional side effects may result such as muscle weakness, cataracts, increased fat deposition at the base of the neck, osteoporosis, diabetes, and impaired ability to fight infections. In addition, chronic use of corticosteroids causes suppression of the adrenal gland's ability to manufacturer cortisone in response to physical stress.

USE DURING PREGNANCY: Corticosteroids have been used extensively during pregnancy. There have been a few reports of an increased risk of cleft lip in infants whose mothers took corticosteroids during the first trimester. However, in a large study of women with asthma treated with corticosteroids no association with any birth defects could be established. Most authorities believe these drugs can be safely taken throughout pregnancy.

During pregnancy betamethasone is frequently given to women at risk of delivering prematurely in order to stimulate the lungs of the fetus to mature more rapidly. Giving betamethasone before 34 weeks gestation has been shown to reduce the risk of respiratory distress syndrome in premature infants.

Some women treated with corticosteroids during pregnancy will need to be given an increased dosage during early labor and for several days after delivery to compensate for the inability of the adrenal glands to produce enough corticosteroid to meet the extra demands of labor and delivery.

USE DURING BREASTFEEDING: Corticosteroids enter breast milk in very small amounts and their effect in the newborn is probably insignificant. The American Academy of Pediatrics considers corticosteroids compatible with breastfeeding.

ALTERNATIVES TO MEDICATIONS: There is no nonpharmacologic alternative to corticosteroids. However, these drugs are usually reserved for conditions that have not responded to less potent medications.

Coumarin anticoagulants (Warfarin)

COMMON BRANDS: Coumadin

TYPE OF DRUG: (Prescription) Anticoagulant

FDA RISK CATEGORY FOR PREGNANCY: X

GENERAL INFORMATION: Coumarin anticoagulants are used in non-pregnant patients to treat acute blood clots in the deep (large) veins of the leg or blood clots that have traveled to the lungs (pulmonary embolism). In some cases coumarin anticoagulants are given to prevent blood clots in individuals who are known to be at great risk of forming a clot in the leg. These drugs can also be used to prevent the formation of a blood clot on an artificial heart valve.

POSSIBLE MATERNAL SIDE EFFECTS: Because these drugs interfere with the natural ability of blood to clot, patients treated with anticoagulants are at risk of prolonged bleeding from lacerations or injuries. Bleeding can range from mild gum bleeding to major hemorrhage.

USE DURING PREGNANCY: Coumarin anticoagulants should not be used during the first trimester of pregnancy. They can cause a variety of birth defects including abnormal bone growth, hydrocephalus, abnormalities of the eyes, growth retardation, and developmental delay. Taken near the time of delivery, coumarin anticoagulants can subject the baby to the risk of severe hemorrhage during birth.

USE DURING BREASTFEEDING: Coumarin anticoagulants have been shown to enter breast milk in small amounts. However, when they were studied in a group of breastfed infants, there was no evidence of increased risk of bleeding. The American Academy of Pediatrics considers coumarin anticoagulants compatible with breastfeeding.

ALTERNATIVES TO MEDICATIONS: There is no way to achieve anticoagulation without medication. However, if anticoagulation during pregnancy is necessary for treatment or prevention of blood clots, heparin (p. 166) given by subcutaneous injection is the treatment of choice throughout pregnancy.

GENERIC NAME: Cromolyn

COMMON BRANDS: Intal

TYPE OF DRUG: (Prescription) Antiasthma

FDA RISK CATEGORY FOR PREGNANCY: B

GENERAL INFORMATION: Cromolyn is administered by inhalation for the prevention of asthma attacks. It is particularly effective for patients whose attacks are triggered by pollens or by exercise. The drug is not useful, however, to stop an attack of asthma once wheezing has begun.

POSSIBLE MATERNAL SIDE EFFECTS: Since very little of the drug is absorbed systemically, side effects are rare. Occasionally, cromolyn can worsen wheezing if taken in the midst of an asthma attack.

USE DURING PREGNANCY: Cromolyn is particularly well suited for use during pregnancy since very little of the drug is absorbed systemically. There have been no reports of birth defects or fetal harm associated with its use during pregnancy.

USE DURING BREASTFEEDING: Cromolyn can be safely used during breastfeeding.

ALTERNATIVES TO MEDICATIONS: In some cases asthma can be prevented by avoidance of known allergens, particularly animals. In many cases, however, cromolyn can prevent asthma and eliminate the need to take other medications associated with more side effects.

GENERIC NAME: Cyclobenzaprine

COMMON BRANDS: Flexeril

TYPE OF DRUG: (Prescription) Muscle relaxant

FDA RISK CATEGORY FOR PREGNANCY: B

GENERAL INFORMATION: Cyclobenzaprine is used for the relief of skeletal muscle spasm. It is generally prescribed for no longer than a few days following muscular strain or injury.

POSSIBLE MATERNAL SIDE EFFECTS: Common side effects include nausea, drowsiness, dry mouth, and dizziness.

USE DURING PREGNANCY: Reproductive studies have been performed in rats, mice, and rabbits at doses up to 20 times the human dose and have revealed no evidence of impaired fertility or harm to the fetus due to cyclobenzaprine. There are, however, no adequate studies in pregnant women.

USE DURING BREASTFEEDING: No information is available.

ALTERNATIVES TO MEDICATIONS: Musculoskeletal pain can often be relieved with warm baths and massage. Acetaminophen (p. 63) is probably the safest medication to take during pregnancy for relief of minor pain and if possible should be substituted for cyclobenzaprine.

GENERIC NAME: Cyclophosphamide

COMMON BRANDS: Cytoxan

TYPE OF DRUG: (Prescription) Anticancer

FDA RISK CATEGORY FOR PREGNANCY: D

GENERAL INFORMATION: Cyclophosphamide is used in combination with other drugs for the treatment of some kinds of cancer. The drug works by interfering with cell division in cancer cells as well as normal cells. Cyclophosphamide also has the ability to interfere with normal antibody production (immunosuppression) and can be used to treat certain chronic diseases such as systemic lupus erythematosus and rheumatoid arthritis.

POSSIBLE MATERNAL SIDE EFFECTS: Side effects of cyclophosphamide are common and often severe. Relatively minor side effects include nausea, loss of appetite, diarrhea, abdominal cramps, and hair loss. More severe adverse effects include suppression of the bone marrow's ability to produce red and white blood cells. The drug can also interfere with normal sperm production in men and normal menstruation in women treated for cancer.

USE DURING PREGNANCY: Malformed infants have been reported following the use of cyclophosphamide during the first trimester. Use of cyclophosphamide during the second and third trimesters probably does not place the fetus at risk for congenital malformations, but it does increase the risk of abnormal growth. Cyclophosphamide should only be used during pregnancy if it is critical to maternal survival. Ideally, its use should be delayed until after the first trimester.

USE DURING BREASTFEEDING: Cyclophosphamide is excreted into breast milk and can have several adverse effects on breastfed infants including abnormal growth, suppression of the immune system, and possibly development of cancer in the future. Women who must be treated with this drug should not breastfeed.

ALTERNATIVES TO MEDICATIONS: There are no nonpharmacologic alternatives to cyclophosphamide. However, treatment of some cancers can be postponed until after pregnancy or at least until after the first trimester.

GENERIC NAME: Cyclosporine

COMMON BRANDS: Sandimmune

TYPE OF DRUG: (Prescription) Immunosuppressive

FDA RISK CATEGORY FOR PREGNANCY: C

GENERAL INFORMATION: Cyclosporine is prescribed to prevent rejection of transplanted organs such as kidney, liver, and heart. Use of this drug is generally limited to medical centers experienced with its use and equipped to deal with potential complications.

POSSIBLE MATERNAL SIDE EFFECTS: Side effects include low red and white blood cell count, headache, mouth ulcers, thickening of the gums, nausea, diarrhea, and kidney damage.

USE DURING PREGNANCY: Cyclosporine has been shown to be harmful to animal fetuses when given in a dosage 2 to 5 times the human dosage. Since there are no adequate human studies to ensure its safety, its use during pregnancy should be limited to situations where the drug is necessary for maternal survival.

USE DURING BREASTFEEDING: The drug enters breast milk in significant amounts. Mothers who must take cyclosporine should not breastfeed their newborns.

ALTERNATIVES TO MEDICATIONS: There are no nonpharmacologic alternatives to cyclosporine for the prevention of organ transplant rejection.

GENERIC NAME: Danazol

COMMON BRANDS: Danocrine

TYPE OF DRUG: (Prescription) Hormone

FDA RISK CATEGORY FOR PREGNANCY: X

GENERAL INFORMATION: Danazol is a derivative of the male sex hormone, testosterone. The drug is used for the treatment of endometriosis, a painful gynecological disease in which tissue normally found in the uterus grows in other places.

POSSIBLE MATERNAL SIDE EFFECTS: Side effects include headache, dizziness, sleep disturbance, irritability, elevated blood pressure, nausea, changes in appetite, jaundice, acne, male-pattern hair growth, and weight gain.

USE DURING PREGNANCY: Danazol has no use during pregnancy and should not be taken. Female fetuses exposed to the drug have had abnormalities of the external genitalia such as fused labia and enlargement of the clitoris.

USE DURING BREASTFEEDING: Because of potential serious adverse effects to the breastfed infant, it is recommended that either breastfeeding or danazol be discontinued.

ALTERNATIVES TO MEDICATIONS: There is no use for danazol during pregnancy. Typically, the pain associated with endometriosis disappears during pregnancy.

GENERIC NAME: Desipramine

COMMON BRANDS: Norpramin

TYPE OF DRUG: (Prescription) Antidepressant

FDA RISK CATEGORY FOR PREGNANCY: C

GENERAL INFORMATION: Desipramine is an antidepressant used for the treatment of chronic depression. The drug often takes several weeks to produce its desired effect.

POSSIBLE MATERNAL SIDE EFFECTS: Possible side effects include drowsiness, lethargy, confusion, blurred vision, dry mouth, a fall in blood pressure associated with standing up quickly, and difficulty urinating.

USE DURING PREGNANCY: There have been no reports of congenital malformations caused by desipramine in human pregnancies. However, the newborns of women treated with this medication can manifest withdrawal symptoms including rapid heart rate, poor feeding, and weight loss. Desipramine is also capable of interfering with sperm motility possibly resulting in male infertility.

USE DURING BREASTFEEDING: The drug enters breast milk in low concentrations. Its effect on the newborn is not known.

ALTERNATIVES TO MEDICATIONS: Depression often gives rise to hopelessness, negativity toward oneself, and at times an inability to carry out normal activities of daily living. Some individuals may become intensely sad or grief-stricken over the loss of someone or something close to them. Others may suffer from chronic depression unrelated to a specific event. In many cases counseling is necessary to truly understand the cause and extent of depression. There are, however, a number of things you can do to deal with depression on your own:

1. Try to identify the specific situation or personal interaction that has caused your sense of hopelessness and negativity.
2. Make a fresh start at correcting the problem. Talk it through. If necessary, repair relationships with previously available support systems. Often family or close friends can serve to reduce your distress.
3. Realize that there are options for most situations. Seldom is there truly "no choice."
4. Understand some of the warning signs that indicate you have severe depression requiring professional counseling. Such signs include
   - Intense sadness, frequent bouts of crying, or depressed mood most of the day,
   - Uncharacteristically negative thoughts about yourself,

- Markedly diminished interest or pleasure in most activities,
- Diminished appetite and weight loss,
- Chronic insomnia or sleeping excessively,
- Feelings of worthlessness or guilt,
- Persistent fatigue or lack of energy,
- Inability to think or concentrate,
- Thoughts or plans for suicide.

5. Patients with severe depression should not stop taking antidepressant medications without careful psychiatric supervision.

GENERIC NAME: Dextromethorphan

COMMON BRANDS: Benylin, Cheracol, Comtrex, Contac, Co-Tylenol, Cremacoat, Dimacol, Hold, Mediquell, Naldecon, Robitussin DM, St. Joseph Nighttime Cold Medicine, Sudafed Cough Syrup, Triaminic, Triaminicol, Vicks Formula 44, Vicks Nyquil Nighttime Colds Medicine

TYPE OF DRUG: (Over-the-counter) Cough suppressant

FDA RISK CATEGORY FOR PREGNANCY: B

GENERAL INFORMATION: Dextromethorphan is moderately effective for the relief of coughing associated with the common cold. It should not be used for coughing caused by asthma. Dextromethorphan is usually given in liquid form and frequently combined with another cough suppressant, guaifenesin (p. 63). Many cough preparations also contain significant amounts of alcohol (p. 67).

POSSIBLE MATERNAL SIDE EFFECTS: Side effects are usually minimal. Occasionally, drowsiness or dizziness can occur. Other side effects may result from additional active ingredients, including alcohol, in combination cold products.

USE DURING PREGNANCY: Dextromethorphan is safe for use during pregnancy. However, chronic use of preparations containing alcohol should be avoided. Abuse of alcohol-containing cough syrups has been shown to cause fetal alcohol syndrome (p. 67). Several over-the-counter cough preparations are free of alcohol. Combination products containing iodine (p. 183) should also be avoided during pregnancy. Preparations that contain sugar should be avoided by women with diabetes.

USE DURING BREASTFEEDING: Dextromethorphan is safe for use during breastfeeding, but alcohol-containing products should be avoided.

ALTERNATIVES TO MEDICATIONS: Over-the-counter cold preparations provide purely symptomatic relief and have no influence on the course of the illness. Minor coughs can often be relieved by cool mist or steam. Cough caused by asthma may require bronchodilating medication and should not be treated with cough suppressants.

GENERIC NAME: Diazepam

COMMON BRANDS: Valium, Valrelease

TYPE OF DRUG: (Prescription) Antianxiety, sedative

FDA RISK CATEGORY FOR PREGNANCY: D

GENERAL INFORMATION: Diazepam is a member of a group of antianxiety medications called benzodiazepines. These drugs are used for the treatment of anxiety and insomnia and as anticonvulsants for control of certain kinds of seizures. They work by relaxing skeletal muscles and by a direct action on the brain. Benzodiazepines can be abused if taken indiscriminately or for a long period of time. Withdrawal symptoms including tremor, agitation, insomnia, muscle cramps, nausea, and seizures can occur if these drugs are discontinued abruptly after chronic use. Benzodiazepines should not be taken without careful medical supervision.

POSSIBLE MATERNAL SIDE EFFECTS: Common side effects with all benzodiazepines include sedation, depression, mental confusion, dizziness, unsteady gait, nightmares, fatigue, dry mouth, and low blood pressure. These drugs can interfere with the ability to safely drive a car or operate dangerous equipment. Physical and psychological dependence can occur with chronic use.

USE DURING PREGNANCY: All benzodiazepines rapidly cross the placenta and enter the fetal circulation. Blood levels in the fetus equal that of the mother's within one hour of taking a pill. Several studies have demonstrated a link between first-trimester use of benzodiazepines and birth defects. The most commonly reported malformations are cleft lip and cleft palate. Used near term benzodiazepines have been associated with lethargy, respiratory problems, and withdrawal symptoms in the newborn. Most authorities believe that it is best to avoid these medications during the first trimester and if possible throughout pregnancy.

USE DURING BREASTFEEDING: Benzodiazepines are excreted into breast milk in significant quantities. They can cause sedation in the newborn and should be avoided during breastfeeding.

ALTERNATIVES TO MEDICATIONS: Before using medications to control anxiety or stress consider the following strategy:

1. Identify the source of your anxiety. Worry often persists because of an inability to identify a problem and take action to solve it. Visualization can begin the process. Close your eyes and take a few deep breaths. Allow an image of the problem to arise.
2. Once you've defined the source of your anxiety, gather information. For example, if you are worried about the outcome of your pregnancy because of a possible hereditary problem or a medication you took before you knew you were pregnant, get information from your physician or a genetic counselor. In most cases what you discover will be very comforting.
3. After obtaining information, decide on a plan of action. Do what you can to deal with the problem, but once you've done all you can, change your focus and move on to other parts of life. Instead of worrying, concentrate on your life beyond the worry. Exercise or take walks. Plan how you will spend the evening or the weekend. Treat yourself to something pleasant, or think up a surprise for someone you care about. As your mind gets busy with other thoughts, you'll find that stress will begin to fade.
4. If anxiety persists despite your best efforts, see a therapist. Often only a few counseling sessions can effectively reduce anxiety and stress and eliminate the need for medication.

GENERIC NAME: Diclofenac

COMMON BRANDS: Voltaren

TYPE OF DRUG: (Prescription) Anti-inflammatory

FDA RISK CATEGORY FOR PREGNANCY: B

GENERAL INFORMATION: Diclofenac is a member of a class of drugs called nonsteroidal anti-inflammatory drugs (NSAIDs). It is indicated for the treatment of arthritis, muscle pain, headache, and pain associated with menstruation.

POSSIBLE MATERNAL SIDE EFFECTS: The most common side effects are nausea and abdominal pain. Rarely, diclofenac can irritate the stomach and cause an ulcer or bleeding from the stomach.

USE DURING PREGNANCY: There have been no reports linking diclofenac to birth defects when the drug was used during the first trimester. However, experience with the drug during early pregnancy is limited.

Used near term diclofenac can have potential effects on pregnancy and the fetus. First, the drug can cause premature closure of an important blood vessel in the fetus called the ductus arteriosus. Normally, this blood vessel does not close until after delivery. Premature closure could result in a serious condition called pulmonary hypertension. Second, diclofenac and other NSAIDs can inhibit labor and prolong pregnancy.

USE DURING BREASTFEEDING: Diclofenac apparently does enter human breast milk, but its effect on the newborn is unknown.

ALTERNATIVES TO MEDICATIONS: Musculoskeletal pain can often be relieved with warm baths, and massage. Painful arthritis can be alleviated by rest, heat, and physical therapy. Nonweight-bearing exercise such as swimming may offer some comfort while enhancing muscle tone. If medication is necessary, acetaminophen (p. 63) is probably the safest medication to take during pregnancy for relief of minor pain.

GENERIC NAME: Dicloxacillin

COMMON BRANDS: Dynapen, Pathocil

TYPE OF DRUG: (Prescription) Antibiotic

FDA RISK CATEGORY FOR PREGNANCY: B

GENERAL INFORMATION: Dicloxacillin is a penicillin-type antibiotic effective against infections caused by streptococci, staphylococci, and pneumococci. The drug is usually reserved for infections caused by organisms resistant to ordinary penicillin.

POSSIBLE MATERNAL SIDE EFFECTS: Side effects are uncommon, but diarrhea may result from treatment with any antibiotic and should be reported to your physician if it lasts longer than 48 hours. A rash can occur at any time in individuals allergic to penicillin.

USE DURING PREGNANCY: Dicloxacillin crosses the placenta, but less readily than penicillin. This antibiotic has not been shown to cause birth defects or any other fetal harm and is considered safe for use during any stage of pregnancy.

USE DURING BREASTFEEDING: Similar to other penicillin-type antibiotics, dicloxacillin enters breast milk. Although it is considered safe for use during breastfeeding, small amounts in breast milk are capable of causing diarrhea in the newborn. Nevertheless, dicloxacillin is one of the most commonly prescribed antibiotics for the treatment of acute mastitis (infection of the breast).

ALTERNATIVES TO MEDICATIONS: Dicloxacillin is usually reserved for serious infections due to penicillin-resistant staphylococci. There are no nonpharmacologic alternatives to it for serious infections, but for some infections less expensive antibiotics may be substituted.

GENERIC NAME: Diethylpropion hydrochloride

COMMON BRANDS: Tenuate, Tepanil

TYPE OF DRUG: (Prescription) Appetite suppressant, stimulant

FDA RISK CATEGORY FOR PREGNANCY: C

GENERAL INFORMATION: Diethylpropion is used primarily as an appetite suppressant. It has several chemical properties similar to amphetamines and other stimulants. Therefore, it has considerable potential for abuse.

POSSIBLE MATERNAL SIDE EFFECTS: Possible side effects of the drug include rapid heart rate, irregular rhythms of the heart, and elevation of blood pressure. Chronic use of diethylpropion can lead to drug dependency.

USE DURING PREGNANCY: The drug has not been shown to cause birth defects in animals or humans. Nevertheless, it should not be used during pregnancy. Since calorie-restricted diets are not recom-

131

mended during pregnancy, there is no need to take any medication designed to suppress appetite. Additionally, use of diethylpropion near the time of delivery can result in withdrawal symptoms in the newborn.

USE DURING BREASTFEEDING: Diethylpropion is excreted into breast milk and can cause poor feeding and rapid heart rate in breastfed infants. This drug should not be used during breastfeeding.

ALTERNATIVES TO MEDICATIONS: Careful nutritional counseling and planning before pregnancy should allow most women to attain ideal body weight before conception. Pregnancy is not the time to begin a calorie-restricted diet. Weight loss during pregnancy can have seriously detrimental effects on the growth and development of the baby. Excessive weight gain during pregnancy can be managed with a carefully planned diet complete with the nutrients essential for you and your baby.

GENERIC NAME: Diethylstilbestrol

COMMON BRANDS: DES

TYPE OF DRUG: (Prescription) Hormone

FDA RISK CATEGORY FOR PREGNANCY: X

GENERAL INFORMATION: Diethylstilbestrol is an estrogen hormone. In the past the drug was given to prevent miscarriage during the first trimester of pregnancy. Subsequent studies revealed that it does not reduce the risk of miscarriage.

POSSIBLE MATERNAL SIDE EFFECTS: Side effects include headache, dizziness, nausea, acne, and high blood pressure, and in some women the risk of blood clotting may be increased.

USE DURING PREGNANCY: Diethylstilbestrol, as well as other estrogen hormones, should not be taken during pregnancy. Several careful studies have shown that diethylstilbestrol can cause significant birth defects. Additionally, there is a twofold risk of vaginal cancer in daughters of women who took the drug during pregnancy. It has also been reported that male offspring of women who took diethylstilbes-

132

trol are more likely to have abnormal sperm production and possibly testicular cancer later in life.

USE DURING BREASTFEEDING: Diethylstilbestrol and other estrogens may reduce the production of breast milk and should be avoided in women who wish to breastfeed.

ALTERNATIVES TO MEDICATIONS: In the past diethylstilbestrol was used to prevent miscarriage. Studies have since shown that it did not work for this purpose. Slight bleeding or spotting of dark blood may signal an impending miscarriage. Since some miscarriages are completely painless, any vaginal bleeding during pregnancy is an indication to call the doctor.

GENERIC NAME: Digoxin

COMMON BRANDS: Lanoxin, Lanoxicaps

TYPE OF DRUG: (Prescription) Heart drug

FDA RISK CATEGORY FOR PREGNANCY: C

GENERAL INFORMATION: Digoxin is used to increase the force of heart muscle contraction in patients with heart failure. It is also used to slow or correct abnormal rhythms of the heart.

POSSIBLE MATERNAL SIDE EFFECTS: Possible side effects include diminished appetite, nausea, and blurred vision. Side effects can usually be prevented by monitoring blood levels of the drug to ensure that the dosage is not excessive.

USE DURING PREGNANCY: Digoxin readily crosses the placenta to reach the fetus. There have been no reports of birth defects in humans. For women with abnormal heart rhythms, especially atrial fibrillation, digoxin is considered safe for use during pregnancy. In some cases digoxin has been used to treat abnormal heart rhythms in the fetus by giving the drug to the mother and calculating the amount that will enter the fetal circulation.

USE DURING BREASTFEEDING: Digoxin is excreted into breast milk but does not appear to cause any harm to the newborn. The American Academy of Pediatrics considers digoxin compatible with breastfeeding.

ALTERNATIVES TO MEDICATIONS: For many women with serious heart problems there is no alternative to taking heart medication. Since pregnancy may place an addition burden on the heart, medications should not be discontinued without consulting a physician. However, some patients with mild heart problems can control symptoms with dietary salt restriction and adequate rest.

GENERIC NAME: Diltiazem

COMMON BRANDS: Cardizem

TYPE OF DRUG: (Prescription) Antihypertensive, antiarrhythmic

FDA RISK CATEGORY FOR PREGNANCY: C

GENERAL INFORMATION: Diltiazem is a member of a class of medications known as calcium-channel blockers. Calcium-channel blockers are used to treat hypertension (high blood pressure), abnormal rhythms of the heart, and angina pectoris (heart pain). These drugs are also capable of suppressing spontaneous contractions of the uterus in women with premature labor.

POSSIBLE MATERNAL SIDE EFFECTS: The most common side effects are constipation, drowsiness, headache, and fatigue. Blood pressure must be checked frequently to ensure that it does not fall too low.

USE DURING PREGNANCY: Diltiazem and other calcium-channel blockers have not been used extensively during pregnancy in the United States. Other antihypertensive medications that have been used for many years during pregnancy are usually given in preference to this newer class of drugs. Recent studies have suggested that calcium-channel blockers may be useful for treatment of premature labor.

USE DURING BREASTFEEDING: Experience with calcium-channel blockers in breastfeeding is limited. However, there are no reports of adverse effects.

ALTERNATIVES TO MEDICATIONS: With a program of weight loss, mild salt restriction, exercise, and cessation of smoking many women can successfully decrease their blood pressure before pregnancy and remain off medications throughout at least the first trimester. However, if antihypertensive medication is necessary, another drug with a proven record of safety during pregnancy (such as methyldopa, p. 215) should be substituted for diltiazem.

GENERIC NAME: Diphenoxylate

COMMON BRANDS: Lomotil (combined with atropine)

TYPE OF DRUG: (Prescription) Antidiarrheal

FDA RISK CATEGORY FOR PREGNANCY: C

GENERAL INFORMATION: Diphenoxylate is chemically similar to the narcotic meperidine (p. 206). It is used for the treatment of acute diarrhea. Use of this medication should be limited to no longer than 24 to 48 hours. Diarrhea that persists longer than 48 hours requires evaluation by a physician.

POSSIBLE MATERNAL SIDE EFFECTS: Possible side effects include drowsiness, nausea, headache, and blurred vision. The duration of diarrhea caused by some bacteria can even be prolonged by the use of diphenoxylate.

USE DURING PREGNANCY: Experience with diphenoxylate during pregnancy has been limited. However, there have been no reports of birth defects caused by the drug. Diphenoxylate should not be used for longer than 48 hours without consulting a physician.

USE DURING BREASTFEEDING: The drug is excreted in breast milk and is not recommended for use during breastfeeding.

ALTERNATIVES TO MEDICATIONS: With acute diarrhea solid foods may be discontinued for 12 to 24 hours. When diarrhea abates, start eating again with dry bread or toast and small amounts of vegetables. Since it is essential to avoid dehydration, be sure to drink plenty of liquids that contain sugar. Soup can also provide some nutrition and hydration without aggravating diarrhea. Symptoms of dehydration include thirst, dry mouth, fast breathing, and sometimes fever. An early sign of dehydration is reduction in the amount and frequency of urination. Drink enough to keep up normal urine output. If adequate hydration cannot be maintained, call the doctor.

During pregnancy consideration should be given to avoiding trips to countries where traveler's diarrhea is known to be common.

GENERIC NAME: Disulfiram

COMMON BRANDS: Antabuse

TYPE OF DRUG: (Prescription) Prevention of alcohol abuse

FDA RISK CATEGORY FOR PREGNANCY: X

GENERAL INFORMATION: Disulfiram is useful in programs to motivate individuals with a history of alcohol abuse to avoid alcohol consumption. When disulfiram is combined with the consumption of even small amounts of alcohol, nausea and vomiting results.

POSSIBLE MATERNAL SIDE EFFECTS: Possible side effects include drowsiness, headache, metallic after-taste, nausea, palpitations, and hyperventilation (rapid breathing).

USE DURING PREGNANCY: Disulfiram has been shown to cause birth defects in laboratory animals and humans. The drug should not be taken during pregnancy.

USE DURING BREASTFEEDING: No information is available.

ALTERNATIVES TO MEDICATIONS: Alcohol (p. 67) is clearly harmful to the baby. For pregnant women who suffer from alcoholism, counseling and an alcohol treatment program is essential. Ideally, every effort should be made to enter an alcohol treatment program before pregnancy.

GENERIC NAME: Docusate sodium, docusate calcium, docusate potassium

COMMON BRANDS:

Docusate sodium: Colace, Correctol, Extra Gentle Ex-Lax, Feen-A-Mint pills, Modane, Peri-Colace, Phillips' LaxCaps, Regutol, Senokot-S, Therevac

Docusate calcium: Doxidan, Surfak
Docusate potassium: Dialose, Kasof

TYPE OF DRUG: (Over-the-counter) Laxative

FDA RISK CATEGORY FOR PREGNANCY: C

GENERAL INFORMATION: Docusate is a common ingredient in many laxatives available over-the-counter. They function primarily as stool softeners and can be useful for people with hemorrhoids or rectal fissures. Chronic laxative use, however, should be avoided.

POSSIBLE MATERNAL SIDE EFFECTS: Docusate is usually well tolerated. Overuse, however, may lead to diarrhea.

USE DURING PREGNANCY: There have been no reports linking the use of docusate-containing laxatives with birth defects in animals or humans. There is some concern, however, that chronic use of these laxatives by a pregnant woman can cause a low blood magnesium level.

USE DURING BREASTFEEDING: Docusate-containing laxatives are safe for use during breastfeeding. However, chronic laxative use should be avoided.

ALTERNATIVES TO MEDICATIONS: Constipation is one of the most common gastrointestinal complaints during pregnancy even for women who were previously very regular. It is likely caused by the combined factors of pressure from the enlarging uterus and relaxation of intestinal muscle due to pregnancy hormones. Most women can control this problem by the following measures:

- Include some high fiber cereal, prunes, or figs with breakfast. Do not, however, eat excessive amounts of fiber. It may be irritating to the stomach.
- Drink hot liquid with breakfast. This often has a stimulating effect on the colon.
- Allow plenty of time for appropriate bowel habits in the morning.
- With your doctor's consent milk of magnesia (p. 78) can be used sparingly at night, but harsh laxatives should be avoided. Some laxatives can cause the uterus to contract.

GENERIC NAME: Doxepin

COMMON BRANDS: Adapin, Sinequan

TYPE OF DRUG: (Prescription) Antidepressant

FDA RISK CATEGORY FOR PREGNANCY: D

GENERAL INFORMATION: Doxepin is a member of a group of drugs called tricyclic antidepressants. It is effective for the treatment of chronic depression. The drug can elevate mood, improve appetite, relieve insomnia, and increase physical activity. Therapy is usually begun with a low dosage and gradually increased to a therapeutic level. Beneficial effects are not usually seen until two to four weeks after treatment has begun.

POSSIBLE MATERNAL SIDE EFFECTS: Side effects include drowsiness, blurred vision, dry mouth, constipation, weight gain, low blood pressure, and abnormal rhythms of the heart.

USE DURING PREGNANCY: Like other tricyclic antidepressants, doxepin has been associated with a variety of birth defects. These drugs should be avoided during pregnancy unless major depression cannot be satisfactorily managed in any other way.

USE DURING BREASTFEEDING: Doxepin enters breast milk in small quantities, but its effect on the newborn is not known.

ALTERNATIVES TO MEDICATIONS: Depression often gives rise to hopelessness, negativity toward oneself, and at times, an inability to carry out normal activities of daily living. Some individuals may become intensely sad or grief-stricken over the loss of someone or something close to them. Others may suffer from chronic depression unrelated to a specific event. In many cases counseling is necessary to truly understand the cause and extent of depression. There are, however, a number of things you can do to deal with depression on your own:

1. Try to identify the specific situation or personal interaction that has caused your sense of hopelessness and negativity.
2. Make a fresh start at correcting the problem. Talk it through. If necessary, repair relationships with previously available support systems. Often family or close friends can serve to reduce your distress.
3. Realize that there are options for most situations. Seldom is there truly "no choice."
4. Understand some of the warning signs that indicate you have

138

severe depression requiring professional counseling. Such signs include

- Intense sadness, frequent bouts of crying, or depressed mood most of the day,
- Uncharacteristically negative thoughts about yourself,
- Markedly diminished interest or pleasure in most activities,
- Diminished appetite and weight loss,
- Chronic insomnia or sleeping excessively,
- Feelings of worthlessness or guilt,
- Persistent fatigue or lack of energy,
- Inability to think or concentrate,
- Thoughts or plans for suicide.

5. Patients with severe depression should not stop taking antidepressant medications without careful psychiatric supervision.

GENERIC NAME: Doxycycline

COMMON BRANDS: Doxy-Caps, Doxy-Tabs, Vibramycin, Vibra-Tabs

TYPE OF DRUG: (Prescription) Antibiotic

FDA RISK CATEGORY FOR PREGNANCY: X

GENERAL INFORMATION: Doxycycline is a tetracycline antibiotic used in nonpregnant individuals for treatment of a variety of infections including gonorrhea, respiratory tract infections, Rocky Mountain spotted fever, and traveler's diarrhea. In some cases doxycycline has been given to travelers to prevent diarrhea.

POSSIBLE MATERNAL SIDE EFFECTS: Common side effects include nausea, loss of appetite, and diarrhea.

USE DURING PREGNANCY: Like other tetracycline antibiotics, doxycycline can cause permanent yellow-brown staining of teeth and abnormal bone development. Staining of teeth is most likely to occur when tetracycline antibiotics are administered after the twenty-fifth week of pregnancy. In addition, there have been a few reports of fetal malformations when doxycycline was administered during the first trimester.

USE DURING BREASTFEEDING: Doxycycline is excreted into breast milk and can stain the teeth of breastfed infants. Neither doxycycline nor any tetracycline antibiotic should be administered during breastfeeding.

ALTERNATIVES TO MEDICATIONS: Like other tetracycline antibiotics, doxycycline should be avoided during pregnancy. Other safer antibiotics are available for the treatment of bacterial infections. Viral illnesses do not require antibiotic therapy.

GENERIC NAME: **Enalapril**

COMMON BRANDS: Vaseretic, Vasotec

TYPE OF DRUG: (Prescription) Antihypertensive

FDA RISK CATEGORY FOR PREGNANCY: C

GENERAL INFORMATION: Enalapril is used for the treatment of hypertension. It belongs to a group of drugs called angiotensin converting enzyme (ACE) inhibitors.

POSSIBLE MATERNAL SIDE EFFECTS: Side effects are usually minimal. Occasionally, dizziness, headache, nausea, or persistent cough can occur.

USE DURING PREGNANCY: Enalapril is a relatively new drug; consequently, there is very little experience with its use during pregnancy. Studies in laboratory animals have shown an increased risk of fetal death related to the drug.

A similar antihypertensive, captopril (p. 98), has been suspected of causing birth defects in a few patients given the drug during the first trimester. Enalapril and other ACE inhibitors have also been shown to damage the baby's kidneys.

USE DURING BREASTFEEDING: Enalapril is secreted into breast milk, but its effects on the newborn are not known.

ALTERNATIVES TO MEDICATIONS: With a program of weight loss, mild salt restriction, exercise, and cessation of smoking many women can successfully decrease their blood pressure before pregnancy and remain off medications throughout at least the first trimester. However, if antihypertensive medication is necessary, another drug with a proven record of safety during pregnancy (such as methyldopa, p. 215) should be substituted for enalapril.

140

GENERIC NAME: Encainide

COMMON BRANDS: Enkaid

TYPE OF DRUG: (Prescription) Antiarrhythmic

FDA RISK CATEGORY FOR PREGNANCY: C

GENERAL INFORMATION: Encainide is a medication used for the treatment of abnormal rhythms of the heart called ventricular arrhythmias.

POSSIBLE MATERNAL SIDE EFFECTS: The most serious side effect of encainide is a paradoxical worsening of the abnormal heart rhythm. Other less severe side effects include blurred vision, dizziness, nausea, and headache.

USE DURING PREGNANCY: Reproductive studies have been performed in laboratory animals at dosages many times the usual human dosage without evidence of harm to the fetus. However, experience with encainide during pregnancy has been limited.

USE DURING BREASTFEEDING: Encainide is excreted into breast milk, but its effect on the newborn is not known.

ALTERNATIVES TO MEDICATIONS: For women with serious rhythm disturbances of the heart there may be no alternative to medications. However, there are other drugs available with a longer record of safety during pregnancy.

GENERIC NAME: Ephedrine

COMMON BRANDS: Broncholate, Bronkaid, Bronkotabs, Marax, Mudrane, Primatene, Quadrinal, Tedral, Theofedral

TYPE OF DRUG: (Over-the-counter and prescription) Bronchodilator

FDA RISK CATEGORY FOR PREGNANCY: C

GENERAL INFORMATION: Ephedrine is found in several over-the-counter and prescription medications used for the treatment of asthma. It is rapidly absorbed after oral administration and usually

141

begins to work within 15 to 60 minutes. The drug works by relaxing and dilating the smooth muscles of the bronchial tubes.

Ephedrine can also be given intravenously to correct the low blood pressure that sometimes occurs from spinal or epidural anesthesia during labor.

POSSIBLE MATERNAL SIDE EFFECTS: Possible side effects include rapid heart rate, palpitations, shakiness, nervousness, and insomnia. There are several newer medications for relief of wheezing which are less likely to cause side effects.

USE DURING PREGNANCY: The Collaborative Perinatal Project found no link between ephedrine and major malformations in newborns exposed to the drug during the first trimester. Ephedrine is considered safe for use during pregnancy, but it should not be used indiscriminately. Use of an over-the-counter ephedrine pill without supervision of a doctor is not an appropriate substitute for proper medical management of asthma.

USE DURING BREASTFEEDING: Ephedrine is excreted into breast milk when taken by pill and can cause irritability in the newborn. It is not known whether significant amounts of ephedrine enter breast milk when it is taken by inhalation.

ALTERNATIVES TO MEDICATIONS: In some cases asthma can be prevented by avoidance of known allergens, particularly animals. If you smoke, stop. It is generally a good rule, however, to use a bronchodilating inhaler at the earliest indication of wheezing. Often prompt effective relief of asthma can prevent episodes from becoming more severe and prolonged.

GENERIC NAME: **Epinephrine**

COMMON BRANDS: Ana-Kit, Bronkaid, Epi-Pen, Primatene Mist, Sus-Phrine

TYPE OF DRUG: (Over-the-counter and prescription) Antiallergy, bronchodilator, sympathomimetic

FDA RISK CATEGORY FOR PREGNANCY: C

GENERAL INFORMATION: Epinephrine is a naturally occurring substance in humans. When used as a medication the drug can relieve symptoms of acute wheezing, allergic reactions, and shock. Small amounts of epinephrine are included in several over-the-counter inhalers used for relief of asthma. The drug can also be given by injection for the treatment of acute, severe allergic reactions (including shock). Individuals known to have severe allergy to insect bites or stings can carry a preloaded device or syringe containing epinephrine for immediate use in the event of a severe reaction.

POSSIBLE MATERNAL SIDE EFFECTS: Common side effects include rapid heart rate, palpitations, anxiety, shakiness, and elevated blood pressure.

USE DURING PREGNANCY: There have been a few reports of fetal malformations associated with the use of epinephrine during the first trimester. Nevertheless, the link to any fetal harm has not been confirmed by any large study. Epinephrine can be potentially life-saving in the event of a severe allergic reaction and should not be withheld because of pregnancy.

USE DURING BREASTFEEDING: Epinephrine is excreted into breast milk and may cause irritability in the infant. It would be a good idea to wait several hours after an injection of epinephrine before breastfeeding.

ALTERNATIVES TO MEDICATIONS: An injection of epinephrine for the treatment of a severe allergic reaction may be life-saving. There is no nonpharmacologic alternative, so treatment should not be delayed.

GENERIC NAME: **Ergotamine**

COMMON BRANDS: Bellergal-S, Cafergot, Ergomar, Ergostat, Medihaler Ergotamine Aerosol, Wigraine

TYPE OF DRUG: (Prescription) Antimigraine

FDA RISK CATEGORY FOR PREGNANCY: X

GENERAL INFORMATION: Drugs containing ergotamine are frequently used in nonpregnant patients to prevent or relieve the symptoms of migraine headaches. Many ergotamine-containing preparations also contain caffeine (p. 96) or phenobarbital (p. 247).

143

POSSIBLE MATERNAL SIDE EFFECTS: Possible side effects include transient rapid heart rate, nausea, vomiting, diarrhea, and numbness in the fingers or toes.

USE DURING PREGNANCY: Use of ergotamine-containing medications has been shown to cause miscarriage, as well as abnormal growth and development in laboratory animals. In addition, ergotamine can cause forceful and prolonged contractions of the uterus. Drugs containing ergotamine should not be used at any time during pregnancy.

Often a safer medication, such as acetaminophen (p. 63), can adequately control the pain of a migraine. However, many migraines are so severe that it is necessary to take a narcotic pain killer such as codeine (p. 118) or meperidine (p. 206) to obtain relief. The occasional use of a narcotic analgesic under the care of a physician to treat severe migraines has not been linked to any fetal harm.

USE DURING BREASTFEEDING: Ergotamine probably enters breast milk. Its effect on breastfed infants is not known. The drug should generally be avoided during breastfeeding.

ALTERNATIVES TO MEDICATIONS: Attempt to identify any specific events, foods, or medications that trigger your migraines and avoid them. Avoid alcohol and excessive fatigue. At the onset of a migraine rest in a quiet, darkened room. Following sleep the pain of a migraine usually abates.

GENERIC NAME: **Erythromycin**

COMMON BRANDS: E.E.S., E-Mycin, ERYC, Ery Ped, Ery-Tab, Erythrocin, Ilosone, PCE Dispertab, Pediamycin, Pediazole, Robimycin, Wyamycin

TYPE OF DRUG: (Prescription) Antibiotic

FDA RISK CATEGORY FOR PREGNANCY: B

GENERAL INFORMATION: Erythromycin is a commonly used antibiotic for the treatment of infections of the respiratory tract, ears, sinuses, and skin. It is also used to treat several sexually transmitted diseases. The drug is often substituted for penicillin-type antibiotics in individuals allergic to penicillin.

144

POSSIBLE MATERNAL SIDE EFFECTS: The most common side effects are nausea and abdominal cramps. the one form of erythromycin, estolate (Ilosone), can cause liver damage and jaundice.

USE DURING PREGNANCY: Erythromycin is considered safe for use during pregnancy. However, the estolate form of the drug can cause damage to the liver and should be avoided during pregnancy.

USE DURING BREASTFEEDING: Erythromycin is excreted into breast milk but is considered safe for use during breastfeeding.

ALTERNATIVES TO MEDICATIONS: Most viral infections do not require treatment with an antibiotic.

GENERIC NAME: Estrogens

COMMON BRANDS: Estratab, Mediatric, Menrium, Ogen, PMB 200, PMB 400, Premarin

TYPE OF DRUG: (Prescription) Hormone

FDA RISK CATEGORY FOR PREGNANCY: X

GENERAL INFORMATION: Estrogens are used for the treatment of symptoms related to menopause—prevention and treatment of osteoporosis.

POSSIBLE MATERNAL SIDE EFFECTS: Common side effects include headache, nausea, vomiting, weight gain, and possibly an increased risk of blood clotting.

USE DURING PREGNANCY: Estrogens of all kinds (see birth control pills, p. 89, and diethylstilbestrol p. 132) should not be taken during pregnancy. Their use has been associated with serious abnormalities of genital organs in female offspring, including future development of cancer of the vagina and cervix.

USE DURING BREASTFEEDING: Estrogens inhibit production of breast milk and should be avoided during breastfeeding.

ALTERNATIVES TO MEDICATIONS: There is no indication for the use of estrogens during pregnancy.

GENERIC NAME: **Ethosuximide**

COMMON BRANDS: Zarontin

TYPE OF DRUG: (Prescription) Anticonvulsant

FDA RISK CATEGORY FOR PREGNANCY: Not classified

GENERAL INFORMATION: Ethosuximide is used for the prevention of petit mal seizures (absence attacks), most commonly found in children. The drug can often be discontinued when women reach reproductive age. It is not effective for prevention of grand mal (major) seizures.

POSSIBLE MATERNAL SIDE EFFECTS: Possible serious adverse effects include interference with the ability of the bone marrow to produce red and white blood cells, and a severe skin reaction called Stevens-Johnson syndrome. Less severe side effects include drowsiness, headache, fatigue, nausea, diarrhea, swelling of the gums, and diminished appetite.

USE DURING PREGNANCY: Ethosuximide is thought by some neurologists to be safe for use during pregnancy. However, there has been only limited experience with ethosuximide during pregnancy. An increased risk of birth defects has been associated with the use of all anticonvulsant medications.

USE DURING BREASTFEEDING: Ethosuximide is excreted into breast milk but has not been shown to cause any harm to the newborn.

ALTERNATIVES TO MEDICATIONS: In many cases there is no alternative to the use of medications for the prevention of seizures during pregnancy. Patients with epilepsy should not discontinue medications without consulting their physician. All women with epilepsy should avoid alcohol and be sure to get plenty of sleep.

GENERIC NAME: **Etretinate**

COMMON BRANDS: Tegason

TYPE OF DRUG: (Prescription) Vitamin (for treatment of psoriasis)

FDA RISK CATEGORY FOR PREGNANCY: X

GENERAL INFORMATION: Etretinate is a member of a class of drugs derived from vitamin A called retinoids (also see isotretinoin, p. 187). The drug is used for the treatment of severe psoriasis unresponsive to other forms of therapy. This drug has the unusual property of being stored in fat tissue for many months or years after its use has been discontinued. Significant amounts of the drug have been detected in fat as long as three years after it was taken.

POSSIBLE MATERNAL SIDE EFFECTS: Side effects include dry, cracking lips, sore mouth, red face, joint pain, headache, fatigue, and irritation of the eyes.

USE DURING PREGNANCY: Like other retinoids, etretinate has been shown to cause major birth defects in animals. This drug **must not** be administered during pregnancy for any reason. Furthermore, the manufacturer and many authorities recommend that the drug not be given to any woman capable of becoming pregnant because of its unusual ability to remain in the body for many years after being used.

USE DURING BREASTFEEDING: The drug probably enters breast milk and should be avoided during breastfeeding.

ALTERNATIVES TO MEDICATIONS: For the treatment of severe psoriasis consult a dermatologist. In some cases this chronic skin condition can be kept under adequate control with limited exposure to sunlight and topical medication.

GENERIC NAME: **Famotidine**

COMMON BRANDS: Pepcid

TYPE OF DRUG: (Prescription) Antiulcer

FDA RISK CATEGORY FOR PREGNANCY: B

GENERAL INFORMATION: Famotidine is used for the treatment of gastric or duodenal ulcers. It works by inhibiting the production of acid by the cells of the stomach. The drug can be administered orally or intravenously.

POSSIBLE MATERNAL SIDE EFFECTS: Famotidine is generally well tolerated. There are no common side effects.

USE DURING PREGNANCY: There has been no evidence of fetal harm in animals. However, there has not been enough experience with the drug to ensure its safety in human pregnancy.

USE DURING BREASTFEEDING: Famotidine is excreted into breast milk. Its safety has not been established.

ALTERNATIVES TO MEDICATIONS: A program of dietary restriction alone is generally not adequate for treatment of stomach or intestinal ulcers. However, an alternative to famotidine during pregnancy is the regular use of antacids (p. 78) between meals.

GENERIC NAME: Fenoprofen

COMMON BRANDS: Nalfon

TYPE OF DRUG: (Prescription) Anti-inflammatory

FDA RISK CATEGORY FOR PREGNANCY: B

GENERAL INFORMATION: Fenoprofen is a member of a group of drugs called nonsteroidal anti-inflammatory drugs (NSAIDs). It is primarily used to reduce the pain and inflammation of acute or chronic arthritis.

POSSIBLE MATERNAL SIDE EFFECTS: Possible side effects include stomach irritation or bleeding, nausea, and fluid retention.

USE DURING PREGNANCY: There have been no reports linking fenoprofen to birth defects when the drug was used during the first trimester. However, experience with the drug during early pregnancy is limited.

Used near term fenoprofen can have potential effects on pregnancy and the fetus. First, the drug can cause premature closure of an important blood vessel in the fetus called the ductus arteriosus. Normally, this blood vessel does not close until after delivery.

Premature closure could result in a serious condition called pulmonary hypertension. Second, fenoprofen and other NSAIDs can inhibit labor and prolong pregnancy.

USE DURING BREASTFEEDING: Fenoprofen enters breast milk in small amounts. Its significance to the breastfed infant is not known.

ALTERNATIVES TO MEDICATIONS: Musculoskeletal pain can often be relieved with warm baths, and massage. Painful arthritis can be alleviated by rest, heat, and physical therapy. Nonweight-bearing exercise such as swimming may offer some comfort while enhancing muscle tone. If medication is necessary, acetaminophen (p. 63) is probably the safest medication to take during pregnancy for relief of minor pain.

GENERIC NAME: Fentanyl

COMMON BRANDS: Innovar, Sublimaze

TYPE OF DRUG: (Prescription) Narcotic analgesic

FDA RISK CATEGORY FOR PREGNANCY: C

GENERAL INFORMATION: Fentanyl is a potent narcotic analgesic administered only by injection. Its use is primarily to induce effective pain control during surgery.

POSSIBLE MATERNAL SIDE EFFECTS: Common side effects include sedation, confusion, dry mouth, nausea, constipation, and pain at the site of injection. Chronic use can lead to drug dependence.

USE DURING PREGNANCY: There have been no reports of birth defects in laboratory animals given very large dosages of fentanyl. Experience with fentanyl during human pregnancy, however, is limited. Similar to other narcotics, use during labor can produce respiratory depression in the newborn.

USE DURING BREASTFEEDING: It is not known whether fentanyl is excreted into breast milk.

ALTERNATIVES TO MEDICATIONS: Techniques of natural childbirth such as Lamaze may eliminate the need for narcotics during labor. However, fentanyl can be safely used to control pain following surgery or after cesarean delivery.

GENERIC NAME: Flunisolide

COMMON BRANDS: AeroBid, Nasalide

TYPE OF DRUG: (Prescription) Corticosteroid inhaler

FDA RISK CATEGORY FOR PREGNANCY: C

GENERAL INFORMATION: Flunisolide inhaler is used for the treatment of chronic asthma. The drug is a form of corticosteroid (p. 119) effective for prevention of wheezing when used in a regular dosage twice each day. It is not effective for relief of acute wheezing.

POSSIBLE MATERNAL SIDE EFFECTS: Possible side effects include hoarseness, thrush (yeast infection of the mouth), and a dry, irritated throat.

USE DURING PREGNANCY: In recommended dosages flunisolide has not been shown to cause malformations in humans. However, when given in extremely high dosages corticosteroids have been associated with an increased risk of cleft palate in laboratory rabbits and rats.

USE DURING BREASTFEEDING: It is not known if flunisolide is excreted into breast milk.

ALTERNATIVES TO MEDICATIONS: In some cases asthma can be prevented by avoidance of known allergens, particularly animals. If you smoke, stop. It is generally a good rule, however, to use a bronchodilating inhaler at the earliest indication of wheezing. Often prompt effective relief of asthma can prevent episodes from becoming more severe and prolonged.

GENERIC NAME: Fluoxetine

COMMON BRANDS: Prozac

TYPE OF DRUG: (Prescription) Antidepressant

FDA RISK CATEGORY FOR PREGNANCY: C

GENERAL INFORMATION: Fluoxetine is a relatively new antidepressant. It is chemically different from other antidepressant medications currently on the market. Its exact mechanism of action is not known.

POSSIBLE MATERNAL SIDE EFFECTS: The most common side effects include headache, nervousness, insomnia, and nausea. Unlike many other antidepressants, fluoxetine does not usually cause drowsiness or increased appetite.

USE DURING PREGNANCY: Reproductive studies have been performed in laboratory animals at dosages approximately 10 times the maximum daily human dosage and have not demonstrated any evidence of fetal harm. Since the drug is relatively new, there has been very little experience with its use during human gestation. Fluoxetine may diminish appetite and cause weight loss. Weight loss is not desirable during pregnancy even for women who are overweight.

USE DURING BREASTFEEDING: No information is available.

ALTERNATIVES TO MEDICATIONS: Depression often gives rise to hopelessness, negativity toward oneself, and at times an inability to carry out normal activities of daily living. Some individuals may become intensely sad or grief-stricken over the loss of someone or something close to them. Others may suffer from chronic depression unrelated to a specific event. In many cases counseling is necessary to truly understand the cause and extent of depression. There are, however, a number of things you can do to deal with depression on your own:

1. Try to identify the specific situation or personal interaction that has caused your sense of hopelessness and negativity.
2. Make a fresh start at correcting the problem. Talk it through. If necessary, repair relationships with previously available support systems. Often family or close friends can serve to reduce your distress.
3. Realize that there are options for most situations. Seldom is there truly "no choice."
4. Understand some of the warning signs that indicate you have severe depression requiring professional counseling. Such signs include
   - Intense sadness, frequent bouts of crying, or depressed mood most of the day,
   - Uncharacteristically negative thoughts about yourself,
   - Markedly diminished interest or pleasure in most activities,
   - Diminished appetite and weight loss,
   - Chronic insomnia or sleeping excessively,
   - Feelings of worthlessness or guilt,
   - Persistent fatigue or lack of energy,
   - Inability to think or concentrate,
   - Thoughts or plans for suicide.
5. Patients with severe depression should not stop taking antidepressant medications without careful psychiatric supervision.

151

GENERIC NAME: Flurazepam

COMMON BRANDS: Dalmane

TYPE OF DRUG: (Prescription) Sedative

FDA RISK CATEGORY FOR PREGNANCY: D

GENERAL INFORMATION: Flurazepam is a member of a group of antianxiety medications called benzodiazepines. These drugs are used for the treatment of anxiety and insomnia. They work by relaxing skeletal muscles and by a direct action on the brain. Benzodiazepines can be abused if taken indiscriminately or for a long period of time. Withdrawal symptoms including tremor, agitation, insomnia, muscle cramps, nausea, and seizures can occur if these drugs are discontinued abruptly after chronic use. Benzodiazepines should not be taken without careful medical supervision.

POSSIBLE MATERNAL SIDE EFFECTS: Common side effects with all benzodiazepines include sedation, depression, mental confusion, dizziness, unsteady gait, nightmares, fatigue, dry mouth, and low blood pressure. These drugs can interfere with the ability to safely drive a car or operate dangerous equipment. Physical and psychological dependence can occur with chronic use.

USE DURING PREGNANCY: All benzodiazepines rapidly cross the placenta and enter the fetal circulation. Blood levels in the fetus equal that of the mother's within one hour of taking a pill. Several studies have demonstrated a link between first-trimester use of benzodiazepines and birth defects. The most commonly reported malformations are cleft lip and cleft palate. Used near term benzodiazepines have been associated with lethargy, respiratory problems, and withdrawal symptoms in the newborn. Most authorities believe that it is best to avoid these medications during the first trimester and if possible throughout pregnancy.

USE DURING BREASTFEEDING: Benzodiazepines are excreted into breast milk in significant quantities. They can cause sedation in the newborn and should be avoided during breastfeeding.

ALTERNATIVES TO MEDICATIONS: Insomnia may be relieved by some of the following techniques:

- Generally, try to avoid daytime naps. However, for some women sleeping patterns change during pregnancy, and a nap may be necessary to supplement abbreviated nighttime sleep.
- Go to bed only when tired. Instead of lying in bed when you are wide awake, get up, do something, and then return to bed when you feel tired.
- Try to establish a regular sleep pattern. Recognize when you *are* able to sleep and build on that.
- Exercise daily. Even a 30-minute walk will aid relaxation.
- Learn techniques of progressive relaxation. These techniques are simple to learn and effective.
- Avoid stimulant drinks such as coffee, tea, and caffeine-containing colas. On the other hand, warm milk may help make you sleepy.
- Never use alcohol to induce sleep.
- If you awaken during the night, recall the dream just before you awoke. Reentering the dream can return you to sleep.
- Make love. Sex is relaxing and often ends with sleep.
- If you are lying awake because a problem is on your mind, talk it through with someone until it's resolved.

GENERIC NAME: Folic acid

COMMON BRANDS: Fero-Folic-500, Folvite, Iberet-Folic, Materna, Optivite, Prenate 90, Stuartnatal 1 + 1, Trinsicon, Vitafol

TYPE OF DRUG: (Over-the-counter) Vitamin

FDA RISK CATEGORY FOR PREGNANCY: A

GENERAL INFORMATION: Folic acid is a water-soluble B complex vitamin essential for the normal production of red blood cells. The American Required Daily Allowance (RDA) of folic acid for nonpregnant individuals is 0.8 mg.

POSSIBLE MATERNAL SIDE EFFECTS: There are generally no side effects.

USE DURING PREGNANCY: Folic acid deficiency is common during pregnancy. Consequently, this vitamin must be supplemented in most diets. Inadequate intake of folic acid during pregnancy can result in anemia in the mother and an infant born smaller than expected. Most authorities recommend that 1 milligram (mg) of folic acid be given by supplement each day to all pregnant women. Not all prenatal multiple vitamin preparations contain 1 mg of folic acid. Therefore, additional supplements may be required. There are no known harmful effects of excessive folic acid intake.

USE DURING BREASTFEEDING: The RDA for folic acid during breastfeeding is 0.5 mg. Supplements to meet the RDA for folic acid are important during breastfeeding for those women with inadequate nutritional intake. If a woman's diet provides adequate folic acid, supplements are not necessary.

ALTERNATIVES TO MEDICATIONS: Foods rich in folic acid include brewer's yeast, liver, green leafy vegetables, and beets.

GENERIC NAME: Furosemide

COMMON BRANDS: Lasix

TYPE OF DRUG: (Prescription) Diuretic

FDA RISK CATEGORY FOR PREGNANCY: C

GENERAL INFORMATION: Furosemide is a potent diuretic used primarily for the treatment of congestive heart failure or severe hypertension. It is not appropriate for common fluid retention.

POSSIBLE MATERNAL SIDE EFFECTS: The most significant side effect is loss of potassium from the body. It is usually necessary to take potassium supplements while being treated with furosemide.

USE DURING PREGNANCY: Furosemide should generally be avoided during pregnancy unless it is needed to treat the rare conditions of congestive heart failure, pulmonary edema (fluid in the lungs), or some cases of chronic kidney disease. This potent diuretic can markedly decrease maternal blood volume and compromise blood flow to the fetus. Neither furosemide nor any other diuretic should be given to relieve the fluid retention that accompanies most normal pregnancies.

USE DURING BREASTFEEDING: Furosemide is excreted into breast milk. While no reports of adverse effects in nursing infants have been reported, the manufacturer recommends against breastfeeding if the drug must be given to the mother.

ALTERNATIVES TO MEDICATIONS: The use of diuretics during pregnancy is usually reserved for women with heart problems or kidney disease. Mild edema (fluid retention) is a common occurrence during pregnancy and does not require treatment. If edema becomes uncomfortable, it can usually be relieved by lying on your side for periods of 30 to 60 minutes. In some cases mild restriction of dietary salt intake may be necessary. Severe salt restriction, however, is not appropriate and may even be harmful. There is no evidence that so-called natural diuretics found in health food stores are effective, and their safety during pregnancy cannot be assured.

GENERIC NAME: Gamma Benzene Hexachloride (Lindane)

COMMON BRANDS: Kwell, Scabene

TYPE OF DRUG: (Prescription) Antiparasite

FDA RISK CATEGORY FOR PREGNANCY: C

GENERAL INFORMATION: Gamma benzene hexachloride (lindane), available as a lotion or shampoo, is used for the treatment of lice and scabies. Neither the lotion nor shampoo is effective for prevention of lice. Instructions for use of the drug should be followed carefully.

POSSIBLE MATERNAL SIDE EFFECTS: Gamma benzene hexachloride can be irritating if it is left on the skin too long, and significant amounts can be absorbed into the bloodstream. Very high dosages applied to the skin or taken orally have caused convulsions in children.

USE DURING PREGNANCY: Gamma benzene hexachloride should generally be avoided during pregnancy. This warning is based on evidence that the drug can be toxic to the neurologic system when used in large quantities. Excessive use of gamma benzene hexachloride has been reported to cause convulsions in children treated with excessive amounts. If it is necessary to treat scabies during pregnancy, only a thin layer of lotion should be applied to the involved area and washed off after eight hours. Simultaneous application of other oils or lotions may enhance systemic absorption and should be avoided. Repeat application of the lotion should not be performed without consulting a physician. One treatment may be enough. For the treatment of lice in the scalp or pubic hair, two tablespoons (30 ml) of shampoo should be worked into a lather for approximately four minutes, then rinsed thoroughly. After consultation with a physician, treatment with shampoo may be repeated in 24 hours but not more than twice in 1 week. Relief of symptoms usually occurs within 24 hours.

USE DURING BREASTFEEDING: It appears that only small amounts of the drug are excreted into breast milk. However, there is not sufficient information to ensure its safety.

ALTERNATIVES TO MEDICATIONS: Pubic lice are usually transmitted sexually. It is important to be sure that sexual partners practice good hygiene. In many cases treatment of lice can be postponed until after pregnancy or at least until after the first trimester.

GENERIC NAME: Gemfibrozil

COMMON BRANDS: Lopid

TYPE OF DRUG: (Prescription) Lipid (fat) lowering drug

FDA RISK CATEGORY FOR PREGNANCY: B

GENERAL INFORMATION: Gemfibrozil is used for the treatment of elevated levels of triglycerides and cholesterol. The drug is usually reserved for individuals whose serum lipids (fats) have not been satisfactorily reduced following a program of dietary restriction and exercise.

POSSIBLE MATERNAL SIDE EFFECTS: Common side effects include nausea, abdominal pain, dry mouth, and gas. In some cases liver tests may become elevated.

USE DURING PREGNANCY: Reproductive studies in rats and rabbits have not shown any adverse fetal effects due to use of gemfibrozil during gestation. However, there have been no careful studies or extensive reports in humans to ensure its safety. Gemfibrozil should only be used during pregnancy in women with extremely elevated levels of triglyceride and cholesterol unresponsive to other forms of therapy.

USE DURING BREASTFEEDING: There is no information available about the use of gemfibrozil during breastfeeding.

ALTERNATIVES TO MEDICATIONS: In most cases high levels of tri-glyceride and cholesterol can be satisfactorily managed throughout pregnancy by a program of restricted dietary fats, exercise, and added dietary fiber. Since elevated lipids do not require urgent medical care, medication is usually not necessary during the relatively brief duration of pregnancy.

GENERIC NAME: Gentian violet

COMMON BRANDS: Genapax Tampons

TYPE OF DRUG: (Prescription) Disinfectant

FDA RISK CATEGORY FOR PREGNANCY: C

GENERAL INFORMATION: Gentian violet can be applied by solution or medicated tampon to the vagina or cervix for the treatment of candida (yeast) vaginitis. Newer and more effective medications are available for treatment of vaginal yeast infections.

POSSIBLE MATERNAL SIDE EFFECTS: Solutions and tampons are usually well tolerated, but they are messy and can stain skin or clothing.

USE DURING PREGNANCY: There have been no careful studies of the use of gentian violet during pregnancy. More convenient treatment is available.

USE DURING BREASTFEEDING: No information is available.

ALTERNATIVES TO MEDICATIONS: To help avoid vaginal yeast infections do not take antibiotics unnecessarily, wear loose cotton underwear, avoid harsh soaps and irritants, and be sure your partner does not have a chronic yeast infection. During pregnancy it is not always necessary to treat mild yeast infections.

GENERIC NAME: Glipizide

COMMON BRANDS: Glucotrol

TYPE OF DRUG: (Prescription) Oral hypoglycemic agent (blood sugar–lowering drug)

FDA RISK CATEGORY FOR PREGNANCY: D

GENERAL INFORMATION: Glipizide is one of several drugs effective for lowering blood sugar levels in patients with type II diabetes mellitus (adult-onset diabetes). Similar to other oral hypoglycemic agents, glipizide acts by increasing the production of insulin in the pancreas and by enhancing the effect of insulin in the cells. The vast majority of individuals with type I diabetes (juvenile-onset) and some people with type II diabetes cannot achieve satisfactory control of their blood sugar levels with oral hypoglycemic agents and must take daily injections of insulin.

POSSIBLE MATERNAL SIDE EFFECTS: The most significant adverse effect of glipizide is hypoglycemia—that is, a blood sugar level that is excessively low. Individuals allergic to sulfa-containing medications will likely be allergic to glipizide.

USE DURING PREGNANCY: Like other oral hypoglycemic agents, glipizide crosses the placenta. Other drugs in this class (sulfonylureas) have been shown to cause birth defects when given during the first trimester. When used near term oral hypoglycemic agents can cause severe hypoglycemia in the newborn immediately after delivery. Neither glipizide nor any other oral hypoglycemic agents should be used during pregnancy. Women treated with these medications who are planning pregnancy should consult their physician and discontinue the drug before attempting to conceive. Some women will be able to satisfactorily control blood sugar levels with diet alone. Others will need to take daily injections of insulin. All patients who discontinue their diabetes medication will need frequent blood tests performed to ensure that blood sugars do not increase to dangerous levels.

USE DURING BREASTFEEDING: It is not known how much glipizide enters breast milk. Because of the theoretical risk that even a small amount of the drug in breast milk could cause hypoglycemia in the newborn, glipizide should generally be avoided during breastfeeding. Some patients can achieve adequate control of their blood sugars by careful diet. Other individuals, however, may require injections of insulin.

ALTERNATIVES TO MEDICATIONS: Some women with type II diabetes treated with glipizide before pregnancy can satisfactorily control their blood sugars by following a strict diet. Most pregnant women, however, will have to take injections of insulin to maintain their blood sugar levels in the range appropriate for pregnancy.

GENERIC NAME: Glucagon

COMMON BRANDS: Glucagon

TYPE OF DRUG: (Prescription) Hormone

FDA RISK CATEGORY FOR PREGNANCY: B

GENERAL INFORMATION: Injection of glucagon causes a rapid increase in blood sugar level and is used for the treatment of severe hypoglycemia (low blood sugar) in individuals with diabetes taking insulin or oral hypoglycemic agents. Glucagon must be administered by injection, since it is rapidly destroyed in the stomach before it can be absorbed. Use of this drug is usually reserved for patients with diabetes who have lost consciousness due to hypoglycemia and are unable to ingest sugar-containing food or liquid. Patients taking insulin should have a glucagon kit (medication and syringe) available at home at all times. It is essential that a family member or someone living at home be instructed how to inject glucagon in an emergency.

POSSIBLE MATERNAL SIDE EFFECTS: There are very few side effects associated with injection of glucagon. Mild nausea and dizziness can occur.

USE DURING PREGNANCY: Injection of glucagon can be life-saving for the treatment of severe hypoglycemia accompanied by loss of consciousness.

 Because the goal in pregnant patients with diabetes is near-normal blood sugar levels, hypoglycemia is always a risk. Glucagon should be available for injection in insulin-treated diabetics. Use of glucagon has not been associated with birth defects or harm to the fetus.

USE DURING BREASTFEEDING: There is no evidence that injection of glucagon to a diabetic woman with severe hypoglycemia causes any harm to the breastfed infant. Use of glucagon for treatment of severe hypoglycemia should not be withheld because of breastfeeding or pregnancy.

ALTERNATIVES TO MEDICATIONS: Mild hypoglycemia can be treated with juice, candy, soda pop, or glucose tablets. However, a woman with insulin-dependent diabetes who is unconscious and unable to take any food or liquid by mouth should be presumed to be suffering from severe hypoglycemia and given an immediate injection of glucagon.

GENERIC NAME: Glyburide

COMMON BRANDS: DiaBeta, Micronase

TYPE OF DRUG: (Prescription) Oral hypoglycemic agent (blood sugar–lowering drug)

FDA RISK CATEGORY FOR PREGNANCY: D

GENERAL INFORMATION: Glyburide is one of several drugs effective for lowering blood sugar levels in patients with type II diabetes mellitus (adult-onset diabetes). Similar to other oral hypoglycemic agents, glyburide acts by increasing the production of insulin in the pancreas and by enhancing the effect of insulin in the cells. The vast majority of individuals with type I diabetes (juvenile-onset) and some people with type II diabetes cannot achieve satisfactory control of their blood sugar levels with oral hypoglycemic agents and must take daily injections of insulin.

POSSIBLE MATERNAL SIDE EFFECTS: The most significant adverse effect of glyburide is hypoglycemia—that is, a blood sugar level that is excessively low. Individuals allergic to sulfa-containing medications may also be allergic to glyburide.

USE DURING PREGNANCY: Like other oral hypoglycemic agents, glyburide crosses the placenta. Other drugs in this class (sulfonylureas) have been shown to cause birth defects when given during the first trimester. When used near term oral hypoglycemic agents can cause severe hypoglycemia in the newborn immediately after delivery. Neither glyburide nor any other oral hypoglycemic agents should be used during pregnancy. Women treated with these medications who are planning pregnancy should consult their physician and discontinue the drug before attempting to conceive. Some women will be able to satisfactorily control blood sugar levels with diet alone. Others will need to take daily injections of insulin. All patients who discontinue their diabetes medication will need frequent blood tests performed to ensure that blood sugars do not increase to dangerous levels.

USE DURING BREASTFEEDING: It is not known how much glyburide

160

enters breast milk. Because of the theoretical risk that even a small amount of the drug in breast milk could cause hypoglycemia in the newborn, glyburide should generally be avoided during breastfeeding. Some patients can achieve adequate control of their blood sugars by careful diet. Other individuals, however, may require injections of insulin.

ALTERNATIVES TO MEDICATIONS: Some women with type II diabetes treated with glyburide before pregnancy can satisfactorily control their blood sugars by following a strict diet. Most pregnant women, however, will have to take injections of insulin to maintain their blood sugar levels in the range appropriate for pregnancy.

GENERIC NAME: Gold

COMMON BRANDS: Myochrysine, Ridaura, Solganal

TYPE OF DRUG: (Prescription) Anti-inflammatory

FDA RISK CATEGORY FOR PREGNANCY: C

GENERAL INFORMATION: Gold salts can be administered orally or by injection for the treatment of rheumatoid arthritis. Treatment with gold is usually reserved for patients who have not responded satisfactorily to aspirin (p. 82) or other antiinflammatory drugs. The drug is most effective when used before rheumatoid arthritis has caused severe, irreversible joint deformity.

POSSIBLE MATERNAL SIDE EFFECTS: Adverse reactions to gold therapy are common and can be potentially severe. They include severe skin rashes, destruction of normal red blood cells, white blood cells, and platelets, kidney damage, and liver damage. It is because of these severe adverse reactions that gold is not used until other less toxic drugs have been shown to be ineffective.

USE DURING PREGNANCY: Gold has been shown to cause birth defects in rats and rabbits. However, use during human gestation has not been clearly linked to adverse effects. Because of the theoretical risk of severe adverse effects and potential fetal harm, gold should not be given during pregnancy. Furthermore, gold may be stored for months in various tissues of the body even after its use has been discontinued. Consult your physician if you are contemplating pregnancy to see how long you should wait before attempting to conceive.

USE DURING BREASTFEEDING: Gold is excreted into breast milk. Because of its potential for causing severe skin rashes, kidney damage, and liver damage, the drug should not be given during breastfeeding. Women with severe rheumatoid arthritis who must take gold should discontinue breastfeeding.

ALTERNATIVES TO MEDICATIONS: Fortunately, many women with rheumatoid arthritis demonstrate significant improvement in joint pain during pregnancy. The reason for diminished symptoms during pregnancy is not known. Nevertheless, many women are able to discontinue potentially hazardous drugs without having to endure severe pain. Adequate rest plus a program of physical therapy may be enough to achieve satisfactory control of rheumatoid arthritis during pregnancy.

GENERIC NAME: Griseofulvin

COMMON BRANDS: Fulvicin-U/F, Grifulvin V, Grisactin, Gris-PEG

TYPE OF DRUG: (Prescription) Antifungal

FDA RISK CATEGORY FOR PREGNANCY: C

GENERAL INFORMATION: Griseofulvin is used to treat fungal infections of hair, skin, and nails. Oral preparations are usually reserved for infections that do not respond to topical creams or lotions.

POSSIBLE MATERNAL SIDE EFFECTS: Mild side effects include headache, nausea, and skin rash. The drug can also cause more significant damage to the kidneys and liver, as well as a reduction in the normal white blood cell count.

USE DURING PREGNANCY: Griseofulvin has been shown to cause birth defects in laboratory animals. Although human studies are lacking, the drug should not be given during pregnancy because of its potential harm to the fetus.

USE DURING BREASTFEEDING: No information is available. However, even a small amount of the drug in breast milk could be harmful to the newborn. It is best avoided during breastfeeding.

ALTERNATIVES TO MEDICATIONS: Although there is no nonpharmacologic alternative to griseofulvin, treatment of most fungal infections of hair, skin, and nails can be postponed until after pregnancy.

GENERIC NAME: Guaifenesin

COMMON BRANDS: Ambenyl-D, Anti-Tuss, Baytussin, Benylin, Breonesin, Cheracol D, Colrex Expectorant, Contac Cough Formula, Cremacoat 2, Dimacol, Fedahist, Glycotuss, Guiatuss, Halotussin, Humibid, Hytuss, Isoclor, Medi-Tuss, Naldecon, Novahistine, Nortussin, Robitussin, Sudafed Cough Syrup, Triaminic, Vicks, Zephrex

TYPE OF DRUG: (Over-the-counter) Expectorant

FDA RISK CATEGORY FOR PREGNANCY: C

GENERAL INFORMATION: Guaifenesin is a common ingredient in many over-the-counter cough and cold preparations. The drug theoretically works by thinning secretions in the respiratory tract and thereby facilitating their removal. In recent years studies have suggested that guaifenesin provides little, if any, benefit. Many of the commercial cold products also contain antihistamines, decongestants, aspirin, acetaminophen, and alcohol.

POSSIBLE MATERNAL SIDE EFFECTS: Side effects are generally minimal. Occasionally nausea can occur. Side effects are more likely from other constituents of multiple ingredients cold preparations.

USE DURING PREGNANCY: The Collaborative Perinatal Project reported a slight excess in the expected number of congenital hernias found in the newborns of mothers who took guaifenesin-containing preparations during the first trimester. Other studies have not confirmed any risk to the fetus. It should be kept in mind that many cough and cold syrups contain significant amounts of alcohol, which should be avoided throughout pregnancy.

USE DURING BREASTFEEDING: No information is available.

ALTERNATIVES TO MEDICATIONS: Expectorants such as guaifenesin are probably of little value. Cool mist or steam should provide some assistance in loosening thick mucous secretions.

GENERIC NAME: Halazepam

COMMON BRANDS: Paxipam

TYPE OF DRUG: (Prescription) Antianxiety, sedative

FDA RISK CATEGORY FOR PREGNANCY: D

GENERAL INFORMATION: Halazepam is a member of a group of antianxiety medications called benzodiazepines. These drugs are used for the treatment of anxiety and insomnia. They work by relaxing skeletal muscles and by a direct action on the brain. Benzodiazepines can be abused if taken indiscriminately or for a long period of time. Withdrawal symptoms including tremor, agitation, insomnia, muscle cramps, nausea, and seizures can occur if these drugs are discontinued abruptly after chronic use. Benzodiazepines should not be taken without careful medical supervision.

POSSIBLE MATERNAL SIDE EFFECTS: Common side effects with all benzodiazepines include sedation, depression, mental confusion, dizziness, unsteady gait, nightmares, fatigue, dry mouth, and low blood pressure. These drugs can interfere with the ability to safely drive a car or operate dangerous equipment. Physical and psychological dependence can occur with chronic use.

USE DURING PREGNANCY: All benzodiazepines rapidly cross the placenta and enter the fetal circulation. Blood levels in the fetus equal that of the mother's within one hour of taking a pill. Several studies have demonstrated a link between first-trimester use of benzodiazepines and birth defects. The most commonly reported malformations are cleft lip and cleft palate.

Used near term benzodiazepines have been associated with lethargy, respiratory problems, and withdrawal symptoms in the newborn. Most authorities believe that it is best to avoid these medications during the first trimester and if possible throughout pregnancy.

USE DURING BREASTFEEDING: Benzodiazepines are excreted into breast milk in significant quantities. They can cause sedation in the newborn and should be avoided during breastfeeding.

ALTERNATIVES TO MEDICATIONS: Before using medications to control anxiety or stress consider the following strategy:

164

1. Identify the source of your anxiety. Worry often persists because of an inability to identify a problem and take action to solve it. Visualization can begin the process. Close your eyes and take a few deep breaths. Allow an image of the problem to arise.
2. Once you've defined the source of your anxiety, gather information. For example, if you are worried about the outcome of your pregnancy because of a possible hereditary problem or a medication you took before you knew you were pregnant, get information from your physician or a genetic counselor. In most cases what you discover will be very comforting.
3. After obtaining information, decide on a plan of action. Do what you can to deal with the problem, but once you've done all you can, change your focus and move on to other parts of life. Instead of worrying, concentrate on your life beyond the worry. Exercise or take walks. Plan how you will spend the evening or the weekend. Treat yourself to something pleasant, or think up a surprise for someone you care about. As your mind gets busy with other thoughts, you'll find that stress will begin to fade.
4. If anxiety persists despite your best efforts, see a therapist. Often only a few counseling sessions can effectively reduce anxiety and stress and eliminate the need for medication.

GENERIC NAME: Haloperidol

COMMON BRANDS: Haldol

TYPE OF DRUG: (Prescription) Antipsychotic

FDA RISK CATEGORY FOR PREGNANCY: C

GENERAL INFORMATION: Haloperidol has been effectively used to control psychotic delusions, agitation, paranoid behavior, and hallucinations. The drug is also capable of controlling persistent nausea and vomiting.

POSSIBLE MATERNAL SIDE EFFECTS: Side effects are common including sedation, dizziness, fatigue, blurred vision, dry mouth, and a movement disorder called tardive dyskinesia.

USE DURING PREGNANCY: There have been a few reports of birth defects presumably associated with exposure to haloperidol during the first trimester. No large studies have confirmed these isolated observations. Because of the theoretical risk, the drug should be avoided during the first trimester. Haloperidol has been safely used, however, during the second and third trimesters to treat an unusual movement disorder associated with pregnancy called chorea gravidarum.

USE DURING BREASTFEEDING: Haloperidol is excreted into breast milk and could theoretically cause sedation in the newborn. The American Academy of Pediatrics considers haloperidol compatible with breastfeeding.

ALTERNATIVES TO MEDICATIONS: For patients with serious psychotic disorders haloperidol should not be discontinued without careful consultation by a psychiatrist. In some cases it is possible to stop the drug or reduce the dosage by increasing the frequency of counseling sessions and by living in a controlled, well-supervised home or hospital setting.

GENERIC NAME: Heparin

COMMON BRANDS: Heparin

TYPE OF DRUG: (Prescription) Anticoagulant

FDA RISK CATEGORY FOR PREGNANCY: C

GENERAL INFORMATION: Heparin is an anticoagulant used for the treatment or prevention of deep vein thrombophlebitis (blood clot in a deep vein of the leg) or pulmonary embolism (blood clot in the lung). Since heparin is not absorbed from the gastrointestinal tract, it must be administered by subcutaneous or intravenous injection. The effect of heparin lasts no longer than 8 to 12 hours. Therefore, subcutaneous injections must be given two or three times daily. The dosage of heparin should be determined by performing a test called the partial thromboplastin time (PTT). Women who are known to have a high risk of forming a blood clot are often treated with a relatively low dose of heparin to prevent clotting. Other women who have already formed a clot in a leg vein or a clot in the lung will require full-dose heparin therapy for several weeks.

POSSIBLE MATERNAL SIDE EFFECTS: The most serious side effect of heparin is hemorrhage usually due to administration of an excessive dosage. Other potential side effects include a reduction in the number of platelets in the blood (thrombocytopenia) that may increase the risk of hemorrhage. Softening of the bones (osteoporosis) may occur after several months of treatment with high dose heparin.

USE DURING PREGNANCY: Heparin does not cross the placenta and has no direct effect on the fetus. It is the safest anticoagulant to use during pregnancy. Nevertheless, the drug must be used with great caution. The dosage should be checked frequently by performing the blood clotting test called the PTT. At the onset of labor some obstetricians will omit or decrease the dosage of heparin to minimize the risk of bleeding associated with vaginal or cesarean delivery. In most cases heparin can be resumed shortly after delivery.

USE DURING BREASTFEEDING: Heparin does not enter breast milk and can be used safely during breastfeeding.

ALTERNATIVES TO MEDICATIONS: In some cases blood clots can be prevented from forming in the legs without an anticoagulant by using special pulsating boots that promote the flow of blood through the leg veins. This device is used primarily in women confined to bed rest in a hospital.

GENERIC NAME: Hepatitis B vaccine

COMMON BRANDS: Heptavax B, Recombivax HB

TYPE OF DRUG: (Prescription) Viral vaccine (inactivated)

FDA RISK CATEGORY FOR PREGNANCY: C

GENERAL INFORMATION: Hepatitis B vaccine promotes active immunity to hepatitis B. It can be given to individuals exposed to the virus by an accidental needle stick or from sexual contact with an infected partner. The vaccine can also be given to persons at risk of contacting the disease. Individuals at substantial risk of acquiring hepatitis B who should be vaccinated include

- Health-care workers exposed to blood or blood products,
- Clients and staff of institutions for people who are mentally retarded,
- Hemodialysis patients,
- Women with bisexual male partners (homosexual women are not at increased risk of sexually transmitted hepatitis B infection),

- Patients with blood clotting disorders who receive clotting factor concentrates,
- Household and sexual contacts of hepatitis B carriers,
- Inmates of long-term correctional facilities,
- International travelers who plan to reside more than six months in areas with high levels of endemic hepatitis B infection and who will have close contact with the local population,
- Newborns whose mothers have active hepatitis B or are known carriers of the virus.

POSSIBLE MATERNAL SIDE EFFECTS: Side effects are minimal. There may be some soreness at the site of injection and possibly a low-grade fever.

USE DURING PREGNANCY: The safety of hepatitis B vaccine during pregnancy remains to be established. To date there have been no reports of adverse effects on the fetus. On the other hand, acute hepatitis B infection can pose a significant risk to both mother and fetus. The Centers for Disease Control has stated that hepatitis B vaccine may be given to pregnant women who are at risk of acquiring the disease.

Newborns exposed to hepatitis B by an infected mother should be treated with the vaccine immediately after birth.

USE DURING BREASTFEEDING: Hepatitis B vaccine is safe for use during breastfeeding.

ALTERNATIVES TO MEDICATIONS: The only alternative to hepatitis B vaccine for the prevention of hepatitis B is careful avoidance of the virus. High-risk situations to avoid include sexual partners likely to have hepatitis B such as intravenous drug abusers and bisexual men, some nursing duties such as close contact with hemodialysis patients or patients receiving multiple blood transfusions, staff positions involving close contact with inmates at correctional institutions, and close contact with children in institutions for the mentally retarded.

In many obstetric clinics and practices all pregnant women are tested for the presence of hepatitis B virus as part of their routine prenatal blood tests.

GENERIC NAME: Heroin

COMMON BRANDS: Not commercially available.

168

TYPE OF DRUG: (Illicit) Narcotic

FDA RISK CATEGORY FOR PREGNANCY: X

GENERAL INFORMATION: Heroin is a commonly abused narcotic. There are no legitimate indications for this drug. It is highly addictive and often adulterated with toxic chemicals such as strychnine.

POSSIBLE MATERNAL SIDE EFFECTS: Addiction, respiratory arrest, cardiovascular collapse.

USE DURING PREGNANCY: Heroin is absolutely contraindicated during pregnancy. The drug readily crosses the placenta. The fetus can experience withdrawal and die in the uterus if the mother stops the drug abruptly. Use of heroin near term will result in an infant born addicted to the drug. The effects of maternal heroin addiction can last in the offspring up to six years.

USE DURING BREASTFEEDING: Heroin is secreted into breast milk in sufficient quantities to cause addiction in the newborn.

ALTERNATIVES TO MEDICATIONS: Heroin addicts should seek skilled professional counseling to begin a supervised withdrawal program. Reasonably safe medications are available to assist with withdrawal from the drug.

GENERIC NAME: **Hydralazine**

COMMON BRANDS: Apresoline

TYPE OF DRUG: (Prescription) Antihypertensive

FDA RISK CATEGORY FOR PREGNANCY: C

GENERAL INFORMATION: Hydralazine can be used alone or in combination with another antihypertensive drug to control high blood pressure. It can be administered orally or intravenously. Hydralazine works by relaxing the muscle in the walls of arteries, thus reducing blood pressure.

POSSIBLE MATERNAL SIDE EFFECTS: The most common side effects of hydralazine are rapid heart rate and dizziness when changing position from lying, sitting, or bending to standing. Additional minor side effects include nausea, headaches, and dizziness.

USE DURING PREGNANCY: Hydralazine enjoys a record of being one of the safest antihypertensive medications used during pregnancy. There have been no reports of malformations associated with use of the drug during the first trimester. Hydralazine is most often used for the reduction of high blood pressure associated with preeclampsia (toxemia). If hydralazine is used for longer than a few weeks, it often loses its effectiveness and requires the addition of another medication. Since treatment of preeclampsia is usually only a matter of days before delivery, hydralazine is well suited for that purpose.

USE DURING BREASTFEEDING: Hydralazine is secreted into breast milk, but it does not appear to have any adverse effect on the newborn. The American Academy of Pediatrics considers hydralazine compatible with breastfeeding.

ALTERNATIVES TO MEDICATIONS: With a program of weight loss, mild salt restriction, exercise, and cessation of smoking many women can successfully decrease their blood pressure before pregnancy and remain off medications throughout at least the first trimester. However, if antihypertensive medication is necessary, hydralazine is considered safe for use during pregnancy.

GENERIC NAME: Hydrochlorothiazide

COMMON BRANDS: Esidrix, HCTZ, HydroDIURIL, Hyperetic, Oretic

TYPE OF DRUG: (Prescription) Diuretic

FDA RISK CATEGORY FOR PREGNANCY: B

GENERAL INFORMATION: Hydrochlorothiazide is a diuretic used for the treatment of chronic hypertension, heart failure, and edema due to certain types of kidney disorders. It works by increasing the urinary excretion of sodium and water. For the treatment of high blood pressure the drug may be used alone or in combination with other antihypertensive medications. Many combination antihypertensive medications contain hydrochlorothiazide.

POSSIBLE MATERNAL SIDE EFFECTS: The most significant side effect is urinary loss of potassium, which may require taking potassium supplements. Other side effects are generally mild, including nausea and loss of appetite.

USE DURING PREGNANCY: The use of hydrochlorothiazide during pregnancy is controversial. Some authorities feel that women treated with this diuretic before pregnancy may safely continue taking the drug throughout pregnancy. Others are concerned about potential loss of fluid and electrolytes (potassium and sodium) and the possibility of decreased blood flow to the fetus. Treatment of hypertension should be reevaluated before attempting pregnancy, and if possible, medications considered safer for use during pregnancy can be substituted for hydrochlorothiazide. If, however, treatment of heart disease, kidney disease, or hypertension necessitates the use of this drug during pregnancy, most authorities believe it is relatively safe. Hydrochlorothiazide should not be given to alleviate the normal water retention that accompanies most pregnancies during the third trimester.

USE DURING BREASTFEEDING: Hydrochlorothiazide enters breast milk but probably has little effect on the newborn. On the other hand, the medication can theoretically interfere with the production of breast milk.

ALTERNATIVES TO MEDICATIONS: The use of diuretics during pregnancy is usually reserved for women with heart problems, chronic hypertension, or kidney disease. Mild edema (fluid retention) is a common occurrence during pregnancy and does not require treatment. If edema becomes uncomfortable, it can usually be relieved by lying on your side for periods of 30 to 60 minutes. In some cases mild restriction of dietary salt intake may be necessary. Severe salt restriction, however, is not appropriate and may even be harmful. There is no evidence that so-called natural diuretics found in health food stores are effective, and their safety during pregnancy cannot be assured.

GENERIC NAME: Hydrocodone

COMMON BRANDS: Codan Syrup, Codimal DH, Donatussin, Entuss, Hycodan, Hycomine, Hycotuss, Hydrocet, Kwelcof, Lortab, Ru-Tuss, Triaminic Expectorant DH, Tussend, Vicodin, Zydone

171

TYPE OF DRUG: (Prescription) Narcotic antitussive (anticough), analgesic

FDA RISK CATEGORY FOR PREGNANCY: C

GENERAL INFORMATION: Hydrocodone can be used by itself or in combination with other medications for the suppression of coughing associated with viral upper-respiratory-tract infections. Used chronically the drug has the potential for addiction.

POSSIBLE MATERNAL SIDE EFFECTS: Side effects include nausea, vomiting, dizziness, and drowsiness.

USE DURING PREGNANCY: There have been no reports linking the use of hydrocodone with birth defects. Theoretically, if the drug were used extensively near term, the baby might experience narcotic withdrawal symptoms.

USE DURING BREASTFEEDING: Hydrocodone probably enters breast milk and could have a sedative effect on the newborn.

ALTERNATIVES TO MEDICATIONS: Cough suppressants provide purely symptomatic relief and have no influence on the course of upper-respiratory infections.

Minor coughs can often be relieved by cool mist or steam. Cough caused by asthma may require bronchodilating medication and should not be treated with cough suppressants.

GENERIC NAME: Hydromorphone

COMMON BRANDS: Dilaudid

TYPE OF DRUG: (Prescription) Narcotic analgesic

FDA RISK CATEGORY FOR PREGNANCY: C

GENERAL INFORMATION: Hydromorphone is an oral narcotic analgesic for relief of moderate to severe pain. Because of its narcotic properties, the drug has potential for abuse and addiction.

POSSIBLE MATERNAL SIDE EFFECTS: Side effects include sedation,

172

dizziness, mental confusion, dry mouth, nausea, and constipation. Chronic use can lead to addiction.

USE DURING PREGNANCY: Use of hydromorphone during pregnancy is usually confined to labor or postoperative period. First-trimester use has not been associated with birth defects. However, prolonged use near term may result in withdrawal symptoms in the newborn. Even limited use near term can cause respiratory depression in the newborn.

USE DURING BREASTFEEDING: It is not known whether hydromorphone is excreted into breast milk. If even a small amount reaches the nursing infant, sedation might result. The drug should be used only for severe pain during breastfeeding.

ALTERNATIVES TO MEDICATIONS: Techniques of natural childbirth such as Lamaze may eliminate the need for narcotics during labor. However, hydromorphone can be safely used to control pain following surgery or after cesarean delivery.

GENERIC NAME: Hydroxychloroquine

COMMON BRANDS: Plaquenil

TYPE OF DRUG: (Prescription) Antiarthritis, antimalaria

FDA RISK CATEGORY FOR PREGNANCY: D

GENERAL INFORMATION: Hydroxychloroquine is indicated for treatment of acute attacks of malaria. It is also used for treatment of painful joints due to rheumatoid arthritis or systemic lupus erythematosis. In patients with rheumatoid arthritis, the drug can halt the progression of joint destruction.

POSSIBLE MATERNAL SIDE EFFECTS: The most common side effects include rash, nausea, vomiting, abdominal cramps, hair loss, and retinopathy (eye problems).

USE DURING PREGNANCY: Hydroxychloroquine has been shown to damage eye tissue in fetal mice. Its use should be avoided during pregnancy unless a physician determines that the benefit of treating acute malaria outweighs any risk of the drug. During pregnancy other medications should be substituted for hydroxychloroquine to treat rheumatoid arthritis or systemic lupus erythematosus.

USE DURING BREASTFEEDING: Children are particularly sensitive to the side effects of hydroxychloroquine. It should not be used during breastfeeding.

ALTERNATIVES TO MEDICATIONS: Travel to areas of the world where the risk of malaria is high should be avoided during pregnancy.

Rheumatoid arthritis often improves spontaneously during pregnancy. Effective physical therapy may offer adequate relief from painful arthritis for many pregnant women.

GENERIC NAME: Hyoscyamine sulfate

COMMON BRANDS: Anaspaz, Bellaspaz, Cystospaz-M, Donnatal, Levsin, Levsinex Timecaps, Neoquess

TYPE OF DRUG: (prescription) Antidiarrheal, gastrointestinal antispasmodic, urinary antispasmodic

FDA RISK CATEGORY FOR PREGNANCY: C

GENERAL INFORMATION: Hyoscyamine is a member of the belladonna (p. 89) group of medications. By decreasing spasm of the colon (large intestine), hyoscyamine is effective in the treatment of irritable bowel syndrome, also called spastic colon or functional bowel syndrome.

POSSIBLE MATERNAL SIDE EFFECTS: The most common side effects include dry mouth, blurred vision, drowsiness, difficulty urinating, and palpitations.

USE DURING PREGNANCY: The Collaborative Perinatal Project found a slight increase in the number of birth defects following first-trimester exposure to belladonna. Since hyoscyamine is a form of belladonna, the drug should generally be avoided during the first trimester. Use during the second and third trimesters, however, appears to be safe.

USE DURING BREASTFEEDING: Belladonna and hyoscyamine enter breast milk and could cause lethargy or poor feeding in the newborn.

ALTERNATIVES TO MEDICATIONS: Alternatives to taking hyoscyamine for treatment of irritable bowel syndrome include additional dietary fiber, regular exercise, and avoidance of gas-forming foods such as beans, onions, cabbage, dried fruits (apricots, dates, raisins), apple juice, and foods made with all-purpose refined white flour.

GENERIC NAME: Ibuprofen

COMMON BRANDS: Advil, Medipren, Midol 200, Motrin, Motrin IB, Nuprin, Rufen

TYPE OF DRUG: (Over-the-counter and prescription) Anti-inflammatory

FDA RISK CATEGORY FOR PREGNANCY: Not classified

GENERAL INFORMATION: Ibuprofen is a member of a class of drugs called nonsteroidal anti-inflammatory drugs (NSAIDs). It is indicated for the treatment of arthritis, muscle pain, headache, and pain associated with menstruation.

POSSIBLE MATERNAL SIDE EFFECTS: The most common side effects are nausea and abdominal pain. Rarely, ibuprofen can irritate the stomach and cause an ulcer or bleeding from the stomach.

USE DURING PREGNANCY: There have been no reports linking ibuprofen to birth defects when the drug was used during the first trimester. However, experience with the drug during early pregnancy is limited. The manufacturer does not recommend its use during pregnancy.

Used near term ibuprofen can have potential effects on pregnancy and the fetus. First, the drug can cause premature closure of an important blood vessel in the fetus called the ductus arteriosus. Normally, this blood vessel does not close until after delivery. Premature closure could result in a serious condition called pulmonary hypertension. Second, ibuprofen and other NSAIDs can inhibit labor and prolong pregnancy.

USE DURING BREASTFEEDING: Ibuprofen apparently does not enter human breast milk in significant amounts.

ALTERNATIVES TO MEDICATIONS: Musculoskeletal pain can often be relieved with warm baths and massage. Painful arthritis can be alleviated by rest, heat, and physical therapy. Nonweight-bearing exercise such as swimming may offer some comfort while enhancing muscle tone. If medication is necessary, acetaminophen (p. 63) is probably the safest medication to take during pregnancy for relief of minor pain.

GENERIC NAME: Imipramine

COMMON BRANDS: Janimine, Tofranil

TYPE OF DRUG: (Prescription) Antidepressant

FDA RISK CATEGORY FOR PREGNANCY: D

GENERAL INFORMATION: Imipramine is a member of a group of drugs called tricyclic antidepressants. It is effective for the treatment of chronic depression. The drug can elevate mood, improve appetite, relieve insomnia, and increase physical activity. Therapy is usually begun with a low dosage and gradually increased to a therapeutic level. Beneficial effects are not usually seen until two to four weeks after treatment has begun.

POSSIBLE MATERNAL SIDE EFFECTS: Side effects include drowsiness, blurred vision, dry mouth, constipation, weight gain, low blood pressure, and abnormal rhythms of the heart.

USE DURING PREGNANCY: Like other tricyclic antidepressants, imipramine has been associated with a variety of birth defects. These drugs should be avoided during pregnancy unless major depression cannot be satisfactorily managed in any other way.

USE DURING BREASTFEEDING: Imipramine enters breast milk in small quantities, but its effect on the newborn is not known.

ALTERNATIVES TO MEDICATIONS: Depression often gives rise to hopelessness, negativity toward oneself, and at times an inability to carry out normal activities of daily living. Some individuals may become intensely sad or grief-stricken over the loss of someone or something close to them. Others may suffer from chronic depression unrelated to a specific event. In many cases counseling is necessary to truly understand the cause and extent of depression. There are, however, a number of things you can do to deal with depression on your own:

1. Try to identify the specific situation or personal interaction that has caused your sense of hopelessness and negativity.
2. Make a fresh start at correcting the problem. Talk it through. If necessary, repair relationships with previously available support systems. Often family or close friends can serve to reduce your distress.
3. Realize that there are options for most situations. Seldom is there truly "no choice."
4. Understand some of the warning signs that indicate you have severe depression requiring professional counseling. Such signs include
   - Intense sadness, frequent bouts of crying, or depressed mood most of the day,
   - Uncharacteristically negative thoughts about yourself,
   - Markedly diminished interest or pleasure in most activities,
   - Diminished appetite and weight loss,
   - Chronic insomnia or sleeping excessively,
   - Feelings of worthlessness or guilt,
   - Persistent fatigue or lack of energy,
   - Inability to think or concentrate,
   - Thoughts or plans for suicide.
5. Patients with severe depression should not stop taking antidepressant medications without careful psychiatric supervision.

GENERIC NAME: Immune globulin

COMMON BRANDS: Gamastan, Gamimune N, Gammagard, H-BIG, Hep-B-Gammagee, MICRhoGAM, RhoGAM

TYPE OF DRUG: (Prescription) Immune serum

FDA RISK CATEGORY FOR PREGNANCY: B

GENERAL INFORMATION: Immune globulin is prepared from the serum of animals or volunteer human donors. These preparations contain antibodies capable of preventing or minimizing the symptoms of an illness. Immune globulin preparations are available for the prevention of chicken pox, hepatitis A, hepatitis B, measles (rubeola), rabies, and tetanus. They are most effective if given immediately before exposure or within 72 hours after exposure. They are of minimal benefit if given longer than two weeks after exposure to an illness.

POSSIBLE MATERNAL SIDE EFFECTS: The most significant risk to treatment with immune globulin is an allergic reaction. Patients with a history of an allergic reaction to human or animal serum should not be treated with immune globulin. If hives or difficulty breathing occurs during the intravenous infusion of immune globulin, the drug should be discontinued immediately.

All plasma used in the preparation of immune globulin is tested by an FDA-approved method for the presence of HIV (AIDS virus) as well as for the hepatitis B virus, and all donors are carefully screened to eliminate those who are in high-risk groups for disease transmission.

USE DURING PREGNANCY: There has been no evidence that use of immune globulin during pregnancy causes any harm to the fetus. Most authorities recommend that the appropriate immune globulin be given to pregnant women clearly exposed to chicken pox, hepatitis A, hepatitis B, measles, rabies, or tetanus.

An immune globulin preparation called RhoGam is also used during pregnancy for prevention of hemolytic disease (anemia) in an Rh-positive baby whose mother is Rh-negative.

USE DURING BREASTFEEDING: It is not known whether immune globulin has any adverse effect on breastfed infants.

ALTERNATIVES TO MEDICATIONS: With the exception of avoidance, there is no nonpharmacologic alternative to immune globulin for prevention of the viral diseases discussed above.

GENERIC NAME: **Indigo carmine**

COMMON BRANDS: Indigo carmine

TYPE OF DRUG: (Prescription) Dye

FDA RISK CATEGORY FOR PREGNANCY: B

GENERAL INFORMATION: Indigo carmine is a dye that can be injected into the amniotic fluid to determine whether the membranes have ruptured. It can also be used to identify the presence of more than one amniotic sac in the case of twins or triplets.

POSSIBLE MATERNAL SIDE EFFECTS: Indigo carmine injected into the amniotic sac generally causes no side effects. If, however, it is injected intravenously, the dye can cause a sudden rise in blood pressure.

USE DURING PREGNANCY: Indigo carmine has been safely used during pregnancy to identify ruptured membranes or multiple gestational sacs (twins).

USE DURING BREASTFEEDING: There is no use for indigo carmine during breastfeeding.

ALTERNATIVES TO MEDICATIONS: For some diagnostic tests there is no alternative to the use of indigo carmine.

GENERIC NAME: Indomethacin

COMMON BRANDS: Indocin

TYPE OF DRUG: (Prescription) Anti-inflammatory

FDA RISK CATEGORY FOR PREGNANCY: Not classified

GENERAL INFORMATION: Indomethacin is a member of a class of drugs called nonsteroidal anti-inflammatory drugs (NSAIDs). It is indicated for the treatment of arthritis, muscle pain, headache, and pain associated with menstruation.

POSSIBLE MATERNAL SIDE EFFECTS: The most common side effects are nausea and abdominal pain. Rarely, indomethacin can irritate the stomach and cause an ulcer or bleeding from the stomach.

USE DURING PREGNANCY: There have been no reports linking indomethacin to birth defects when the drug was used during the first trimester. However, experience with the drug during early pregnancy is limited.

Used near term indomethacin can have potential effects on pregnancy and the fetus. First, the drug can cause premature closure of an important blood vessel in the fetus called the ductus arteriosus. Normally, this blood vessel does not close until after delivery. Premature closure could result in a serious condition called pulmonary hypertension. Second, indomethacin and other NSAIDs can inhibit labor and prolong pregnancy. Some obstetricians have effectively used indomethacin to halt premature labor.

USE DURING BREASTFEEDING: Indomethacin enters human breast milk, but its effect on the newborn is not known. The drug's safety during breastfeeding cannot be ensured.

ALTERNATIVES TO MEDICATIONS: Musculoskeletal pain can often be relieved with warm baths and massage. Painful arthritis can be alleviated by rest, heat, and physical therapy. Nonweight-bearing exercise such as swimming may offer some comfort while enhancing muscle tone. If medication is necessary, acetaminophen (p. 63) is probably the safest medication to take during pregnancy for relief of minor pain.

GENERIC NAME: Influenza virus vaccine

COMMON BRANDS: Fluogen, Fluzone

TYPE OF DRUG: (Prescription) Viral vaccine (inactivated)

FDA RISK CATEGORY FOR PREGNANCY: C

GENERAL INFORMATION: This vaccine promotes active immunity to influenza by inducing production of antibodies. Protection is provided only against the viral strain contained in the vaccine. There is no activity against the common cold. The vaccine is produced from an inactivated virus and is free of any live virus.

Protection from influenza generally occurs within 14 to 28 days of vaccination and lasts for approximately 6 months. Vaccination must be repeated yearly.

POSSIBLE MATERNAL SIDE EFFECTS: Side effects include soreness at the site of inoculation, mild fever, and muscle aches. Individuals allergic to egg proteins should not be vaccinated with influenza vaccine. Also, anyone with a history of Guillain-Barré syndrome should avoid vaccination.

USE DURING PREGNANCY: Ideally, women who are candidates for vaccination against influenza should be inoculated before pregnancy. Nevertheless, the vaccine has been used throughout pregnancy and has not been linked to fetal harm. In most cases vaccination can be postponed until the completion of the first trimester. On the other hand, acute influenza can significantly complicate pregnancy. Individuals with chronic illnesses such as diabetes, heart disease, lung disease, kidney disorders, and disorders of the immune system should be inoculated with influenza vaccine during pregnancy. During an epidemic of influenza candidates for vaccination might reasonably include all pregnant women.

USE DURING BREASTFEEDING: Inoculation with the influenza virus vaccine is not thought to pose any risk to the nursing infant.

ALTERNATIVES TO MEDICATIONS: Not all individuals need to be vaccinated against influenza. People for whom the vaccine is usually recommended include the elderly and those with chronic diseases such as diabetes, heart disease, chronic lung disease, and disorders of the immune system. Certain individuals whose occupation places them at high risk for infection with the influenza virus such as school teachers and health-care professionals may also wish to consider vaccination. The vaccine will not prevent the common cold.

GENERIC NAME: **Insulin**

COMMON BRANDS: Humulin, Iletin, Mixtard, Novolin, Velosulin

TYPE OF DRUG: (Prescription) Hormone

FDA RISK CATEGORY FOR PREGNANCY: B

GENERAL INFORMATION: Insulin is a hormone normally produced by the pancreas. The pancreas of individuals with type I diabetes mellitus (previously called juvenile diabetes) fails to produce insulin. As a result these patients must take daily injections of insulin to maintain their blood glucose (sugar) levels in an acceptable range. There are many different types of insulin.

Insulin may be produced from beef or pork pancreas. Recently, preparations identical to human insulin have been produced by biochemically altering pork insulin or by genetically programing bacteria to produce human insulin. These human insulins are seen by the body as identical to normal human insulin. As a result no antibodies to these preparations are formed. Insulin preparations also vary according to their onset and duration of action. Some preparations work quickly but for relatively brief periods. Others take longer to begin working, but their duration of action may last up to 12 to 24 hours. A patient may be treated with one or a combination of insulin types.

POSSIBLE MATERNAL SIDE EFFECTS: The most significant side effect of insulin treatment is hypoglycemia (low blood sugar). Hypoglycemia can be profound and even result in loss of consciousness. All patients treated with insulin must carry some form of rapid-glucose tablet or candy to treat the symptoms of hypoglycemia before blood sugars fall to critical levels.

USE DURING PREGNANCY: Insulin is the preferred medical treatment of diabetes during pregnancy for women whose blood sugars cannot be satisfactorily controlled with diet alone. Those who took pills before pregnancy to control their blood sugars must be switched to insulin before conception.

The amount of insulin necessary to control blood sugar levels will vary throughout pregnancy. Often during early gestation the need for insulin decreases, therefore the dosage of each injection must be decreased. From the middle of the second trimester until the time of delivery, the dosage of insulin must usually be increased. Immediately after delivery the dosage will again be decreased. Adjustment of insulin throughout pregnancy requires the expert guidance of an internist or specialist in diabetes.

Insulin has not been shown to cause birth defects. On the other hand, poorly controlled diabetes has been clearly linked to congenital malformations. Therefore, diabetes must be carefully controlled from the very moment of conception to ensure the best outcome for both mother and baby.

USE DURING BREASTFEEDING: Insulin does not enter breast milk. Use during breastfeeding poses no risk to the newborn.

ALTERNATIVES TO MEDICATIONS: For women with type I diabetes (juvenile diabetes) there is no alternative to daily injections of insulin. Some women with type II diabetes (adult-onset diabetes) or gestational diabetes can satisfactorily control their blood sugar levels by careful attention to diet.

GENERIC NAME: **Intrauterine device (IUD)**

COMMON BRANDS: Cu-7, Lippes Loop, ParaGard T380A, Progestasert, Tatum-T

TYPE OF DRUG: (Prescription) Contraceptive device

FDA RISK CATEGORY FOR PREGNANCY: X

GENERAL INFORMATION: The IUD is a small device that can be inserted into the uterus by a physician. It is believed to work by blocking implantation of the fertilized egg in the uterus. In recent years IUDs have been used much less frequently for contraception. If pregnancy is desired, an IUD must be removed by your doctor.

POSSIBLE MATERNAL SIDE EFFECTS: Side effects of the IUD can be serious, including infection in the uterus, perforation of the uterus, severe menstrual bleeding, interference with the ability to become pregnant in the future, and miscarriage of a pregnancy that occurred with the IUD in place (see below).

USE DURING PREGNANCY: Becoming pregnant with the IUD in place is uncommon, but it can occur. The odds of this happening are between 1 and 5 in 100. If pregnancy does occur with the IUD in place there are essentially two choices—leaving the IUD in place or having it removed by your doctor as soon as possible. Most obstetricians feel that the chance of delivering a healthy full-term baby are best if the IUD is removed as soon as pregnancy is confirmed. If the IUD is removed, the risk of spontaneous miscarriage is approximately 20 percent. This risk may sound high, but the rate of miscarriage in all known pregnancies is estimated to be approximately 15 to 20 percent. Most obstetricians have concluded that the risk of miscarriage after removal of an IUD is less than the risk of leaving it in place.

If you decide to continue your pregnancy without removing the IUD, you should be especially alert for such signs as bleeding, cramps, or fever during the first trimester. Any of these signs may indicate an acute complication and should be immediately brought to the attention of your physician. Leaving an IUD in place also increases the risk of premature labor.

USE DURING BREASTFEEDING: The IUD may be used during breastfeeding.

ALTERNATIVES TO MEDICATIONS: The IUD should be removed several months prior to attempting pregnancy. In the interim you may use some form of barrier contraception such as a condom or diaphragm.

GENERIC NAME: Iodide

COMMON BRANDS: Elixophyllin-KI, Iodo-Niacin, Mudrane, Organidin, Pediacof, Pima Syrup, Quadrinal, SSKI, Theo-Organidin, Tuss-Organidin, Tussi-Organidin DM

TYPE OF DRUG: (Over-the-counter and prescription) Expectorant

FDA RISK CATEGORY FOR PREGNANCY: X

GENERAL INFORMATION: The effectiveness of iodide as an expectorant in various combination cold and asthma medications is controversial. In theory, iodinated glycerol or potassium iodide may reduce the thickness of mucus secretions and promote effective removal of mucus by coughing. Many authorities doubt that iodide-containing preparations are effective.

POSSIBLE MATERNAL SIDE EFFECTS: The most common side effect is mild nausea. Occasionally a skin rash may develop.

USE DURING PREGNANCY: Iodide-containing preparations should not be used during pregnancy because these drugs freely cross the placenta and can be taken up by the fetal thyroid gland. Iodide can cause the fetal thyroid to enlarge resulting in a goiter (enlarged thyroid). Since a large number of prescription and over-the-counter drugs contain iodide, a physician or pharmacist should be consulted before taking any cold or asthma preparation.

USE DURING BREASTFEEDING: Iodide enters breast milk and is absorbed by the newborn. The significance of high levels of iodide in breast milk is not known. Nevertheless, iodide-containing medications should be avoided during breastfeeding.

ALTERNATIVES TO MEDICATIONS: Iodide-containing cold and cough preparations should not be used during pregnancy. Often steam or cool mist will satisfactorily loosen bronchial mucous secretions and facilitate removal by coughing.

GENERIC NAME: **Ipratropium**

COMMON BRANDS: Atrovent

TYPE OF DRUG: (Prescription) Bronchodilator

FDA RISK CATEGORY FOR PREGNANCY: B

GENERAL INFORMATION: Ipratropium is a aerosol preparation used for the prevention of bronchial spasm in patients with chronic lung disease and asthma. The drug is only minimally absorbed from the bronchial tubes into the circulation.

POSSIBLE MATERNAL SIDE EFFECTS: Because the drug is not well absorbed there are few side effects. With repeated high doses nervousness and palpitations can occur.

USE DURING PREGNANCY: Since ipratropium has only been on the market in the United States for a few years, there has been relatively little experience with the drug in pregnant women. Animal studies, however, demonstrated no evidence of harm to the fetus.

USE DURING BREASTFEEDING: No information is available, but it is unlikely that ipratropium taken by inhalation enters breast milk in significant amounts or is taken up by the newborn.

ALTERNATIVES TO MEDICATIONS: In some cases asthma can be prevented by avoidance of known allergens, particularly animals. If you smoke, stop. It is generally a good rule, however, to use a bronchodilating inhaler such as albuterol (p. 66) at the earliest indication of wheezing. Often prompt effective relief of asthma can prevent minor episodes from becoming more severe and prolonged.

GENERIC NAME: Iron supplements

COMMON BRANDS: Chromagen, Femiron, Feosol, Feostat, Fergon, Fero-Folic-500, ferrous fumarate, ferrous gluconate, ferrous sulfate, Hemaspan, Hemocyte, Iberet, Irospan, Natalins, Pramilet, Prenate, Slow Fe, Stuartinic, various multiple vitamin and mineral supplements

TYPE OF DRUG: (Over-the-counter) Iron supplement

FDA RISK CATEGORY FOR PREGNANCY: A

GENERAL INFORMATION: Iron is an essential part of hemoglobin, the oxygen-carrying component of red blood cells. Because of monthly blood loss, it is common for menstruating women to be at least mildly iron deficient. Oral iron supplements are indicated for the prevention and treatment of iron-deficiency anemia. Various iron preparations are available over-the-counter. Preparations provide different amounts of elemental iron: ferrous fumarate provides 33 percent of elemental iron, ferrous gluconate provides 12 percent of elemental iron, and ferrous sulfate provides 20 percent of elemental iron. The usual American diet provides approximately 15 mg of elemental iron daily.

POSSIBLE MATERNAL SIDE EFFECTS: Possible side effects include nausea, loss of appetite, and constipation. Bowel movements will usually become dark or black.

USE DURING PREGNANCY: Since most women are at least mildly iron deficient at the start of pregnancy, iron supplements are usually advised. Daily oral supplementation of 30 to 60 mg of elemental iron is recommended during pregnancy. A 100 mg tablet of ferrous fumarate provides approximately 33 mg of elemental iron, a 435 mg tablet of ferrous gluconate provides approximately 50 mg of elemental iron, and a 325 mg tablet of ferrous sulfate provides approximately 65 mg of elemental iron. The dosage of iron supplement needed for pregnancy varies for different women and should be determined by a physician.

USE DURING BREASTFEEDING: Iron supplements may be safely taken during breastfeeding. There are no risks for the nursing infant.

ALTERNATIVES TO MEDICATIONS: Foods containing substantial amounts of iron include liver and other organ meats, lean meats, dark-green leafy vegetables, beets, dried fruits (apricots, prunes, and figs), egg yolks, shellfish, molasses, and whole grains. Many breads and cereals are fortified with iron.

GENERIC NAME: # Isoniazid (INH)

COMMON BRANDS: INH, Laniazid, Rifamate

TYPE OF DRUG: (Prescription) Antituberculous

FDA RISK CATEGORY FOR PREGNANCY: C

GENERAL INFORMATION: Isoniazid is used for the treatment or prevention of tuberculosis (TB). When the drug is used for treatment of active TB, it is usually combined with one or two other antituberculous drugs.

Isoniazid may also be recommended for patients thought to be at high risk of developing active TB, so-called prophylactic therapy. In these persons treatment is usually continued for one year. Individuals at high risk of TB include

- Persons whose TB skin test has converted from negative (no reaction) to positive within the last two years,
- Persons under age 35, especially children, with a positive skin test,
- Family members and close contacts of a patient with active TB,
- Patients with a positive skin test and lowered immunity from cancer, diabetes, or other chronic diseases,
- Patients with a positive skin test and lowered immunity from long-term treatment with corticosteroids.

POSSIBLE MATERNAL SIDE EFFECTS: Side effects from isoniazid can be significant, including anemia, liver damage, and nerve damage (neuropathy). Concomitant treatment with vitamin B_6 (pyridoxine) is thought to decrease the risk of neuropathy.

USE DURING PREGNANCY: Several large studies have shown that isoniazid can be given safely during pregnancy. Evidence of active TB requires drug therapy at any stage of pregnancy. Prophylactic treatment of women thought to be at high risk might be postponed until after the first trimester or even until after pregnancy.

USE DURING BREASTFEEDING: Isoniazid has been shown to enter breast milk and could theoretically cause some damage to the infant's liver. Although the American Academy of Pediatrics considers isoniazid compatible with breastfeeding, the drug should be used with caution.

ALTERNATIVES TO MEDICATIONS: For the treatment of active tuberculosis there is no alternative to taking medications.

GENERIC NAME: Isotretinoin

COMMON BRANDS: Accutane

TYPE OF DRUG: (Prescription) Antiacne

FDA RISK CATEGORY FOR PREGNANCY: X

GENERAL INFORMATION: Isotretinoin is a vitamin A derivative used in nonpregnant individuals for the treatment of severe, cystic acne that has been unresponsive to other forms of therapy. Treatment with the drug may be necessary for up to six months.

POSSIBLE MATERNAL SIDE EFFECTS: Side effects are common, including nausea, headache, dryness and irritation of the lips and gums, inflammation of the liver, and an elevation in the serum concentration of triglycerides.

USE DURING PREGNANCY: Isotretinoin has been clearly shown to cause birth defects in humans and **must not** be used during pregnancy. Prior to beginning treatment with isotretinoin in any woman of reproductive potential a pregnancy test should be negative and adequate contraception must be ensured. Women who inadvertently became pregnant while taking the drug should consult a physician immediately and consider termination of the pregnancy.

USE DURING BREASTFEEDING: It is not known if isotretinoin is excreted into breast milk, but breastfeeding is not advised while taking the drug.

ALTERNATIVES TO MEDICATIONS: Meticulous cleansing and limited exposure to sunlight may help prevent acne. Avoid heavy oil-based cosmetics.

GENERIC NAME: Kaolin and pectin mixtures

COMMON BRANDS: Donnagel PG, Kaopectate, K-P, K-Pec, Parepectolin, Pectokay

TYPE OF DRUG: (Over-the-counter) Antidiarrheal

FDA RISK CATEGORY FOR PREGNANCY: C

GENERAL INFORMATION: Preparations that combine kaolin and pectin are used to treat acute uncomplicated diarrhea. Kaolin adsorbs irritants and forms a protective coating on the intestinal lining. Pectin acts to consolidate the stool. Some prescription products also include the narcotic antidiarrheal drug, paregoric.

Any antidiarrheal medication, including kaolin and pectin, should be discontinued and the doctor notified if diarrhea persists for more than 48 hours or if fever develops.

POSSIBLE MATERNAL SIDE EFFECTS: Side effects are usually minimal. However, excessive use can cause constipation.

USE DURING PREGNANCY: Kaolin and pectin are not absorbed from the stomach or intestine. They are considered safe for use during pregnancy. However, careful studies in humans have not been performed.

USE DURING BREASTFEEDING: Because kaolin and pectin are not absorbed, they pose no significant risk to nursing infants.

ALTERNATIVES TO MEDICATIONS: With acute diarrhea solid foods may be discontinued for 12 to 24 hours. When diarrhea abates, start eating again with dry bread or toast and small amounts of vegetables. Since it is essential to avoid dehydration, be sure to drink plenty of liquids that contain sugar. Soup can also provide some nutrition and hydration without aggravating diarrhea. Symptoms of dehydration include thirst, dry mouth, fast breathing, and sometimes fever. An early sign of dehydration is reduction in the amount and frequency of urination. Drink enough to keep up normal urine output. If adequate hydration cannot be maintained, call the doctor.

GENERIC NAME: **Ketoconazole**

COMMON BRANDS: Nizoral

TYPE OF DRUG: (Prescription) Antifungal

FDA RISK CATEGORY FOR PREGNANCY: C

GENERAL INFORMATION: Ketoconazole can be applied topically as a cream or taken by pill for the treatment of fungal skin infections.

POSSIBLE MATERNAL SIDE EFFECTS: Side effects from use of ketoconazole cream are minimal. Mild itching can occur. Treatment with ketoconazole tablets, however, can be associated with nausea and vomiting, at times severe. The drug has also been shown to cause liver damage, and therefore blood tests of liver function must be performed frequently during therapy. The drug should be discontinued immediately if there is any sign of jaundice.

USE DURING PREGNANCY: Ketoconazole has been shown to cause birth defects in rats when taken orally. These observations have not been confirmed in humans, nor is it known if there is any risk to using the cream. The drug should be used only if absolutely necessary during pregnancy. The oral preparation should not be taken during the first trimester.

USE DURING BREASTFEEDING: It is not known whether ketoconazole cream is sufficiently absorbed and excreted into breast milk to pose any risk to the newborn. Taken by pill the drug likely enters breast milk and should be avoided during breastfeeding.

ALTERNATIVES TO MEDICATIONS: Treatment of mild fungal skin infections can usually be postponed until after pregnancy or at least until after the first trimester.

GENERIC NAME: Ketoprofen

COMMON BRANDS: Orudis

TYPE OF DRUG: (Prescription) Anti-inflammatory

FDA RISK CATEGORY FOR PREGNANCY: B

GENERAL INFORMATION: Ketoprofen is a member of a class of drugs called nonsteroidal anti-inflammatory drugs (NSAIDs). It is indicated for the treatment of arthritis, muscle pain, headache, and pain associated with menstruation.

POSSIBLE MATERNAL SIDE EFFECTS: The most common side effects are nausea and abdominal pain. Rarely, ketoprofen can irritate the stomach and cause an ulcer or bleeding from the stomach.

USE DURING PREGNANCY: There have been no reports linking ketoprofen to birth defects when the drug was used during the first trimester. However, experience with the drug during early pregnancy is limited.

Used near term ketoprofen can have potential effects on pregnancy and the fetus. First, the drug can cause premature closure of an important blood vessel in the fetus called the ductus arteriosus. Normally, this blood vessel does not close until after delivery. Premature closure could result in a serious condition called pulmonary hypertension. Second, ketoprofen and other NSAIDs can inhibit labor and prolong pregnancy.

USE DURING BREASTFEEDING: Ketoprofen enters human breast milk, but its effect on the newborn is not known. The drug's safety during breastfeeding cannot be ensured.

ALTERNATIVES TO MEDICATIONS: Musculoskeletal pain can often be relieved with warm baths and massage. Painful arthritis can be alleviated by rest, heat, and physical therapy. Nonweight-bearing exercise such as swimming may offer some comfort while enhancing muscle tone. If medication is necessary, acetaminophen (p. 63) is probably the safest medication to take during pregnancy for relief of minor pain.

GENERIC NAME: Labetalol

COMMON BRANDS: Normodyne, Normozide, Trandate

TYPE OF DRUG: (Prescription) Antihypertensive

FDA RISK CATEGORY FOR PREGNANCY: C

GENERAL INFORMATION: Labetalol is used for the treatment of chronic hypertension. It is combination medication comprised of a beta blocker and an alpha blocker. Beta blockers work by inhibiting a major effect of the nervous system on blood pressure, and alpha blockers lower blood pressure by dilating the arteries.

POSSIBLE MATERNAL SIDE EFFECTS: Possible side effects include fatigue, slow heart rate, and worsening of asthma. Theoretically, the alpha-blocking component of the drug is included to minimize some of the side effects commonly caused by a beta blocker (such as asthma and slow heart rate).

USE DURING PREGNANCY: In recent years labetalol has been used for the treatment of hypertension during pregnancy. Although there are no reports of birth defects associated with the drug, extensive experience during the first trimester is still lacking. Labetalol has also been used intravenously for rapid reduction of blood pressure associated with toxemia (preeclampsia).

USE DURING BREASTFEEDING: Labetalol enters breast milk. Although it is believed that the drug is safe for use during breastfeeding, the infant should be observed for slow heart rate, low blood pressure, and signs of abnormal behavior.

ALTERNATIVES TO MEDICATIONS: With a program of weight loss, mild salt restriction, exercise, and cessation of smoking many women can successfully decrease their blood pressure before pregnancy and remain off medications throughout at least the first trimester. However, if antihypertensive medication is necessary, another drug with a proven record of safety during pregnancy (such as methyldopa, p. 215) should be considered.

GENERIC NAME: Levothyroxine

COMMON BRANDS: Euthroid, Levothroid, Synthroid, Synthrox, Thyrolar

TYPE OF DRUG: (Prescription) Thyroid hormone

FDA RISK CATEGORY FOR PREGNANCY: A

GENERAL INFORMATION: Levothyroxine is a naturally occurring hormone produced by the thyroid gland in adults, children, and fetuses. It is the treatment of choice for hypothyroidism (an underactive thyroid gland) (p. 14). It is usually given in the form of a pill once daily. The appropriate dosage can be determined and adjusted by measuring the level of thyroid hormone in the blood.

POSSIBLE MATERNAL SIDE EFFECTS: When levothyroxine is given in the appropriate dosage there are no significant side effects. An excessive dosage may result in tremulousness, insomnia, weight loss, rapid heart rate, palpitations, and diarrhea.

USE DURING PREGNANCY: Levothyroxine should be given to pregnant women with hypothyroidism. Although levothyroxine may cross the placenta, it has no adverse effect on the fetus. The dosage may need to be adjusted during pregnancy, and therefore blood levels should be checked at least once each trimester.

USE DURING BREASTFEEDING: Levothyroxine enters breast milk in small amounts but probably has no effect on the baby. Excessive dosages, however, should be avoided.

ALTERNATIVES TO MEDICATIONS: There is no nonpharmacologic alternative to levothyroxine for the treatment of hypothyroidism.

GENERIC NAME: Lisinopril

COMMON BRANDS: Prinivil, Zestril

TYPE OF DRUG: (Prescription) Antihypertensive

FDA RISK CATEGORY FOR PREGNANCY: C

GENERAL INFORMATION: Lisinopril is used for the treatment of hypertension. It belongs to a group of drugs called angiotensin converting enzyme (ACE) inhibitors.

POSSIBLE MATERNAL SIDE EFFECTS: Side effects are usually minimal. Occasionally, dizziness, headache, nausea, or persistent cough can occur.

USE DURING PREGNANCY: Lisinopril is a relatively new drug; consequently, there is very little experience with its use during pregnancy. Studies in laboratory animals have shown an increased risk of fetal death related to the drug. A similar antihypertensive, captopril (p. 98), has been suspected of causing birth defects, and kidney damage in the offspring of mothers given the drug during pregnancy. Lisinopril and other ACE inhibitors should be avoided during pregnancy since there are other antihypertensives with a longer record of safety.

USE DURING BREASTFEEDING: Lisinopril is secreted into breast milk, but its effects on the newborn are not known.

ALTERNATIVES TO MEDICATIONS: With a program of weight loss, mild salt restriction, exercise, and cessation of smoking many women can successfully decrease their blood pressure before pregnancy and remain off medications throughout at least the first trimester. However, if antihypertensive medication is necessary, another drug with a proven record of safety during pregnancy (such as methyldopa, p. 215) should be substituted for lisinopril.

GENERIC NAME: Lithium

COMMON BRANDS: Cibalith-S, Eskalith, Lithane, Lithobid, Lithonate, Lithotabs

TYPE OF DRUG: (Prescription) Antipsychotic

FDA RISK CATEGORY FOR PREGNANCY: D

GENERAL INFORMATION: Lithium is used for the treatment of the manic-depressive illness. It reduces the level of manic episodes and may be effective within a few weeks of beginning therapy. Typical manic symptoms include extreme restlessness, rapid speech, lack of sleep, grandiose ideas, aggressiveness, and poor judgment.

POSSIBLE MATERNAL SIDE EFFECTS: Side effects of lithium are directly related to the dosage and the amount of the drug in the blood. At the usual dosage side effects include excessive urination, thirst, and a fine tremor of the hands. At higher dosages nausea, diarrhea, drowsiness, poor coordination, and blurred vision may occur.

USE DURING PREGNANCY: Lithium has been clearly linked to congenital heart defects when given during the first trimester. If possible the drug should not be given during pregnancy. If, however, discontinuation of lithium would pose a serious threat to a woman with manic-depressive illness, the dosage should be reduced to the lowest effective level.

USE DURING BREASTFEEDING: Lithium is secreted into breast milk and should be avoided during breastfeeding.

ALTERNATIVES TO MEDICATIONS: In some cases manic-depressive illness can be managed by psychotherapy. However, medications should not be discontinued without consulting a physician.

GENERIC NAME: Local anesthetics

COMMON BRANDS: Carbocaine (mepivacaine), Duranest (etidocaine), Marcaine (bupivacaine), Nesacaine (chloroprocaine), Pontocaine (tetracaine), Xylocaine (lidocaine)

TYPE OF DRUG: (Prescription) Anesthetic

FDA RISK CATEGORY FOR PREGNANCY: C

GENERAL INFORMATION: Local anesthetics are used during a variety of minor surgical and dental procedures and for spinal or epidural anesthesia during labor and delivery. They work by blocking the transmission of nerve impulses from sensory nerves.

POSSIBLE MATERNAL SIDE EFFECTS: Side effects of local anesthetics are minimal unless they are inadvertently injected directly into a vein. An inadvertent intravascular injection could result in hypotension (low blood pressure) or in rare instances convulsions.

USE DURING PREGNANCY: Local anesthetics are generally considered safe for use during pregnancy. Lidocaine is frequently employed for minor surgical or dental procedures. Chloroprocaine, lidocaine, and bupivacaine have proved to be the most useful for epidural block during labor and delivery. Epidural or spinal anesthesia must be administered by an obstetrician or specially trained anesthesiologist with experience giving this type of anesthesia.

USE DURING BREASTFEEDING: It is not known whether local anesthetics are excreted into breast milk. However, it is unlikely that they would have any detrimental effect on the newborn.

ALTERNATIVES TO MEDICATIONS: In order to achieve adequate anesthesia for minor surgical procedures, local anesthetics are usually necessary. Occasionally, control of pain during minor procedures has been achieved with acupuncture or hypnosis.

GENERIC NAME: Loperamide

COMMON BRANDS: Imodium, Imodium A-D

TYPE OF DRUG: (Over-the-counter) Antidiarrheal

FDA RISK CATEGORY FOR PREGNANCY: B

GENERAL INFORMATION: Loperamide is used for the treatment of acute, uncomplicated diarrhea. It works by decreasing motility of the intestine. Like all medications employed for control of diarrhea, loperamide should not be used longer than 48 hours. If diarrhea persists longer than 48 hours or if fever develops, a physician should be called.

POSSIBLE MATERNAL SIDE EFFECTS: Side effects are usually mild but may include drowsiness, dry mouth, and constipation.

USE DURING PREGNANCY: There have been no reports linking loperamide with birth defects or other fetal harm.

USE DURING BREASTFEEDING: No information is available.

ALTERNATIVES TO MEDICATIONS: With acute diarrhea solid foods may be discontinued for 12 to 24 hours. When diarrhea abates, start eating again with dry bread or toast and small amounts of vegetables.

Since it is essential to avoid dehydration, be sure to drink plenty of liquids that contain sugar. Soup can also provide some nutrition and hydration without aggravating diarrhea. Symptoms of dehydration include thirst, dry mouth, fast breathing, and sometimes fever. An early sign of dehydration is reduction in the amount and frequency of urination. Drink enough to keep up normal urine output. If adequate hydration cannot be maintained, call the doctor.

GENERIC NAME: Lorazepam

COMMON BRANDS: Ativan

TYPE OF DRUG: (Prescription) Antianxiety, sedative

FDA RISK CATEGORY FOR PREGNANCY: D

GENERAL INFORMATION: Lorazepam is a member of a group of antianxiety medications called benzodiazepines. These drugs are used for the treatment of anxiety and insomnia. They work by relaxing skeletal muscles and by a direct action on the brain. Benzodiazepines can be abused if taken indiscriminately or for a long period of time. Withdrawal symptoms including tremor, agitation, insomnia, muscle cramps, nausea, and seizures can occur if these drugs arc discontinued abruptly after chronic use. Benzodiazepines should not be taken without careful medical supervision.

POSSIBLE MATERNAL SIDE EFFECTS: Common side effects with all benzodiazepines include sedation, depression, mental confusion, dizziness, unsteady gait, nightmares, fatigue, dry mouth, and low blood pressure. These drugs can interfere with the ability to safely drive a car or operate dangerous equipment. Physical and psychological dependence can occur with chronic use.

USE DURING PREGNANCY: All benzodiazepines rapidly cross the placenta and enter the fetal circulation. Blood levels in the fetus equal that of the mother's within one hour of taking a pill. Several studies have demonstrated a link between first-trimester use of benzodiazepines and birth defects. The most commonly reported malformations are cleft lip and cleft palate.

Used near term benzodiazepines have been associated with lethargy, respiratory problems, and withdrawal symptoms in the newborn. Most authorities believe that it is best to avoid these med-

196

ications during the first trimester, and if possible, throughout pregnancy.

USE DURING BREASTFEEDING: Benzodiazepines are excreted into breast milk in significant quantities. They can cause sedation in the newborn and should be avoided during breastfeeding.

ALTERNATIVES TO MEDICATIONS: Before using medications to control anxiety or stress consider the following strategy:

1. Identify the source of your anxiety. Worry often persists because of an inability to identify a problem and take action to solve it. Visualization can begin the process. Close your eyes and take a few deep breaths. Allow an image of the problem to arise.
2. Once you've defined the source of your anxiety, gather information. For example, if you are worried about the outcome of your pregnancy because of a possible hereditary problem or a medication you took before you knew you were pregnant, get information from your physician or a genetic counselor. In most cases what you discover will be very comforting.
3. After obtaining information, decide on a plan of action. Do what you can to deal with the problem, but once you've done all you can, change your focus and move on to other parts of life. Instead of worrying, concentrate on your life beyond the worry. Exercise or take walks. Plan how you will spend the evening or the weekend. Treat yourself to something pleasant, or think up a surprise for someone you care about. As your mind gets busy with other thoughts, you'll find that stress will begin to fade.
4. If anxiety persists despite your best efforts, see a therapist. Often only a few counseling sessions can effectively reduce anxiety and stress and eliminate the need for medication.

GENERIC NAME: Lovastatin

COMMON BRANDS: Mevacor

TYPE OF DRUG: (Prescription) Cholesterol-lowering

FDA RISK CATEGORY FOR PREGNANCY: X

GENERAL INFORMATION: Lovastatin is used to reduce cholesterol in individuals with chronically elevated levels who have not been able to reduce serum cholesterol by dietary and exercise measures. The drug works by inhibiting a chemical step in the production of cholesterol in the body.

POSSIBLE MATERNAL SIDE EFFECTS: Possible side effects include nausea, constipation, muscle aches and abnormal liver function tests (blood tests). Individuals treated with these medications should have blood drawn periodically to check liver function tests.

USE DURING PREGNANCY: Lovastatin has been commercially available for only a relatively short time. The drug interferes with a biochemical reaction that is essential for the formation of cell membranes. Theoretically this drug could interfere with normal cellular development in the fetus and cause birth defects. For this reason lovastatin should not be taken during pregnancy. Women taking the drug should ensure that effective contraception is used or that the drug is discontinued several months before they attempt to conceive.

USE DURING BREASTFEEDING: Lovastatin has been shown to enter breast milk. Although its effects on the newborn are not known, the drug should not be given to nursing mothers because it could have an adverse effect on growing cells.

ALTERNATIVES TO MEDICATIONS: Treatment of elevated serum cholesterol can usually be achieved with dietary restriction of cholesterol and saturated fat. The addition of soluble dietary fiber may also be helpful.

GENERIC NAME: Lysergic acid diethylamide

COMMON BRANDS: LSD, acid

TYPE OF DRUG: (Illicit) Hallucinogen

FDA RISK CATEGORY FOR PREGNANCY: X

GENERAL INFORMATION: LSD has no legitimate medical use. Street preparations contain various amounts of the drug as well as a variety of potentially toxic impurities. The drug can cause severe, prolonged hallucinations. Chronic users can experience "flashback" hallucinations months after discontinuing use.

POSSIBLE MATERNAL SIDE EFFECTS: Severe hallucinations, paranoia, flashbacks, rapid heart rate, abnormal heart rhythms, and a variety of other effects can be due to the drug itself or added impurities.

USE DURING PREGNANCY: LSD should not be used at any time during pregnancy. Theoretically, the drug is capable of damaging chromosomes and causing birth defects. Somewhat surprisingly, however, studies of women who took the drug during early pregnancy have not revealed a clear risk of birth defects. Nevertheless, common sense should dictate that it not be used.

USE DURING BREASTFEEDING: It is not known whether LSD enters breast milk. Even small amounts, however, could have devastating effects on the breastfed infant.

ALTERNATIVES TO MEDICATIONS: Women with substance abuse problems should seek counseling before pregnancy.

GENERIC NAME: Magnesium hydroxide

COMMON BRANDS: Haley's M-O, Phillips' Milk of magnesia

TYPE OF DRUG: (Over-the-counter) Laxative

FDA RISK CATEGORY FOR PREGNANCY: B

GENERAL INFORMATION: Magnesium hydroxide is the active ingredient in several over-the-counter laxative preparations. It works by drawing water into the stool and stimulating the bowel to move. Approximately 15 to 30 percent of magnesium may be absorbed systemically from the gastrointestinal tract.

POSSIBLE MATERNAL SIDE EFFECTS: The most significant adverse effect of magnesium hydroxide is diarrhea and laxative dependence usually caused by overuse. Chronic constipation requires medical evaluation. Neither magnesium hydroxide nor any laxative should be used longer than a few days.

USE DURING PREGNANCY: Magnesium hydroxide is considered safe for use during pregnancy. It has not been linked to adverse fetal effects. However, diarrhea due to magnesium hydroxide can cause premature labor.

USE DURING BREASTFEEDING: Some magnesium may be excreted into breast milk. However, this does not appear to cause any harm to the newborn.

ALTERNATIVES TO MEDICATIONS: Proper diet, including fiber-containing foods, and appropriate exercise will usually relieve mild constipation associated with pregnancy.

GENERIC NAME: Magnesium sulfate

COMMON BRANDS: Magnesium sulfate

TYPE OF DRUG: (Prescription) Anticonvulsant, mineral

FDA RISK CATEGORY FOR PREGNANCY: B

GENERAL INFORMATION: Magnesium is a naturally occurring mineral in the body. Certain illnesses can cause a deficiency of magnesium requiring oral or intravenous replacement of the mineral. Magnesium has also been shown to prevent convulsions, especially in pregnant women with preeclampsia (toxemia) (p. 16).

POSSIBLE MATERNAL SIDE EFFECTS: Excessive intravenous or intramuscular administration of magnesium sulfate can result in lethargy or even stupor. Normal breathing can also be inhibited if too much of the drug is given. Intravenous or intramuscular use of magnesium sulfate should always be carefully supervised in the hospital. Magnesium blood levels can be measured to ensure that the dosage is safe and effective.

USE DURING PREGNANCY: Magnesium sulfate is the most commonly used drug for the prevention of convulsions in women with preeclampsia. The drug may also be used to reduce or eliminate premature uterine contractions. It is usually administered intravenously but may also be given by repeat intramuscular injections. Recently, an oral form of magnesium sulfate has been used to treat patients with premature labor at home. Intravenous or intramuscular use must be carefully monitored to prevent respiratory depression (interference with normal breathing). If the drug is not given excessively, there is little risk to the fetus. However, excessive dosage can result in several complications in the newborn including respiratory depression, lethargy, muscle weakness, and loss of normal reflexes.

USE DURING BREASTFEEDING: In many women with preeclampsia magnesium sulfate is continued for 24 to 72 hours following delivery. A small amount of the drug enters breast milk but does not pose any significant risk to the newborn. The American Academy of Pediatrics considers magnesium sulfate compatible with breastfeeding.

ALTERNATIVES TO MEDICATIONS: Treatment of women with preeclampsia includes bed rest in a quiet, nonstimulating room (usually in a hospital), careful monitoring of blood pressure, and fetal surveillance. In most patients the use of magnesium sulfate will also be necessary.

GENERIC NAME: Marijuana

COMMON BRANDS: Marijuana

TYPE OF DRUG: (Illicit) Hallucinogen

FDA RISK CATEGORY FOR PREGNANCY: X

GENERAL INFORMATION: Marijuana is a commonly used hallucinogen throughout the United States. It is frequently contaminated with various herbicides and adulterated with other chemicals and hallucinogens.

POSSIBLE MATERNAL SIDE EFFECTS: Side effects include hallucinations, dizziness, apathy, impaired judgment, increased appetite, and hypoglycemia. Other side effects are possible if the pure plant has been adulterated with additional chemicals or hallucinogens.

USE DURING PREGNANCY: Marijuana should not be used during any stage of pregnancy. Several studies have implicated regular use of the drug in the cause of birth defects, inadequate fetal growth, and depression of the central nervous system in the newborn. The likelihood of other drugs or herbicides contaminating marijuana place the baby at even greater risk.

Fortunately, occasional use of marijuana, even during the first trimester, is unlikely to cause birth defects. If you smoked marijuana on a few occasions before you found out you were pregnant, your baby is most likely unharmed. Nevertheless, you should make your obstetrician fully aware of your use of the drug so appropriate tests can be performed to be sure the baby is all right.

USE DURING BREASTFEEDING: Tetrahydrocannabinol, the active ingredient in marijuana, has been shown to enter breast milk. Since the drug may have a profound effect on the newborn, it should not be used during breastfeeding.

ALTERNATIVES TO MEDICATIONS: Marijuana should not be used during pregnancy. Women habituated to the drug should receive counseling in a drug rehabilitation program.

GENERIC NAME: Measles (Rubeola) vaccine

COMMON BRANDS: Attenuvax, M-R-Vax II, M-M-R II

TYPE OF DRUG: (Prescription) Virus vaccine (live)

FDA RISK CATEGORY FOR PREGNANCY: X

GENERAL INFORMATION: Measles vaccine is made from inactivated live measles virus. It is often combined with mumps and rubella live virus vaccines. Its use in women should be restricted to those who are definitely not pregnant and do not plan to become pregnant for at least three months.

POSSIBLE MATERNAL SIDE EFFECTS: The most common side effects are pain and redness at the site of injection. Allergic reactions to the vaccine can occur in some individuals.

USE DURING PREGNANCY: Measles vaccine should not be given during pregnancy. The exact risk of inadvertent vaccination during the first trimester is not known. Pregnant women exposed to measles who have never had the disease or have never been immunized may be treated with immune globulin (p. 177) after exposure, preferably within 72 hours. If this is not possible, use of immune globulin within seven days of exposure may prevent or at least modify the disease.

USE DURING BREASTFEEDING: It is not known whether measles vaccine is secreted into breast milk, nor is it known whether it has any effect on the newborn.

ALTERNATIVES TO MEDICATIONS: There is no nonpharmacologic alternative to measles vaccine for achieving active immunity to the disease. A simple blood test can determine whether a woman is immune to the disease from previous exposure. As discussed above, immune globulin may be given safely during pregnancy to nonimmune women exposed to measles.

GENERIC NAME: Mebendazole

COMMON BRANDS: Vermox

TYPE OF DRUG: (Prescription) Antiworm

FDA RISK CATEGORY FOR PREGNANCY: C

GENERAL INFORMATION: Mebendazole is used for the treatment of pinworm, roundworm, whipworm, hookworm, and various intestinal worm infestations.

POSSIBLE MATERNAL SIDE EFFECTS: Side effects are usually mild but nausea or mild abdominal pain can occur.

USE DURING PREGNANCY: Mebendazole has been shown to cause birth defects in laboratory rats. For this reason use of the drug is not advised during pregnancy. Even though the manufacturer reports that first-trimester use in human pregnancy has not been linked with birth defects, treatment should be deferred in most cases until after pregnancy or at least until after the first trimester. In most cases there is no urgency to treat intestinal parasites.

USE DURING BREASTFEEDING: It is not known whether mebendazole is excreted into breast milk.

ALTERNATIVES TO MEDICATIONS: Although there is no non-pharmacologic alternative for the treatment of intestinal parasites, the mere presence of worms is not necessarily an indication for treatment. In most cases treatment can be deferred until after pregnancy or at least until after the first trimester.

GENERIC NAME: Meclofenamate

COMMON BRANDS: Meclomen

TYPE OF DRUG: (Prescription) Anti-inflammatory

FDA RISK CATEGORY FOR PREGNANCY: Not classified

203

GENERAL INFORMATION: Meclofenamate is a member of a class of drugs called nonsteroidal anti-inflammatory drugs (NSAIDs). It is indicated for the treatment of arthritis, muscle pain, headache, and pain associated with menstruation.

POSSIBLE MATERNAL SIDE EFFECTS: The most common side effects are nausea and abdominal pain. Rarely, meclofenamate can irritate the stomach and cause an ulcer or bleeding from the stomach.

USE DURING PREGNANCY: There have been no reports linking meclofenamate to birth defects when the drug was used during the first trimester. However, experience with the drug during early pregnancy is limited.

Used near term meclofenamate can have potential effects on pregnancy and the fetus. First, the drug can cause premature closure of an important blood vessel in the fetus called the ductus arteriosus. Normally, this blood vessel does not close until after delivery. Premature closure could result in a serious condition called pulmonary hypertension. Second, meclofenamate and other NSAIDs can inhibit labor and prolong pregnancy.

USE DURING BREASTFEEDING: Meclofenamate enters human breast milk, but its effect on the newborn is not known. The drug's safety during breastfeeding cannot be ensured.

ALTERNATIVES TO MEDICATIONS: Musculoskeletal pain can often be relieved with warm baths and massage. Painful arthritis can be alleviated by rest, heat, and physical therapy. Nonweight-bearing exercise such as swimming may offer some comfort while enhancing muscle tone. If medication is necessary, acetaminophen (p. 63) is probably the safest medication to take during pregnancy for relief of minor pain.

Generic name: Mefenamic acid

COMMON BRANDS: Ponstel

TYPE OF DRUG: (Prescription) Anti-inflammatory

FDA RISK CATEGORY FOR PREGNANCY: C

GENERAL INFORMATION: Mefenamic acid is a member of a class of drugs called nonsteroidal anti-inflammatory drugs (NSAIDs). It is indicated for the treatment of arthritis, muscle pain, headache, and pain associated with menstruation.

POSSIBLE MATERNAL SIDE EFFECTS: The most common side effects are nausea and abdominal pain. Rarely, mefenamic acid can irritate the stomach and cause an ulcer or bleeding from the stomach.

USE DURING PREGNANCY: There have been no reports linking mefenamic acid to birth defects when the drug was used during the first trimester. However, experience with the drug during early pregnancy is limited.

Used near term mefenamic acid can have potential effects on pregnancy and the fetus. First, the drug can cause premature closure of an important blood vessel in the fetus called the ductus arteriosus. Normally, this blood vessel does not close until after delivery. Premature closure could result in a serious condition called pulmonary hypertension. Second, mefenamic acid and other NSAIDs can inhibit labor and prolong pregnancy.

USE DURING BREASTFEEDING: Mefenamic acid enters human breast milk, but its effect on the newborn is not known. The drug's safety during breastfeeding cannot be ensured.

ALTERNATIVES TO MEDICATIONS: Musculoskeletal pain can often be relieved with warm baths and massage. Painful arthritis can be alleviated by rest, heat, and physical therapy. Nonweight-bearing exercise such as swimming may offer some comfort while enhancing muscle tone. If medication is necessary, acetaminophen (p. 63) is probably the safest medication to take during pregnancy for relief of minor pain.

GENERIC NAME: # Menotropins

COMMON BRANDS: Pergonal

TYPE OF DRUG: (Prescription) Ovulation stimulant, sperm production stimulant

FDA RISK CATEGORY FOR PREGNANCY: X

GENERAL INFORMATION: Menotropins are used to stimulate ovulation in certain women who are infertile. They can also be used to stimulate the manufacture of sperm in men with inadequate sperm production. These medications are not effective in all infertile individuals. Evaluation by a gynecologist or endocrinologist is necessary before treatment.

POSSIBLE MATERNAL SIDE EFFECTS: One of the most significant side effects in women treated with menotropins is the so-called hyperstimulation syndrome characterized by sudden painful ovarian enlargement accompanied by fluid in the abdomen (ascites) or fluid around the lungs (pleural effusion).

The drug should be discontinued immediately if sudden pain in the ovaries or abdomen occurs. Use of the drug to stimulate ovulation results in about a 20 percent incidence of multiple births (most commonly twins).

In men enlargement of the breasts is common.

USE DURING PREGNANCY: The drug should not be used during pregnancy. There has been a clear link to birth defects. Therefore, it is essential that use of menotropins be guided by a physician thoroughly familiar with their use.

USE DURING BREASTFEEDING: There is no indication for menotropins during breastfeeding.

ALTERNATIVES TO MEDICATIONS: There is no nonpharmacologic alternative for stimulation of ovulation.

GENERIC NAME: ## Meperidine

COMMON BRANDS: Demerol

TYPE OF DRUG: (Prescription) Narcotic analgesic

FDA RISK CATEGORY FOR PREGNANCY: Not classified

GENERAL INFORMATION: Meperidine is a narcotic analgesic used for the relief of severe acute pain. It can be administered by pill or injection. Like all narcotics prolonged or indiscriminate use can lead to addiction.

POSSIBLE MATERNAL SIDE EFFECTS: Possible side effects include sedation, dizziness, impaired judgment, agitation, confusion, dry mouth, nausea, and dependence.

USE DURING PREGNANCY: Meperidine has been used safely during pregnancy. There are no reports linking first-trimester use with birth defects. However, the drug rapidly crosses the placenta to reach the fetus. A large dose given at term can cause respiratory depression and lethargy in the newborn. Chronic use can also result in addiction of the newborn and subsequent withdrawal symptoms. Only the lowest possible dosage necessary to control pain should be used.

USE DURING BREASTFEEDING: Meperidine is excreted into breast milk but in relatively small amounts. The risk to the newborn appears to be minimal if the dosage is kept within the usual range needed to achieve pain control. An inappropriately high dosage or chronic use could adversely affect the breastfed newborn.

ALTERNATIVES TO MEDICATIONS: Techniques of natural childbirth such as Lamaze may eliminate the need for narcotics during labor. However, meperidine can be safely used to control pain following surgery or after cesarean delivery.

GENERIC NAME: **Meprobamate**

COMMON BRANDS: Deprol, Equagesic, Equanil, Meprospan, Miltown, PMB 200, PMB 400

TYPE OF DRUG: (Prescription) Sedative, tranquilizer

FDA RISK CATEGORY FOR PREGNANCY: D

GENERAL INFORMATION: Meprobamate is a sedative used for the treatment of acute anxiety. Chronic use of the drug can result in physical dependence and sudden cessation may precipitate withdrawal symptoms.

POSSIBLE MATERNAL SIDE EFFECTS: Possible side effects include drowsiness, dizziness, unsteady gait, slurred speech, nausea, and palpitations.

USE DURING PREGNANCY: Use of meprobamate during the first trimester has been linked to various malformations including congenital heart defects. The drug should not be used during pregnancy. Use of meprobamate at term can cause sedation and abnormal behavior in the newborn.

USE DURING BREASTFEEDING: Meprobamate is excreted into breast milk, but its effect on the nursing infant is not known. In general it is best to avoid meprobamate during breastfeeding.

ALTERNATIVES TO MEDICATIONS: Insomnia may be relieved by some of the following techniques:

- Generally, try to avoid daytime naps. However, for some women sleeping patterns change during pregnancy, and a nap may be necessary to supplement abbreviated nighttime sleep.
- Go to bed only when tired. Instead of lying in bed when you are wide awake, get up, do something, and then return to bed when you feel tired.
- Try to establish a regular sleep pattern. Recognize when you *are* able to sleep and build on that.
- Exercise daily. Even a 30-minute walk will aid relaxation.
- Learn techniques of progressive relaxation. These techniques are simple to learn and effective.
- Avoid stimulant drinks such as coffee, tea, and caffeine-containing colas. On the other hand, warm milk may help make you sleepy.
- Never use alcohol to induce sleep.
- If you awaken during the night, recall the dream just before you awoke. Reentering the dream can return you to sleep.
- Make love. Sex is relaxing and often ends with sleep.
- If you are lying awake because a problem is on your mind, talk it through with someone until it's resolved.

GENERIC NAME: Metaproterenol

COMMON BRANDS: Alupent, Metaprel

TYPE OF DRUG: (Prescription) Bronchial dilator

FDA RISK CATEGORY FOR PREGNANCY: C

GENERAL INFORMATION: Metaproterenol is commonly administered by inhalation for the treatment of bronchial spasm due to asthma. It can also be given by pill, but this form of the drug probably offers no advantage over the aerosol preparation and may result in more side effects. The bronchodilating effect of metaproterenol begins within a few minutes when it is given by inhalation.

POSSIBLE MATERNAL SIDE EFFECTS: Possible side effects include shakiness, palpitations, nervousness, and nausea. These adverse effects are much more likely to occur if the drug is given by pill rather than by inhalation. Since the drug is poorly absorbed when given by inhalation, side effects are usually minimal.

USE DURING PREGNANCY: No birth defects have been linked to the first-trimester use of metaproterenol in human pregnancies. However, large dosages given to rabbits have been shown to cause fetal loss and possibly birth defects.

USE DURING BREASTFEEDING: No information is available.

ALTERNATIVES TO MEDICATIONS: In some cases asthma can be prevented by avoidance of known allergens, particularly animals. If you smoke, stop. It is generally a good rule, however, to use a bronchodilating inhaler at the earliest indication of wheezing. Often prompt effective relief of asthma can prevent minor episodes from becoming more severe and prolonged.

GENERIC NAME: **Methadone**

COMMON BRANDS: Dolophine, Methadone

TYPE OF DRUG: (Prescription) Narcotic

FDA RISK CATEGORY FOR PREGNANCY: Not classified

GENERAL INFORMATION: Methadone is an opiate narcotic primarily used in programs to facilitate withdrawal from heroin addiction. The drug has also been used for the treatment of acute severe pain. As is the case with any narcotic, there can be a serious potential for addiction to methadone.

POSSIBLE MATERNAL SIDE EFFECTS: Maternal side effects are similar to those of any narcotic including sedation, dizziness, euphoria, dry mouth, loss of appetite, and constipation.

USE DURING PREGNANCY: The use of methadone during pregnancy is almost exclusively limited to treatment of heroin addiction. Although there has been no clear link between methadone use during the first trimester and birth defects, current information is not sufficient to ensure its safety. Several reports indicate that infants of methadone-treated women have smaller than normal babies. Nevertheless, it is generally considered that a methadone program for treatment of heroin addiction is preferable to continued use of illicit drugs. Withdrawal from methadone is generally not advised during pregnancy.

When the drug is used near term, there is a possibility of addiction in the newborn. These infants may manifest withdrawal symptoms such as agitation, poor feeding, and poor sleeping.

USE DURING BREASTFEEDING: Methadone has been shown to enter breast milk in significant quantities. It has been suggested that the presence of methadone in breast milk may minimize the withdrawal symptoms in addicted newborns. The drug should be used during breastfeeding only with careful medical supervision of both mother and child.

ALTERNATIVES TO MEDICATIONS: For some women a supervised drug-withdrawal program using limited amounts of methadone may be the only realistic alternative to heroin addiction.

GENERIC NAME: **Methaqualone**

COMMON BRANDS: Quaalude

TYPE OF DRUG: (Prescription) Sedative

FDA RISK CATEGORY FOR PREGNANCY: D

GENERAL INFORMATION: In the past methaqualone has been used as a sleeping pill for the treatment of acute insomnia. Today, the drug is rarely used for legitimate medical reasons. Preparations purchased illegally on the street may be adulterated with other drugs or chemicals.

POSSIBLE MATERNAL SIDE EFFECTS: Side effects include sedation, dizziness, poor judgment, and possible habituation.

USE DURING PREGNANCY: There is no use for methaqualone during pregnancy. Although the drug has not been clearly implicated in the cause of birth defects, its safety during any stage of pregnancy cannot be ensured.

USE DURING BREASTFEEDING: Methaqualone probably enters breast milk and should be avoided during breastfeeding.

ALTERNATIVES TO MEDICATIONS: Insomnia may be relieved by some of the following techniques:

- Generally, try to avoid daytime naps. However, for some women sleeping patterns change during pregnancy, and a nap may be necessary to supplement abbreviated nighttime sleep.
- Go to bed only when tired. Instead of lying in bed when you are wide awake, get up, do something, and then return to bed when you feel tired.
- Try to establish a regular sleep pattern. Recognize when you *are* able to sleep and build on that.
- Exercise daily. Even a 30-minute walk will aid relaxation.
- Learn techniques of progressive relaxation. These techniques are simple to learn and effective.
- Avoid stimulant drinks such as coffee, tea, and caffeine-containing colas. On the other hand, warm milk may help make you sleepy.
- Never use alcohol to induce sleep.
- If you awaken during the night, recall the dream just before you awoke. Reentering the dream can return you to sleep.
- Make love. Sex is relaxing and often ends with sleep.
- If you are lying awake because a problem is on your mind, talk it through with someone until it's resolved.

GENERIC NAME: # Methenamine

COMMON BRANDS: Hiprex and Urex (methenamine hippurate), Mandameth and Mandelamine, Thiacide, Urogid-Acid (methenamine mandelate)

TYPE OF DRUG: (Prescription) Urinary antiseptic

FDA RISK CATEGORY FOR PREGNANCY: C

GENERAL INFORMATION: Methenamine is used to reduce the number of bacteria in the urine of women who suffer from chronic or recurrent urinary tract infections. The drug is converted in the urine to formaldehyde, which is capable of killing bacteria.

POSSIBLE MATERNAL SIDE EFFECTS: Possible side effects include nausea and painful urination.

USE DURING PREGNANCY: Methenamine is absorbed from the gastrointestinal tract and crosses the placenta. Although there have been no reports clearly linking methenamine to birth defects or fetal harm, other antibiotics with proven safety during pregnancy should generally be used in its place.

USE DURING BREASTFEEDING: Methenamine is excreted into breast milk, but no adverse effects on the newborn have been reported.

ALTERNATIVES TO MEDICATIONS: Lower-urinary-tract infections (p. 31) (bladder infections) can lead to serious infections of the kidneys possibly causing severe complications of pregnancy. There is no alternative to effective treatment with an antibiotic.

GENERIC NAME: ## Methimazole

COMMON BRANDS: Tapazole

TYPE OF DRUG: (Prescription) Antithyroid

FDA RISK CATEGORY FOR PREGNANCY: D

GENERAL INFORMATION: Methimazole is given to block the production of thyroid hormone in patients with hyperthyroidism (an overactive thyroid gland) (p. 294). Individuals may be treated with the drug for several months while allowing hyperthyroidism to resolve spontaneously. It may also be used for a shorter period to control symptoms of hyperthyroidism before surgery or radioactive iodine therapy.

POSSIBLE MATERNAL SIDE EFFECTS: Since the drug interferes with the production of thyroid hormone, it is possible to overcompensate and cause symptoms of hypothyroidism (an underactive thyroid). Methimazole can also interfere with the normal production of red and white blood cells. It is essential that a complete blood count be performed periodically during treatment with this medication.

USE DURING PREGNANCY: Methimazole freely crosses the placenta and has been shown to cause several possible adverse effects on the fetus. The drug can be taken up by the fetal thyroid gland, which forms during the first trimester, and cause a goiter (an enlarged thyroid gland). Methimazole has also been shown to cause an abnormal scalp condition in the fetus called aplasia cutis.

USE DURING BREASTFEEDING: Methimazole is excreted into breast milk and can have an adverse effect on the function of the thyroid gland in the newborn. Its use should generally be avoided during breastfeeding.

ALTERNATIVES TO MEDICATIONS: Mild hyperthyroidism is often well tolerated and does not need to be treated in all cases. When the condition is clinically significant, however, treatment with medication may be indicated. If an antithyroid drug is needed during pregnancy, propylthiouracil (p. 266) is the drug of choice.

GENERIC NAME: Methocarbamol

COMMON BRANDS: Robaxin, Robaxisal

TYPE OF DRUG: (Prescription) Muscle relaxant

FDA RISK CATEGORY FOR PREGNANCY: C

GENERAL INFORMATION: Methocarbamol is used for acute relief of muscle spasm usually due to injury or overuse. It appears to work by a sedative action rather than by directly affecting the muscles.

POSSIBLE MATERNAL SIDE EFFECTS: Side effects include drowsiness, light-headedness, low blood pressure, slow heart rate, blurred vision, nausea, diminished appetite, and a metallic taste.

USE DURING PREGNANCY: Since the safety of methocarbamol has not been established, the drug should generally be avoided during pregnancy.

USE DURING BREASTFEEDING: It is not known whether methocarbamol is excreted into breast milk.

ALTERNATIVES TO MEDICATIONS: Acute muscle strain can often be relieved by rest and warm compresses. If medication is needed for pain relief, acetaminophen (p. 63) is the drug of choice during pregnancy.

GENERIC NAME: Methotrexate

COMMON BRANDS: Folex, Mexate

TYPE OF DRUG: (Prescription) Anticancer (chemotherapy)

FDA RISK CATEGORY FOR PREGNANCY: D

GENERAL INFORMATION: Methotrexate is an anticancer drug often used in combination with other anticancer medications. The drug interferes with one of the basic chemical reactions in the formation of new cells. In addition to its action against cancer, methotrexate has also been used in the treatment of severe psoriasis and rheumatoid arthritis.

POSSIBLE MATERNAL SIDE EFFECTS: Methotrexate frequently causes a variety of side effects, some potentially quite serious. Common side effects include hair loss, nausea, inflammation of the gums and tongue, rash, and interference with normal cellular production in the bone marrow resulting in anemia and a low white blood cell count.

USE DURING PREGNANCY: Because methotrexate crosses the placenta and interferes with a basic chemical reaction in the development of normal cells, it has great potential for causing birth defects. Whenever possible the drug should be avoided during the first trimester. Ideally, it should not be used during any stage of pregnancy. If, however, the life of the mother depends on the use of this anticancer drug, it may be used with extreme caution during pregnancy. There have been some reassuring reports of normal children born to women treated with methotrexate during pregnancy.

USE DURING BREASTFEEDING: Methotrexate is excreted into breast milk and may have an adverse effect on the development of nursing infants. Breastfeeding is not recommended if methotrexate therapy is necessary.

ALTERNATIVES TO MEDICATIONS: Unfortunately, there are no proven nonpharmacologic alternatives to methotrexate for the treatment of certain types of cancer. In some cases, however, treatment

214

with chemotherapy can be postponed until after pregnancy or at least until after the first trimester.

GENERIC NAME: Methsuximide

COMMON BRANDS: Celontin

TYPE OF DRUG: (Prescription) Anticonvulsant

FDA RISK CATEGORY FOR PREGNANCY: Not classified

GENERAL INFORMATION: Methsuximide is an anticonvulsant medication used for the prevention of petit mal (minor) seizures. It is generally not effective for the treatment of grand mal (major) seizures.

POSSIBLE MATERNAL SIDE EFFECTS: Possible side effects include dizziness, unsteadiness, insomnia, blurred vision, skin rash, nausea, and decreased appetite.

USE DURING PREGNANCY: Only five patients treated with methsuximide during the first trimester of pregnancy have been reported in the medical literature. Although there have been no reports of associated birth defects, experience with the drug is too limited to ensure its safety. All anticonvulsants appear capable of causing birth defects.

USE DURING BREASTFEEDING: No information is available.

ALTERNATIVES TO MEDICATIONS: Patients free of petit mal seizures since childhood should discuss the possibility of discontinuing the drug prior to pregnancy with their physician.

GENERIC NAME: Methyldopa

COMMON BRANDS: Aldoclor, Aldomet, Aldoril

TYPE OF DRUG: (Prescription) Antihypertensive

FDA RISK CATEGORY FOR PREGNANCY: B

GENERAL INFORMATION: Methyldopa is used to treat chronic hypertension. It is often combined with another medication such as a diuretic to achieve satisfactory control of blood pressure.

POSSIBLE MATERNAL SIDE EFFECTS: Methyldopa is usually well tolerated, but side effects may include drowsiness (especially during the first one to two weeks of therapy), dizziness, nightmares, dry mouth, nasal stuffiness, and diarrhea. The drug should be discontinued immediately if jaundice occurs.

USE DURING PREGNANCY: Methyldopa has been studied during pregnancy more extensively than any other antihypertensive. There has been no link established between use of the drug during any trimester of pregnancy and birth defects or fetal harm. Methyldopa is currently considered the drug of choice for the control of chronic high blood pressure during pregnancy.

USE DURING BREASTFEEDING: Methyldopa is excreted into breast milk, but it does not appear to have any detrimental effect on the fetus. The American Academy of Pediatrics considers methyldopa compatible with breastfeeding.

ALTERNATIVES TO MEDICATIONS: With a program of weight loss, mild salt restriction, exercise, and cessation of smoking many women can successfully decrease their blood pressure before pregnancy and remain off medications throughout at least the first trimester.

GENERIC NAME: **Methylphenidate**

COMMON BRANDS: Ritalin

TYPE OF DRUG: (Prescription) Stimulant

FDA RISK CATEGORY FOR PREGNANCY: C

GENERAL INFORMATION: There are very few medical uses for methylphenidate. In children the drug has been used to control hyperactive behavior. In adults it is effective for the treatment of a rare disorder characterized by excessive sleep called narcolepsy. The drug is also frequently abused by individuals who want to avoid sleep.

POSSIBLE MATERNAL SIDE EFFECTS: The most common side effects of methylphenidate are insomnia, restlessness, headache, palpitations, blurred vision, nausea, and diminished appetite. Drug dependence can result from chronic use.

USE DURING PREGNANCY: There is not sufficient information about the use of methylphenidate during pregnancy to ensure its safety. It should generally be avoided during pregnancy.

USE DURING BREASTFEEDING: It is not known whether methylphenidate enters breast milk in significant quantities. However, small amounts could cause restlessness and poor feeding in newborns.

ALTERNATIVES TO MEDICATIONS: Methylphenidate should not be used during pregnancy. Moreover, there is no need for any stimulant.

GENERIC NAME: Methysergide

COMMON BRANDS: Sansert

TYPE OF DRUG: (Prescription) Antimigraine

FDA RISK CATEGORY FOR PREGNANCY: X

GENERAL INFORMATION: Methysergide can be taken daily to prevent recurrent migraine headaches. It is not effective once an acute migraine attack has begun. Nor is it effective for the treatment of common tension headaches.

POSSIBLE MATERNAL SIDE EFFECTS: Side effects of methysergide can be significant including restlessness, insomnia, and hallucinations similar to those experienced with LSD. The drug can also cause heart pains in patients with coronary heart disease.

USE DURING PREGNANCY: Methysergide can cause miscarriage or premature labor and should not be used during any stage of pregnancy.

USE DURING BREASTFEEDING: Methysergide is excreted into breast milk and should not be taken during breastfeeding.

ALTERNATIVES TO MEDICATIONS: Attempt to identify any specific events, foods, or medications that trigger your migraines and avoid them. Avoid alcohol and excessive fatigue. At the onset of a migraine rest in a quiet, darkened room. Following sleep the pain of a migraine is usually less.

GENERIC NAME: Metoclopramide

COMMON BRANDS: Reglan

TYPE OF DRUG: (Prescription) Antinausea

FDA RISK CATEGORY FOR PREGNANCY: B

GENERAL INFORMATION: Metoclopramide has been used to prevent or reduce nausea and vomiting in patients with esophageal reflux, in diabetics with delayed emptying of the stomach, and in cancer patients receiving chemotherapy.

POSSIBLE MATERNAL SIDE EFFECTS: Possible side effects include restlessness, anxiety, insomnia, and abnormal involuntary movements.

USE DURING PREGNANCY: Experience with metoclopramide in human pregnancy is limited, but animal studies have not demonstrated any unusual risk of birth defects or fetal harm. Other drugs used to control nausea have been studied more extensively during pregnancy.

USE DURING BREASTFEEDING: Metoclopramide is excreted into breast milk. Some studies have suggested that the drug enhances the production of breast milk. However, more research is needed before it is used for this purpose. The effect of metoclopramide on the newborn is not known.

ALTERNATIVES TO MEDICATIONS: Nausea can often be controlled with the following measures:

- Avoid foods that appear or smell offensive to you. This may seem blatantly obvious, but the role of the psyche in nausea is a very important one.
- Avoid an empty stomach. Eat several small meals throughout the day rather than two or three larger ones. If a large meal is necessary, midday is probably the best time for it.
- Avoid greasy or fatty foods. Substitute foods rich in complex carbo-

hydrates such as whole-grain breads, cereals, and pasta. Fresh green leafy vegetables may help alleviate nausea because they are rich in vitamin B$_6$.

- Eat a small snack at bedtime and save two crackers at the bedside. On awakening, eat the crackers before getting out of bed and remain in bed for an additional few minutes.
- Drink plenty of fluids throughout the day to avoid dehydration.
- If nausea does occur, lie down. It helps. In fact, many women find that frequent rest periods forestall the discomfort.

GENERIC NAME: Metoprolol

COMMON BRANDS: Lopressor

TYPE OF DRUG: (Prescription) Antihypertensive

FDA RISK CATEGORY FOR PREGNANCY: C

GENERAL INFORMATION: Metoprolol is a member of a group of drugs called beta blockers. Beta blockers act by inhibiting a major chemical reaction in the nervous system. Each of these drugs is capable of slowing the heart rate and lowering blood pressure. Their uses in the general population include treatment of high blood pressure, control of abnormal rhythms of the heart, control of acute hyperthyroidism (overactive thyroid gland), prevention of angina (heart pain), prevention of migraine headaches, and prevention of acute performance anxiety (stage fright).

POSSIBLE MATERNAL SIDE EFFECTS: Possible side effects include slow heart rate, fatigue, wheezing (in patients with asthma), and depression.

USE DURING PREGNANCY: Beta blockers cross the placenta, but they have not been linked to congenital malformations. A large study of the use of beta blockers during pregnancy revealed no evidence of abnormal fetal growth or development. They are now being used more frequently for the treatment of high blood pressure during pregnancy. Newborn infants of women who took metoprolol near delivery should be checked closely in the newborn nursery for slow heart rate and low blood sugar.

USE DURING BREASTFEEDING: Beta blockers are excreted into breast milk and theoretically could slow the baby's heart rate. Nevertheless, the American Academy of Pediatrics considers metoprolol and other beta blockers compatible with breastfeeding.

ALTERNATIVES TO MEDICATIONS: With a program of weight loss, mild salt restriction, exercise, and cessation of smoking many women can successfully decrease their blood pressure before pregnancy and remain off medications throughout at least the first trimester. However, if antihypertensive medication is necessary, another drug with a proven record of safety during pregnancy (such as methyldopa, p. 215) should be considered.

GENERIC NAME: Metronidazole

COMMON BRANDS: Flagyl, Metric 21, Protostat

TYPE OF DRUG: (Prescription) Antiamoeba

FDA RISK CATEGORY FOR PREGNANCY: B

GENERAL INFORMATION: Metronidazole is an oral medication used for the treatment of amoebic intestinal infections such as giardiasis and vaginal trichomoniasis.

POSSIBLE MATERNAL SIDE EFFECTS: Nausea and vomiting are relatively common side effects. Alcohol must not be consumed while metronidazole is taken. The two may interact to cause severe nausea, vomiting, palpitations, dizziness, and respiratory difficulties.

USE DURING PREGNANCY: The use of metronidazole during pregnancy is controversial. The drug is known to cause mutations in bacteria and cancer in rodents. Although there has been no clear link between the use of metronidazole and birth defects in humans, it would be prudent to avoid the drug at least during the first trimester.

USE DURING BREASTFEEDING: Metronidazole is excreted into breast milk. Although its effect on the newborn is not known, the drug should be used only if necessary during breastfeeding. Consideration should be given to discontinuing breastfeeding.

ALTERNATIVES TO MEDICATIONS: Although there are no non-pharmacologic alternatives to metronidazole for the treatment of parasitic or amoebic infections, not all of these infections require immediate therapy. In some cases treatment can be postponed until after pregnancy or at least until after the first trimester.

GENERIC NAME: Miconazole

COMMON BRANDS: Micatin, Monistat 3, Monistat 7, Monistat-Derm

TYPE OF DRUG: (Prescription) Antifungal

FDA RISK CATEGORY FOR PREGNANCY: B

GENERAL INFORMATION: Miconazole is applied topically for the treatment of vaginal or skin fungal infections. Only a small amount of the drug is absorbed systemically following vaginal application. An intravenous preparation is also available for life-threatening fungal infections.

POSSIBLE MATERNAL SIDE EFFECTS: Topical application rarely causes anything more troubling than vaginal itching.

USE DURING PREGNANCY: Miconazole is considered safe for topical use during pregnancy. There have been no reports linking the drug with birth defects or other fetal harm. The drug should not be used, however, once the membranes have ruptured. Intravenous use of miconazole has not been satisfactorily studied during pregnancy.

USE DURING BREASTFEEDING: Topical application of miconazole during breastfeeding has not been shown to cause any harm to the newborn.

ALTERNATIVES TO MEDICATIONS: To help avoid vaginal yeast infections do not take antibiotics unnecessarily, wear loose cotton underwear, avoid harsh soaps and irritants, and be sure your partner does not have a chronic yeast infection. During pregnancy it is not always necessary to treat mild yeast infections.

GENERIC NAME: Midazolam

COMMON BRANDS: Versed

TYPE OF DRUG: (Prescription) Antianxiety, sedative

FDA RISK CATEGORY FOR PREGNANCY: D

GENERAL INFORMATION: Midazolam is a member of a group of antianxiety medications called benzodiazepines. It can be administered intravenously or by intramuscular injection to achieve anesthesia during surgical procedures. It works by relaxing skeletal muscles and by a direct action on the brain.

POSSIBLE MATERNAL SIDE EFFECTS: Common side effects of Midazolam include sedation, depression, mental confusion, dizziness, unsteady gait, respiratory depression, and low blood pressure.

USE DURING PREGNANCY: All benzodiazepines rapidly cross the placenta and enter the fetal circulation. Blood levels in the fetus equal that of the mother's within one hour of administration. Several studies have demonstrated a link between first-trimester use of benzodiazepines and birth defects. The most commonly reported malformations are cleft lip and cleft palate. Used near term benzodiazepines have been associated with lethargy, respiratory problems, and withdrawal symptoms in the newborn. Most authorities believe that it is best to avoid these medications during the first trimester and if possible throughout pregnancy.

USE DURING BREASTFEEDING: Benzodiazepines are excreted into breast milk in significant quantities. They can cause sedation in the newborn and should be avoided during breastfeeding.

ALTERNATIVES TO MEDICATIONS: Medications other than benzodiazepines are available for anesthesia.

GENERIC NAME: **Mineral oil**

COMMON BRANDS: Agoral, Haley's M-O Kandremul, Milkinol, Neo-Cultol, Nujol, Zymenol

TYPE OF DRUG: (Over-the-counter) Laxative

FDA RISK CATEGORY FOR PREGNANCY: C

GENERAL INFORMATION: Mineral oil works as a laxative by lubricating the intestine and inhibiting fluid absorption from the colon.

Chronic use of mineral oil may interfere with the absorption of certain vitamins such as vitamin K.

POSSIBLE MATERNAL SIDE EFFECTS: The most common side effect is diarrhea when mineral oil is used excessively. Occasionally, diarrhea due to mineral oil can cause premature labor.

USE DURING PREGNANCY: Absorption of mineral oil is minimal and appears to have no adverse effect on the fetus. Chronic or excessive use, however, can cause a deficiency of vitamin K and other fat-soluble vitamins.

USE DURING BREASTFEEDING: Mineral oil appears to have no adverse effects during breastfeeding.

ALTERNATIVES TO MEDICATIONS: Constipation is one of the most common gastrointestinal complaints during pregnancy even for women who were previously very regular. It is likely caused by the combined factors of pressure from the enlarging uterus and relaxation of intestinal muscles due to pregnancy hormones. Most women can control this problem by the following measures:

- Include some high-fiber cereal, prunes, or figs with breakfast. Do not, however, eat excessive amounts of fiber. It may be irritating to the stomach.
- Drink hot liquid with breakfast. This often has a stimulating effect on the colon.
- Allow plenty of time for appropriate bowel habits in the morning.

GENERIC NAME: **Minocycline**

COMMON BRANDS: Minocin

TYPE OF DRUG: (Prescription) Antibiotic

FDA RISK CATEGORY FOR PREGNANCY: X

GENERAL INFORMATION: Minocycline is a tetracycline-antibiotic used in nonpregnant individuals for treatment of a variety of infections including gonorrhea, respiratory tract infections, Rocky Mountain spotted fever, and traveler's diarrhea. In some cases minocycline has been given to travelers to prevent diarrhea.

USE DURING PREGNANCY: Like other tetracycline-antibiotics, minocycline can cause permanent yellow-brown staining of teeth and abnormal bone development. Staining of teeth is most likely to occur when tetracycline-antibiotics are administered after the twenty-fifth week of pregnancy. In addition, there have been a few reports of fetal malformations when minocycline was administered during the first trimester.

USE DURING BREASTFEEDING: Minocycline is excreted into breast milk and can stain the teeth of breastfed infants. Neither minocycline nor any tetracycline antibiotic should be administered during breastfeeding.

ALTERNATIVES TO MEDICATIONS: Like other tetracycline antibiotics, minocycline should be avoided during pregnancy. Other safer antibiotics are available for the treatment of bacterial infections. Viral illnesses do not require antibiotic therapy.

GENERIC NAME: Minoxidil

COMMON BRANDS: Loniten, Rogaine

TYPE OF DRUG: (Prescription) Antihypertensive, hair-growth stimulant

FDA RISK CATEGORY FOR PREGNANCY: C

GENERAL INFORMATION: Minoxidil is a potent antihypertensive generally reserved for patients whose blood pressure has not been satisfactorily controlled on less potent medications. A topical preparation of minoxidil has recently become available to restore hair growth in patients with hair loss.

POSSIBLE MATERNAL SIDE EFFECTS: The most significant side effects include fluid retention (frequently requiring the addition of a diuretic) and excessive hair growth.

USE DURING PREGNANCY: There has been no evidence of birth defects in laboratory animals treated with minoxidil. However, there is very little experience with its use during human pregnancy. Since its safety cannot be ensured, other antihypertensive medications should be used in place of minoxidil. Topical use has not been studied during pregnancy.

USE DURING BREASTFEEDING: No information is available.

ALTERNATIVES TO MEDICATIONS: Minoxidil is generally reserved for treatment of hypertension resistant to other antihypertensive medications. With a program of weight loss, mild salt restriction, exercise, and cessation of smoking many women can successfully decrease their blood pressure before pregnancy and remain off medications throughout at least the first trimester. However, if antihypertensive medication is necessary, another drug with a proven record of safety during pregnancy (such as methyldopa, p. 215) should be substituted for minoxidil.

GENERIC NAME: # Misoprostol

COMMON BRANDS: Cytotec

TYPE OF DRUG: (Prescription) Antiulcer

FDA RISK CATEGORY FOR PREGNANCY: X

GENERAL INFORMATION: Misoprostol is a newly released medication used for prevention of stomach ulcers in patients being treated with nonsteroidal anti-inflammatory drugs.

POSSIBLE MATERNAL SIDE EFFECTS: The most commonly reported side effect is diarrhea.

USE DURING PREGNANCY: Misoprostol should not be used during any stage of pregnancy. The drug has been shown to cause vaginal bleeding and spontaneous miscarriage. Misoprostol should not be used in a woman of childbearing potential unless she is using effective contraception. A pregnancy test should be performed before beginning therapy to ensure that you are not pregnant.

USE DURING BREASTFEEDING: No information is available.

ALTERNATIVES TO MEDICATIONS: Misoprostol should not be used during pregnancy. As an alternative to taking misoprostol for prevention of gastric irritation from nonsteroidal anti-inflammatory drugs, always take anti-inflammatory medications with food.

GENERIC NAME: # Monoamine oxidase inhibitors

COMMON BRANDS: Eutonyl, Nardil, Parnate

TYPE OF DRUG: (Prescription) Antidepressant

FDA RISK CATEGORY FOR PREGNANCY: C

GENERAL INFORMATION: Monoamine oxidase (MAO) inhibitors are used to treat severe, chronic depression unresponsive to other antidepressant medications. There are several foods and beverages that are incompatible with these medications. A list of incompatible foods should be available to anyone treated for depression with MAO inhibitors.

POSSIBLE MATERNAL SIDE EFFECTS: The most serious adverse reaction due to MAO inhibitors is sudden severe hypertension (hypertensive crisis). Ingestion of food rich in tyramine may provoke a sudden rise in blood pressure. Some of the foods and beverages to avoid include aged cheese (cottage cheese and cream cheese are allowed), yogurt, sausage, liver, pickled herring, wine, and beer. Most over-the-counter cold preparations should also be avoided.

USE DURING PREGNANCY: Although these drugs have been used during pregnancy, their safety has not been established.

USE DURING BREASTFEEDING: No information is available.

ALTERNATIVES TO MEDICATIONS: Depression often gives rise to hopelessness, negativity toward oneself, and at times an inability to carry out normal activities of daily living. Some individuals may become intensely sad or grief-stricken over the loss of someone or something close to them. Others may suffer from chronic depression unrelated to a specific event. In many cases counseling is necessary to truly understand the cause and extent of depression. There are, however, a number of things you can do to deal with depression on your own:

1. Try to identify the specific situation or personal interaction that has caused your sense of hopelessness and negativity.
2. Make a fresh start at correcting the problem. Talk it through. If necessary, repair relationships with previously available support systems. Often family or close friends can serve to reduce your distress.
3. Realize that there are options for most situations. Seldom is there truly "no choice."
4. Understand some of the warning signs that indicate you have

severe depression requiring professional counseling. Such signs include
- Intense sadness, frequent bouts of crying, or depressed mood most of the day,
- Uncharacteristically negative thoughts about yourself,
- Markedly diminished interest or pleasure in most activities,
- Diminished appetite and weight loss,
- Chronic insomnia or sleeping excessively,
- feelings of worthlessness or guilt,
- Persistent fatigue or lack of energy,
- Inability to think or concentrate,
- Thoughts or plans for suicide.
5. Patients with severe depression should not stop taking antidepressant medications without careful psychiatric supervision.

GENERIC NAME: Morphine

COMMON BRANDS: Morphine

TYPE OF DRUG: (Prescription) Narcotic analgesic

FDA RISK CATEGORY FOR PREGNANCY: Not classified

GENERAL INFORMATION: Morphine is a narcotic analgesic used for the control of acute, severe pain. Like all narcotics it has the potential for abuse and addiction. Morphine can be administered orally or by intravenous infusion.

POSSIBLE MATERNAL SIDE EFFECTS: Side effects include nausea, vomiting, dry mouth, dizziness, sedation, confusion, and psychic dependance.

USE DURING PREGNANCY: There has been no reported association between first trimester use of morphine and birth defects. Like all narcotics, however, morphine freely and rapidly crosses the placenta. Use near term may result in addiction of the newborn with subsequent withdrawal symptoms.

USE DURING BREASTFEEDING: Morphine is excreted into breast milk. It would be prudent to wait two or three hours after the last dose before breastfeeding to avoid sedation in the infant.

ALTERNATIVES TO MEDICATIONS: Techniques of natural childbirth such as Lamaze may eliminate the need for narcotics during labor. However, morphine can be safely used to control pain following surgery or after cesarean delivery.

GENERIC NAME: **Mumps vaccine**

COMMON BRANDS: Mumpsvax

TYPE OF DRUG: (Prescription) Live virus vaccine

FDA RISK CATEGORY FOR PREGNANCY: X

GENERAL INFORMATION: Mumps is an inactivated live virus vaccine that promotes active immunity to mumps. It is often combined in a preparation containing measles and rubella vaccines. Its use should be restricted to women who are not pregnant and currently using effective contraception.

POSSIBLE MATERNAL SIDE EFFECTS: Side effects are minimal, but pain at the injection site is common.

USE DURING PREGNANCY: Because mumps vaccine is made from a live virus, the vaccine could theoretically have an adverse effect on the fetus. It should not be administered during pregnancy.

USE DURING BREASTFEEDING: It is not known whether mumps vaccine enters breast milk. No adverse effects have been reported in the newborn.

ALTERNATIVES TO MEDICATIONS: Vaccines made from live virus should not be administered during pregnancy. The only alternative is avoiding contact with infected individuals.

GENERIC NAME: **Nadolol**

COMMON BRANDS: Corgard, Corzide

TYPE OF DRUG: (Prescription) Antihypertensive

FDA RISK CATEGORY FOR PREGNANCY: C

GENERAL INFORMATION: Nadolol is a member of a group of drugs called beta blockers. Beta blockers act by inhibiting a major chemical reaction in the nervous system. Each of these drugs is capable of slowing the heart rate and lowering blood pressure. Their uses in the general population include treatment of high blood pressure, control of abnormal rhythms of the heart, control of acute hyperthyroidism (overactive thyroid gland), relief of angina (heart pain), prevention of migraine headaches, and prevention of acute performance anxiety (stage fright).

POSSIBLE MATERNAL SIDE EFFECTS: Possible side effects include slow heart rate, fatigue, wheezing (in patients with asthma), and depression.

USE DURING PREGNANCY: Beta blockers cross the placenta, but they have not been linked to congenital malformations. A large study of the use of beta blockers during pregnancy revealed no evidence of abnormal fetal growth or development. They are now being used more frequently for the treatment of high blood pressure during pregnancy. Newborn infants of women who took nadolol near delivery should be checked closely in the newborn nursery for slow heart rate and low blood sugar.

USE DURING BREASTFEEDING: Beta blockers are excreted into breast milk and theoretically could slow the baby's heart rate. Nevertheless, the American Academy of Pediatrics considers nadolol and other beta blockers compatible with breastfeeding.

ALTERNATIVES TO MEDICATIONS: With a program of weight loss, mild salt restriction, exercise, and cessation of smoking many women can successfully decrease their blood pressure before pregnancy and remain off medications throughout at least the first trimester. However, if antihypertensive medication is necessary, another drug with a proven record of safety during pregnancy (such as methyldopa, p. 215) should be considered.

GENERIC NAME: Nafcillin

COMMON BRANDS: Nafcil, Nallpen, Unipen

TYPE OF DRUG: (Prescription) Antibiotic

FDA RISK CATEGORY FOR PREGNANCY: B

GENERAL INFORMATION: Nafcillin is a penicillin-type antibiotic effective against infections caused by streptococci, staphylococci, and pneumococci. The drug is usually reserved for infections caused by organisms resistant to ordinary penicillin. Individuals allergic to penicillin will also be allergic to nafcillin.

POSSIBLE MATERNAL SIDE EFFECTS: The most common adverse effect of nafcillin is an allergic reaction manifest by itching, hives, or fever. This antibiotic can also cause acute diarrhea. If diarrhea occurs, nafcillin should be discontinued immediately and a physician notified. Rarely, kidney damage can result from treatment with nafcillin. Diagnosis of kidney damage usually requires a blood test or urinalysis.

USE DURING PREGNANCY: Nafcillin crosses the placenta but less readily than penicillin. This antibiotic has not been shown to cause birth defects or any other fetal harm and is considered safe for use during any stage of pregnancy.

USE DURING BREASTFEEDING: Similar to other penicillin-type antibiotics, nafcillin enters breast milk. Although it is considered safe for use during breastfeeding, small amounts in breast milk are capable of causing diarrhea in the newborn.

ALTERNATIVES TO MEDICATIONS: Nafcillin is usually reserved for serious infections due to penicillin-resistant staphylococci. There are no nonpharmacologic alternatives to nafcillin for serious infections, but for some infections less expensive antibiotics may be substituted.

GENERIC NAME: **Nalidixic acid**

COMMON BRANDS: NegGram

TYPE OF DRUG: (Prescription) Antibiotic

FDA RISK CATEGORY FOR PREGNANCY: B

GENERAL INFORMATION: Nalidixic acid is a commonly used antibiotic for the treatment of uncomplicated urinary tract infections.

POSSIBLE MATERNAL SIDE EFFECTS: Side effects are generally mini-

230

mal. However, there are some special circumstances in which the drug should be avoided. The manufacturer advises that nalidixic acid not be given to individuals with epilepsy because the drug can theoretically cause seizures. In addition, blacks with a known enzyme deficiency called glucose-6-phosphate dehydrogenase (G-6-PD) deficiency should avoid this antibiotic because it can cause a sudden destruction of red blood cells in these individuals.

USE DURING PREGNANCY: There are no reports in the medical literature of birth defects caused by the use of nalidixic acid during pregnancy. Consequently, the drug has been classified by the FDA in risk category B for use during pregnancy. Other chemically similar antibiotics (ciprofloxacin, p. 110 and norfloxacin, p. 237), however, have been shown to cause abnormalities of bones and joints when given to immature animals. Because of this theoretical risk and the availability of safer antibiotics, nalidixic acid should generally be avoided during pregnancy.

USE DURING BREASTFEEDING: Nalidixic acid is excreted into breast milk in small amounts. Its effect on the newborn is not known. Safer antibiotics should generally be used.

ALTERNATIVES TO MEDICATIONS: Although there are no non-pharmacologic alternatives to antibiotics for the treatment of acute urinary tract infections, other antibiotics are more appropriate for use during pregnancy.

GENERIC NAME: **Naloxone**

COMMON BRANDS: Narcan

TYPE OF DRUG: (Prescription) Narcotic antagonist

FDA RISK CATEGORY FOR PREGNANCY: B

GENERAL INFORMATION: Naloxone is a narcotic antagonist used to reverse the effects of narcotic overdose. The drug can effectively reverse the effects of illicit narcotics or excessive narcotic administration during surgical anesthesia. It must be administered by injection.

POSSIBLE MATERNAL SIDE EFFECTS: Administration of naloxone to a narcotic addict, including an addicted newborn, can cause acute narcotic withdrawal symptoms. The drug should be given with caution in any individual suspected of addiction. Nevertheless, its use may be life saving in patients whose breathing is impaired by narcotic overdose.

USE DURING PREGNANCY: Naloxone has been approved for the treatment of narcotic overdose during pregnancy. It can also be used for treatment of respiratory distress in a newborn whose mother took illicit narcotics or was treated with narcotic analgesics during labor and delivery. Newborn infants of narcotic addicts may themselves be addicted and manifest signs of withdrawal following treatment with naloxone. Such infants require careful observation.

USE DURING BREASTFEEDING: It is not known whether naloxone is excreted into breast milk. Because the drug can be life saving, it should not be withheld because of breastfeeding.

ALTERNATIVES TO MEDICATIONS: There is no nonpharmacologic alternative to naloxone for the treatment of narcotic overdose.

GENERIC NAME: **Naproxen**

COMMON BRANDS: Anaprox, Naprosyn

TYPE OF DRUG: (Prescription) Anti-inflammatory

FDA RISK CATEGORY FOR PREGNANCY: B

GENERAL INFORMATION: Naproxen is a member of a class of drugs called nonsteroidal anti-inflammatory drugs (NSAIDs). It is indicated for the treatment of arthritis, muscle pain, headache, and pain associated with menstruation.

POSSIBLE MATERNAL SIDE EFFECTS: The most common side effects are nausea and abdominal pain. Rarely, naproxen can irritate the stomach and cause an ulcer or bleeding from the stomach.

USE DURING PREGNANCY: There have been no reports linking naproxen to birth defects when the drug was used during the first trimester. However, experience with the drug during early pregnancy is limited.

Used near term naproxen can have potential effects on pregnancy and the fetus. First, the drug can cause premature closure of an important blood vessel in the fetus called the ductus arteriosus. Normally, this blood vessel does not close until after delivery. Premature closure could result in a serious condition called pulmonary hypertension. Second, naproxen and other NSAIDs can inhibit labor and prolong pregnancy.

USE DURING BREASTFEEDING: Naproxen enters human breast milk, but its effect on the newborn is not known. The drug's safety during breastfeeding cannot be ensured.

ALTERNATIVES TO MEDICATIONS: Musculoskeletal pain can often be relieved with warm baths and massage. Painful arthritis can be alleviated by rest, heat, and physical therapy. Nonweight-bearing exercise such as swimming may offer some comfort while enhancing muscle tone. If medication is necessary, acetaminophen (p. 63) is probably the safest medication to take during pregnancy for relief of minor pain.

GENERIC NAME: Nicotine polacrilex

COMMON BRANDS: Nicorette

TYPE OF DRUG: (Prescription) Smoking cessation aid

FDA RISK CATEGORY FOR PREGNANCY: X

GENERAL INFORMATION: Nicotine gum can be used as a temporary aid in a program of smoking cessation. It should be used only under medical supervision. In general, smokers who have a high "physical" type of dependence are most likely to benefit from the use of nicotine chewing gum.

POSSIBLE MATERNAL SIDE EFFECTS: Side effects include nausea, hiccups, jaw muscle aches, palpitations, and lightheadedness.

USE DURING PREGNANCY: Nicotine gum should be avoided during pregnancy. Nicotine in any form may be harmful to the fetus. Birth defects have been linked to first-trimester use of nicotine. Use during later pregnancy can interfere with normal growth.

USE DURING BREASTFEEDING: Because nicotine freely enters breast milk, nicotine chewing gum should be avoided during breastfeeding.

ALTERNATIVES TO MEDICATIONS: Unfortunately, there is no easy way to stop smoking. Pregnancy should provide the motivation to enroll in a supervised smoking cessation program. Every effort should be made to quit.

GENERIC NAME: **Nifedipine**

COMMON BRANDS: Procardia

TYPE OF DRUG: (Prescription) Antihypertensive, antiarrhythmic

FDA RISK CATEGORY FOR PREGNANCY: C

GENERAL INFORMATION: Nifedipine is a member of a class of medication known as calcium-channel blockers. Calcium-channel blockers are used to treat hypertension (high blood pressure), abnormal rhythms of the heart, and angina pectoris (heart pain). These drugs are also capable of suppressing spontaneous contractions of the uterus.

POSSIBLE MATERNAL SIDE EFFECTS: The most common side effects are constipation, drowsiness, headache, and fatigue. Blood pressure must be checked frequently to ensure that it does not fall too low.

USE DURING PREGNANCY: Nifedipine and other calcium-channel blockers have not been used extensively during pregnancy in the United States. Other antihypertensive medications that have been used for many years during pregnancy are usually given in preference to this newer class of drugs. Nifedipine can be absorbed from under the tongue for rapid reduction of high blood pressure. In addition, recent studies have suggested that calcium-channel blockers may be useful for treatment of premature labor.

USE DURING BREASTFEEDING: Experience with calcium-channel blockers in breastfeeding is limited. However, there are no reports of adverse effects.

ALTERNATIVES TO MEDICATIONS: With a program of weight loss, mild salt restriction, exercise, and cessation of smoking many women can successfully decrease their blood pressure before pregnancy and remain off medications throughout at least the first trimester. However, if antihypertensive medication is necessary, another drug with a proven record of safety during pregnancy (such as methyldopa, p. 215) should be substituted for nifedipine.

GENERIC NAME: Nitrofurantoin

COMMON BRANDS: Furadantin, Macrodantin

TYPE OF DRUG: (Prescription) Antibiotic

FDA RISK CATEGORY FOR PREGNANCY: B

GENERAL INFORMATION: Nitrofurantoin is most often used to treat uncomplicated urinary tract infections. Patients with recurrent infections or infections due to uncommon organisms are usually treated with an antibiotic known to have broader antibacterial coverage.

POSSIBLE MATERNAL SIDE EFFECTS: The most common side effect is nausea. This effect can be minimized by taking the drug with food or milk. Black women with a known enzyme deficiency called glucose-6-phosphate dehydrogenase (G-6-PD) deficiency should avoid this antibiotic because it can cause a sudden destruction of red blood cells in these individuals.

USE DURING PREGNANCY: Use of nitrofurantoin during pregnancy has not been associated with birth defects or other fetal harm. It is considered safe for use during pregnancy.

USE DURING BREASTFEEDING: Nitrofurantoin is excreted into breast milk in small amounts. It is generally considered safe for use during breastfeeding.

ALTERNATIVES TO MEDICATIONS: There is no nonpharmacologic alternative to antibiotics for the treatment of acute urinary tract infection. Nitrofurantoin is considered safe for use during pregnancy.

GENERIC NAME: Nizatidine

COMMON BRANDS: Axid

TYPE OF DRUG: (Prescription) Antiulcer agent

FDA RISK CATEGORY FOR PREGNANCY: C

GENERAL INFORMATION: Nizatidine is used for the treatment of stomach (gastric) and intestinal (duodenal) ulcers. It works by inhibiting the production of acid in the stomach.

POSSIBLE MATERNAL SIDE EFFECTS: The drug is usually well tolerated, but sweating, hives, and drowsiness have been reported in some patients.

USE DURING PREGNANCY: Since nizatidine is a relatively new drug, there is very little experience with its use during human pregnancy. Reproductive studies in rats using dosages up to 300 times the human dosage did not demonstrate any evidence of birth defects or fetal harm. Other drugs, such as antacids (p. 78), are available for treatment of ulcers during pregnancy.

USE DURING BREASTFEEDING: Nizatidine is excreted into breast milk and may inhibit the production of stomach acid in the breastfed infant. The drug should be avoided during breastfeeding.

ALTERNATIVES TO MEDICATIONS: A program of dietary restriction, alone, is generally not adequate for treatment of stomach or intestinal ulcers. However, an alternative to nizatidine during pregnancy is the regular use of antacids (p. 78) between meals.

GENERIC NAME: **Nonoxynol-9**

COMMON BRANDS: Semicid Vaginal Contraceptive, Today Vaginal Contraceptive

TYPE OF DRUG: (Over-the-counter) Contraceptive

FDA RISK CATEGORY FOR PREGNANCY: Not applicable

GENERAL INFORMATION: Spermicides provide a safe, non-systematic form of birth control. These compounds work by killing sperm before they can reach the egg. The most commonly used spermicide—Nonoxynol-9—can be used in a cream combined with a condom or diaphragm, or in a vaginal sponge or insert.

POSSIBLE MATERNAL SIDE EFFECTS: A small number of men and women can be sensitive to spermicides and should not use them if irritation occurs and persists.

USE DURING PREGNANCY: Since spermicides are intended to prevent pregnancy, they have no use once pregnancy is diagnosed. As soon as pregnancy is suspected, even before it is confirmed by a test, use of spermicides should be stopped. It is estimated that between 300,000 and 600,000 women each year use spermicides around the time of conception and during early pregnancy. Fortunately, review of several large studies and the most recent scientific evidence suggest that there is no link between the use of spermicides during the first trimester and birth defects.

USE DURING BREASTFEEDING: Spermicides can be used safely during breastfeeding.

ALTERNATIVES TO MEDICATIONS: If pregnancy is desired, contraception of any kind is not appropriate. However, the use of spermicides in various contraceptive products is safe.

GENERIC NAME: **Norfloxacin**

COMMON BRANDS: Noroxin

TYPE OF DRUG: (Prescription) Antibiotic

FDA RISK CATEGORY FOR PREGNANCY: C

GENERAL INFORMATION: Norfloxacin is a relatively new antibiotic used for the treatment of urinary tract and respiratory infections.

POSSIBLE MATERNAL SIDE EFFECTS: Norfloxacin is generally well tolerated. The most frequently reported side effect is mild nausea.

USE DURING PREGNANCY: There is very little experience with norfloxacin during human pregnancy. Reproductive studies have been performed in mice and rats and have not demonstrated any link between the drug and birth defects. However, norfloxacin and chemically similar antibiotics (ciprofloxacin, p. 110, and nalidixic acid, p. 230) have been shown to cause abnormalities of bones and joints in immature animals. Because of this theoretical risk and the availability of safer antibiotics, norfloxacin should generally be avoided during pregnancy.

USE DURING BREASTFEEDING: It is not known if norfloxacin is excreted into breast milk. Because other safe antibiotics are available, it should generally be avoided during breastfeeding.

ALTERNATIVES TO MEDICATIONS: For the treatment of serious bacterial infections there are no nonpharmacologic alternatives. There are, however, several antibiotics with a longer record of safety during pregnancy that can be substituted for norfloxacin.

GENERIC NAME: Nortriptyline

COMMON BRANDS: Pamelor

TYPE OF DRUG: (Prescription) Antidepressant

FDA RISK CATEGORY FOR PREGNANCY: D

GENERAL INFORMATION: Nortriptyline is a member of a group of drugs called tricyclic antidepressants. It is effective for the treatment of chronic depression. The drug can elevate mood, improve appetite, relieve insomnia, and increase physical activity. Therapy is usually begun with a low dosage and gradually increased to a therapeutic level. Beneficial effects are not usually seen until two to four weeks after treatment has begun.

POSSIBLE MATERNAL SIDE EFFECTS: Side effects include drowsiness, blurred vision, dry mouth, constipation, weight gain, low blood pressure, and abnormal rhythms of the heart.

USE DURING PREGNANCY: Like other tricyclic antidepressants, nortriptyline has been associated with a variety of birth defects. These drugs should be avoided during pregnancy unless major depression cannot be satisfactorily managed in any other way.

USE DURING BREASTFEEDING: Nortriptyline enters breast milk in small quantities, but its effect on the newborn is not known.

ALTERNATIVES TO MEDICATIONS: Depression often gives rise to hopelessness, negativity toward oneself, and at times an inability to carry out normal activities of daily living. Some individuals may become intensely sad or grief-stricken over the loss of someone or something close to them. Others may suffer from chronic depression unrelated to a specific event. In many cases counseling is necessary to truly understand the cause and extent of depression. There are, however, a number of things you can do to deal with depression on your own:

1. Try to identify the specific situation or personal interaction that has caused your sense of hopelessness and negativity.
2. Make a fresh start at correcting the problem. Talk it through. If necessary, repair relationships with previously available support systems. Often family or close friends can serve to reduce your distress.
3. Realize that there are options for most situations. Seldom is there truly "no choice."
4. Understand some of the warning signs that indicate you have severe depression requiring professional counseling. Such signs include
   • Intense sadness, frequent bouts of crying, or depressed mood most of the day,
   • Uncharacteristically negative thoughts about yourself,
   • Markedly diminished interest or pleasure in most activities,
   • Diminished appetite and weight loss,
   • Chronic insomnia or sleeping excessively,
   • Feelings of worthlessness or guilt,
   • Persistent fatigue or lack of energy,
   • Inability to think or concentrate,
   • Thoughts or plans for suicide.
5. Patients with severe depression should not stop taking antidepressant medications without careful psychiatric supervision.

GENERIC NAME: Nystatin

COMMON BRANDS: Mycolog, Mycostatin, Mytrex, Nilstat, Nystatin, Nystex

TYPE OF DRUG: (Prescription) Antifungal

FDA RISK CATEGORY FOR PREGNANCY: B

GENERAL INFORMATION: Nystatin is applied topically for the treatment of vaginal or skin fungal infections. Only a small amount of the drug is absorbed systemically following vaginal application.

POSSIBLE MATERNAL SIDE EFFECTS: Side effects are usually limited to vaginal itching.

USE DURING PREGNANCY: Nystatin is considered safe for topical use during pregnancy. There have been no reports linking the drug with birth defects or other fetal harm. The drug should not be used, however, once the membranes have ruptured. Intravenous use of nystatin has not been satisfactorily studied during pregnancy.

USE DURING BREASTFEEDING: Topical application of nystatin during breastfeeding has not been shown to cause any harm to the newborn.

ALTERNATIVES TO MEDICATIONS: To help avoid vaginal yeast infections do not take antibiotics unnecessarily, wear loose cotton underwear, avoid harsh soaps and irritants, and be sure your partner does not have a chronic yeast infection. During pregnancy it is not always necessary to treat mild yeast infections.

GENERIC NAME: Oxazepam

COMMON BRANDS: Serax

TYPE OF DRUG: (Prescription) Antianxiety, sedative

FDA RISK CATEGORY FOR PREGNANCY: D

GENERAL INFORMATION: Oxazepam is a member of a group of antianxiety medications called benzodiazepines. These drugs are used for the treatment of anxiety and insomnia. They work by relaxing skeletal muscles and by a direct action on the brain.

Benzodiazepines can be abused if taken indiscriminately or for a long period of time. Withdrawal symptoms including tremor, agitation, insomnia, muscle cramps, nausea, and seizures can occur if these drugs are discontinued abruptly after chronic use. Benzodiazepines should not be taken without careful medical supervision.

POSSIBLE MATERNAL SIDE EFFECTS: Common side effects with all benzodiazepines include sedation, depression, mental confusion, dizziness, unsteady gait, nightmares, fatigue, dry mouth, and low blood pressure. These drugs can interfere with the ability to safely drive a car or operate dangerous equipment. Physical and psychological dependence can occur with chronic use.

USE DURING PREGNANCY: All benzodiazepines rapidly cross the placenta and enter the fetal circulation. Blood levels in the fetus equal that of the mother's within one hour of taking a pill. Several studies have demonstrated a link between first-trimester use of benzodiazepines and birth defects. The most commonly reported

240

malformations are cleft lip and cleft palate. Used near term benzodiazepines have been associated with lethargy, respiratory problems, and withdrawal symptoms in the newborn. Most authorities believe that it is best to avoid these medications during the first trimester and if possible throughout pregnancy.

USE DURING BREASTFEEDING: Benzodiazepines are excreted into breast milk in significant quantities. They can cause sedation in the newborn and should be avoided during breastfeeding.

ALTERNATIVES TO MEDICATIONS: Before using medications to control anxiety or stress consider the following strategy:

1. Identify the source of your anxiety. Worry often persists because of an inability to identify a problem and take action to solve it. Visualization can begin the process. Close your eyes and take a few deep breaths. Allow an image of the problem to arise.
2. Once you've defined the source of your anxiety, gather information. For example, if you are worried about the outcome of your pregnancy because of a possible hereditary problem or a medication you took before you knew you were pregnant, get information from your physician or a genetic counselor. In most cases what you discover will be very comforting.
3. After obtaining information, decide on a plan of action. Do what you can to deal with the problem, but once you've done all you can, change your focus and move on to other parts of life. Instead of worrying, concentrate on your life beyond the worry. Exercise or take walks. Plan how you will spend the evening or the weekend. Treat yourself to something pleasant, or think up a surprise for someone you care about. As your mind gets busy with other thoughts, you'll find that stress will begin to fade.
4. If anxiety persists despite your best efforts, see a therapist. Often only a few counseling sessions can effectively reduce anxiety and stress and eliminate the need for medication.

GENERIC NAME: Oxtriphylline

COMMON BRANDS: Choledyl

TYPE OF DRUG: (Prescription) Bronchodilator

FDA RISK CATEGORY FOR PREGNANCY: C

GENERAL INFORMATION: Oxtriphylline is a member of a class of medications called theophyllines (p. 292) commonly used in the management of asthma. It works by relaxing the muscles of the bronchial tubes thereby allowing air to move freely and relieving the wheezing and shortness of breath associated with acute asthma.

POSSIBLE MATERNAL SIDE EFFECTS: The side effects of oxtriphylline are common to all theophylline medications (p. 292). They include restlessness, headache, insomnia, palpitations, and nausea. If any of these side effects continue more than a few days, the drug should be discontinued and a physician notified. Levels of the medications can be measured in the blood to determine if the dosage is excessive. Drinking caffeine-containing beverages may worsen side effects and should be limited or avoided while taking these medications.

USE DURING PREGNANCY: Similar to other theophylline drugs, oxtriphylline crosses the placenta and enters the fetal circulation. A large study of pregnant women with asthma demonstrated no harm to the baby when theophylline was taken during any stage of pregnancy. Immediately after birth, however, newborns will have significant concentrations of the drug in their blood and may manifest restlessness, irritability, rapid heart rate, or nausea. These adverse effects generally last no longer than 24 hours and do not cause any permanent harm.

USE DURING BREASTFEEDING: Theophylline drugs, including oxtriphylline, enter breast milk and can cause irritability, restlessness, and poor feeding in the newborn. Although these symptoms should be looked for in the newborn, it is felt that taking a theophylline medication for asthma is compatible with breastfeeding.

ALTERNATIVES TO MEDICATIONS: In some cases asthma can be prevented by avoidance of known allergens, particularly animals. If you smoke, stop. It is generally a good rule, however, to use a bronchodilating inhaler at the earliest indication of wheezing. Often prompt effective relief of asthma can prevent minor episodes from becoming more severe and prolonged.

GENERIC NAME: Oxycodone

COMMON BRANDS: Percocet, Percodan, Roxicet, Roxicodone, Roxiprin, Tylox

TYPE OF DRUG: (Prescription) Narcotic analgesic

FDA RISK CATEGORY FOR PREGNANCY: C

GENERAL INFORMATION: Oxycodone is a synthetic narcotic analgesic effective when taken orally. It is usually combined with aspirin (Percodan) or acetaminophen (Percocet). Use of oxycodone should be limited to no longer than a few days for the relief of moderate to severe pain.

POSSIBLE MATERNAL SIDE EFFECTS: Common side effects include nausea, lightheadedness, dizziness, insomnia, and blurred vision. Chronic use can result in drug dependence or addiction.

USE DURING PREGNANCY: Although there have been no reports of birth defects caused by first-trimester use of oxycodone, there has been relatively little experience with the drug during pregnancy. Similar to other narcotics, chronic use of oxycodone can result in addiction to the drug and withdrawal symptoms in the newborn. Used near the time of delivery, the drug can interfere with normal breathing in the infant.

USE DURING BREASTFEEDING: Oxycodone probably enters breast milk and can cause sedation in the breastfed infant. If the drug must be taken during breastfeeding, it is best to breastfeed immediately before taking a dose.

ALTERNATIVES TO MEDICATIONS: Use of hypnosis or relaxation techniques may be helpful for controlling pain. However, oxycodone may be used for relief of severe pain.

GENERIC NAME: **Oxytocin**

COMMON BRANDS: Pitocin, Syntocinon

TYPE OF DRUG: (Prescription) Uterine stimulant

FDA RISK CATEGORY FOR PREGNANCY: Not applicable

GENERAL INFORMATION: Oxytocin is used to initiate or improve uterine contractions in certain pregnant women. Its use is indicated when a medical or obstetric problem requires delivery before the onset of spontaneous labor or to improve the strength of spontaneous uterine contractions when they are not adequate for delivery. The drug should not be used merely for the convenience of the patient or obstetrician in selecting the time of delivery.

POSSIBLE MATERNAL SIDE EFFECTS: When oxytocin is carefully supervised by a obstetrician and obstetric nurse, side effects are minimal. Most notable is the discomfort that accompanies uterine contractions.

USE DURING PREGNANCY: Oxytocin is indicated for induction of labor in patients with such disorders as diabetes, Rh problems, and preeclampsia. Many women with these problems need to be delivered before term to prevent harm to the baby or even stillbirth. There are several circumstances where oxytocin may not be effective or cannot be safely used. In such cases cesarean delivery may be necessary.

USE DURING BREASTFEEDING: Minimal amounts of the drug enter breast milk.

ALTERNATIVES TO MEDICATIONS: For most women normal contractions during labor are sufficient to result in delivery. In some cases oxytocin must be used to induce labor or to improve the strength of contractions.

GENERIC NAME: Penicillin

COMMON BRANDS: Amoxil (Amoxicillin), Dynapen (Dicloxacillin), Geopen (Carbenicillin), Omnipen (Ampicillin), Bicillin (Penicillin G), Penicillin V

TYPE OF DRUG: (Prescription) Antibiotic

FDA RISK CATEGORY FOR PREGNANCY: B

GENERAL INFORMATION: There are many natural and synthetic penicillin antibiotics used for the treatment of various infectious diseases. Penicillin is not, however, effective against viruses. Often bacteria responsible for an infection must be cultured and tested in a laboratory to determine the best penicillin preparation or other antibiotic for treatment.

POSSIBLE MATERNAL SIDE EFFECTS: Penicillins are usually well tolerated. Antibiotics should be discontinued immediately if general-

244

ized itching or hives occur. Alternative drugs are available for individuals allergic to penicillin.

USE DURING PREGNANCY: Penicillins have been used extensively to treat infections during pregnancy. They have not been shown to cause any adverse effects in the fetus and are considered safe for use throughout pregnancy.

USE DURING BREASTFEEDING: Penicillins are excreted into breast milk but pose no special problems for the newborn.

ALTERNATIVES TO MEDICATIONS: There are no alternatives to antibiotics for the treatment of bacterial infections. When an antibiotic is needed during pregnancy, penicillin is a safe choice.

GENERIC NAME: Phenazopyridine

COMMON BRANDS: Pyridium, Urobiotic-250

TYPE OF DRUG: (Prescription) Urinary analgesic

FDA RISK CATEGORY FOR PREGNANCY: B

GENERAL INFORMATION: Phenazopyridine is used to reduce the pain, burning, and urinary frequency associated with an acute bladder infection. It does not cure an infection and therefore must be given with an antibiotic. The drug can usually be discontinued after the second day of antibiotic therapy.

POSSIBLE MATERNAL SIDE EFFECTS: Side effects are usually minimal. The drug will color the urine red or orange, which may stain fabrics.

USE DURING PREGNANCY: There have been no reports linking phenazopyridine with birth defects or fetal harm. It is considered safe for use during pregnancy. Effective treatment of urinary infections is especially important during pregnancy. Merely alleviating symptoms with an analgesic like phenazopyridine does not adequately treat an infection. An antibiotic must be used in addition.

USE DURING BREASTFEEDING: No information is available.

ALTERNATIVES TO MEDICATIONS: It is not necessary to take phenazopyridine for the treatment of an acute urinary tract infection, since the drug does not contribute to healing. Symptoms usually abate within 24 to 48 hours of beginning antibiotics.

GENERIC NAME: Phencyclidine

COMMON BRANDS: PCP

TYPE OF DRUG: (Illicit) Hallucinogen

FDA RISK CATEGORY FOR PREGNANCY: X

GENERAL INFORMATION: There is no legitimate use for this hallucinogenic drug.

POSSIBLE MATERNAL SIDE EFFECTS: Adverse effects are common and potentially severe. They include hallucinations and irrational behavior including violence. Overdose can result in death.

USE DURING PREGNANCY: Phencyclidine should not be used during pregnancy. It has been associated with several birth defects including abnormalities of the face. Newborns may manifest a variety of behavioral and feeding problems.

USE DURING BREASTFEEDING: The drug is excreted into breast milk and should not be taken during breastfeeding.

ALTERNATIVES TO MEDICATIONS: Phencyclidine must not be used during pregnancy.

GENERIC NAME: Phenmetrazine

COMMON BRANDS: Preludin

TYPE OF DRUG: (Prescription) Appetite suppressant, stimulant

FDA Risk Category For Pregnancy: C

GENERAL INFORMATION: Phenmetrazine is used primarily as an appetite suppressant. It has several chemical properties similar to amphetamines and other stimulants. Therefore, it has considerable

246

potential for abuse. Possible side effects of the drug include rapid heart rate, irregular rhythms of the heart, and elevation of blood pressure.

POSSIBLE MATERNAL SIDE EFFECTS: Common side effects include nervousness, irritability, insomnia, palpitations, and high blood pressure.

USE DURING PREGNANCY: The drug has not been shown to cause birth defects in animals or humans. Nevertheless, it has no use during pregnancy. Calorie-restricted diets are not recommended during pregnancy; therefore, there is no need to take any medication designed to suppress appetite. Moreover, use of phenmetrazine near the time of delivery can result in withdrawal symptoms in the newborn.

USE DURING BREASTFEEDING: Phenmetrazine is excreted into breast milk and can cause poor feeding and rapid heart rate in breastfed infants. This drug should not be used during breastfeeding.

ALTERNATIVES TO MEDICATIONS: Careful nutritional counseling and planning before pregnancy should allow most women to attain ideal body weight before conception. Pregnancy is not the time to begin a calorie-restricted diet. Weight loss during pregnancy can have seriously detrimental effects on the growth and development of the baby. Excessive weight gain during pregnancy can be managed with a carefully planned diet complete with the nutrients essential for gestation.

GENERIC NAME: Phenobarbital

COMMON BRANDS: Luminal, Solfoton, and various combination products

TYPE OF DRUG: (Prescription) Anticonvulsant, sedative

FDA RISK CATEGORY FOR PREGNANCY: D

GENERAL INFORMATION: Phenobarbital, alone or combined with phenytoin (p. 252), is used to suppress major and minor epileptic seizures. It works by blocking nerve impulses in the brain. The drug can also be used as a sedative for treatment of some anxiety disorders and in patients with preeclampsia. Additionally, several combination drug preparations used to treat functional bowel syndrome (spastic colon) or asthma contain significant amounts of phenobarbital as a secondary ingredient.

POSSIBLE MATERNAL SIDE EFFECTS: The most common side effects are drowsiness, lethargy, and confusion.

USE DURING PREGNANCY: The use of phenobarbital during pregnancy remains controversial. Since 1964 it has been recognized that first-trimester use of the drug can cause a variety of fetal malformations. It is also acknowledged that epileptic seizures (possibly resulting from discontinuing anticonvulsant medication) can be associated with fetal death, birth defects, and harm to the mother. With this dilemma in mind most authorities and the American College of Obstetricians and Gynecologists recommend the following:

1. All women with epilepsy whether or not they are taking anticonvulsant medication should consult their physician before attempting pregnancy or just as soon as pregnancy is suspected.
2. Women who have been free of seizures for several years should consult their physician to see whether medication can be discontinued before pregnancy. Some anticonvulsant medications are considered safer than others, and at least a change in medications may be appropriate.
3. Women with recurrent seizures should not stop taking their medications when they find out they are pregnant without first consulting a physician. The risk to both mother and baby is greater from a major epileptic seizure than from taking medication. Even if phenobarbital must be taken during the first trimester, the chance of having a normal baby is approximately 90 percent.
4. The use of anticonvulsant medications during pregnancy requires careful medical follow-up. Blood levels of the drugs should be checked frequently, generally monthly, to ensure that the dosage is effective and not toxic.
5. The pediatrician should be notified before delivery if anticonvulsants were prescribed during pregnancy so the baby can be checked immediately for any problems.

USE DURING BREASTFEEDING: Phenobarbital is excreted into breast milk in significant amounts and can cause sedation in the newborn. Although the American Academy of Pediatrics considers phenobarbital compatible with breastfeeding, careful follow-up of the baby is essential.

248

ALTERNATIVES TO MEDICATIONS: When phenobarbital is being given to prevent seizures, it should not be discontinued without consulting a physician. If it is being taken for anxiety or sedation, strong consideration should be given to discontinuing the drug during or, ideally, before pregnancy.

Insomnia may be relieved by some of the following techniques:

- Generally, try to avoid daytime naps. However, for some women sleeping patterns change during pregnancy, and a nap may be necessary to supplement abbreviated nighttime sleep.
- Go to bed only when tired. Instead of lying in bed when you are wide awake, get up, do something, and then return to bed when you feel tired.
- Try to establish a regular sleep pattern. Recognize when you *are* able to sleep and build on that.
- Exercise daily. Even a 30-minute walk will aid relaxation.
- Learn techniques of progressive relaxation. These techniques are simple to learn and effective.
- Avoid stimulant drinks such as coffee, tea, and caffeine-containing colas. On the other hand, warm milk may help make you sleepy.
- Never use alcohol to induce sleep.
- If you awaken during the night, recall the dream just before you awoke. Reentering the dream can return you to sleep.
- Make love. Sex is relaxing and often ends with sleep.
- If you are lying awake because a problem is on your mind, talk it through with someone until it's resolved.

GENERIC NAME: **Phenolphthalein**

COMMON BRANDS: Alophen, Correctol, Evac-U-Lax, Ex-Lax, Feen-a-Mint, Modane, Phenolax, Phillips' LaxCaps, Prulet

TYPE OF DRUG: (Over-the-counter) Laxative

FDA RISK CATEGORY FOR PREGNANCY: Not classified

GENERAL INFORMATION: Phenolphthalein is a stimulant laxative that acts primarily on the large intestine to produce a semifluid stool usually in four to eight hours.

POSSIBLE MATERNAL SIDE EFFECTS: The most common side effect is diarrhea from excessive use. Long-term use of phenolphthalein can cause chronic colon problems and malabsorption of important nutrients. Diarrhea due to phenolphthalein can cause premature labor.

USE DURING PREGNANCY: There have been no medical reports of birth defects or fetal harm from occasional use of phenolphthalein during pregnancy. Nevertheless, relief of constipation is best achieved through proper diet and exercise.

USE DURING BREASTFEEDING: Phenolphthalein is excreted into breast milk but has not been demonstrated to cause any harm to the newborn.

ALTERNATIVES TO MEDICATIONS: Constipation is one of the most common gastrointestinal complaints during pregnancy even for women who were previously very regular. It is likely caused by the combined factors of pressure from the enlarging uterus and relaxation of intestinal muscle due to pregnancy hormones. Most women can control this problem by the following measures:

- Include some high-fiber cereal, prunes, or figs with breakfast. Do not, however, eat excessive amounts of fiber. It may be irritating to the stomach.
- Drink hot liquid with breakfast. This often has a stimulating effect on the colon.
- Allow plenty of time for appropriate bowel habits in the morning.

GENERIC NAME: **Phenylephrine (nasal spray)**

COMMON BRANDS: Allerest, Donatussin Drops, Dristan Nasal Spray, Neo-Synephrine, Sinex

TYPE OF DRUG: (Over-the-counter) Nasal decongestant

FDA RISK CATEGORY FOR PREGNANCY: C

GENERAL INFORMATION: Phenylephrine acts topically on the mucosa (lining) of the nose to decrease mucus production. It is frequently used to treat the runny nose associated with a viral respiratory infection. The drug should not be used longer than 48 hours because chronic use can lead to dependency. Therefore, it should not be used to treat chronic allergic rhinitis.

POSSIBLE MATERNAL SIDE EFFECTS: Even nasal preparations of phenylephrine can cause systemic side effects. The most common are restlessness, insomnia, headache, dizziness, palpitations, elevated blood pressure, and nausea. Prolonged or chronic use may result in rebound nasal congestion and chronic swelling of nasal mucosa. To reduce the risk of rebound congestion, nasal drops or sprays should be used sparingly, in the lowest effective concentration, and for no longer than 48 hours.

USE DURING PREGNANCY: The safety of phenylephrine during the first trimester cannot be ensured. The Collaborative Perinatal Project reported a slight increased incidence of minor birth defects in the offspring of women who used phenylephrine during the first trimester. Nevertheless, most authorities believe that occasional use of phenylephrine nasal decongestant is unlikely to harm the fetus. Nasal sprays should not be used to treat persistent nasal congestion frequently associated with normal pregnancy.

USE DURING BREASTFEEDING: It is not known whether phenylephrine in nasal sprays is excreted in breast milk. It should be used with caution during breastfeeding.

ALTERNATIVES TO MEDICATIONS: Saline (salt water) nasal sprays or inhalation of steam can often provide temporary relief of nasal congestion without risk of dependency.

GENERIC NAME: Phenylpropanolamine

COMMON BRANDS: A.R.M. Allergy Relief Medicine, Acutrim, Allerest, Bayer Children's Cough Syrup, Cheracol, Contac, Coricidin, Dexatrim, Dimetapp, Entex, Naldecon, Ornade, Robitussin-CF, Sinarest, Sine-Off, Tavist-D, Triaminic, Triaminicin, Trind, Tuss-Ornade

TYPE OF DRUG: (Over-the-counter and prescription) Appetite suppressant, decongestant

FDA RISK CATEGORY FOR PREGNANCY: C

GENERAL INFORMATION: Phenylpropanolamine, often combined with an antihistamine (p. 79), is an active ingredient in several over-the-counter cold and allergy preparations. The drug has also been shown to suppress appetite and is marketed over-the-counter as a "diet pill" for weight reduction.

POSSIBLE MATERNAL SIDE EFFECTS: Common side effects include dizziness, headache, restlessness, insomnia, loss of appetite, and palpitations. Elevation in blood pressure can also occur.

USE DURING PREGNANCY: There have been several isolated reports of birth defects in infants of mothers who took phenylpropanolamine during the first trimester. However, it has not been possible to clearly establish any link between phenylpropanolamine and malformations since the drug is frequently combined with other active ingredients. Because its safety cannot be ensured, it is best to avoid this medication during the first trimester. Women with chronic hypertension or preeclampsia should not take phenylpropanolamine because it could cause further elevation of blood pressure. Its use as an appetite suppressant for weight reduction has no place during pregnancy.

USE DURING BREASTFEEDING: Phenylpropanolamine probably enters breast milk and could interfere with normal feeding in the newborn. It should be used cautiously.

ALTERNATIVES TO MEDICATIONS: Inhalation of steam or use of saline (salt water) nasal sprays will often provide temporary relief of nasal congestion.

GENERIC NAME: Phenytoin

COMMON BRANDS: Dilantin

TYPE OF DRUG: (Prescription) Anticonvulsant

FDA RISK CATEGORY FOR PREGNANCY: D

GENERAL INFORMATION: By directly stabilizing electrical impulses in the brain, phenytoin can prevent grand mal (major) seizures in individuals with epilepsy. It can be given intravenously for rapid control of seizures or orally for long-term prevention. Phenytoin must be given in a precise dosage to ensure effectiveness and prevent toxicity. Blood levels can be determined to guide your physician in adjusting the dosage. It is important for patients treated with phenytoin not to take any other medications, including over-the-counter preparations, because phenytoin can have several adverse interactions with other drugs. Treatment of epilepsy requires expert medical care. No anticonvulsant should be discontinued without consulting a physician.

POSSIBLE MATERNAL SIDE EFFECTS: Side effects include drowsiness, slurred speech, blurred vision, unsteadiness, nausea, and thickening of the gums. Drowsiness usually disappears after the first week of therapy. Nausea can be alleviated by taking the drug with food or milk. Gum problems can be prevented with excellent dental hygiene. If side effects persist, notify your physician so a blood level of the drug can be measured.

USE DURING PREGNANCY: The use of phenytoin during pregnancy remains controversial. It has been recognized that first-trimester use of the drug can cause a variety of fetal malformations including facial abnormalities, limb defects, and mental retardation. It is also acknowledged that epileptic seizures (possibly resulting from discontinuing anticonvulsant medication) can be associated with fetal death, birth defects, and harm to the mother.

With this dilemma in mind most authorities and the American College of Obstetricians and Gynecologists recommend the following:

1. All women with epilepsy whether or not they are taking anticonvulsant medication should consult their physician before attempting pregnancy or just as soon as pregnancy is suspected.
2. Women who have been free of seizures for several years should consult their physician to see whether medication can be discontinued before pregnancy. Some anticonvulsant medications are considered safer than others, and at least a change in medications may be appropriate.
3. Women with recurrent seizures should not stop taking their medications when they find out they are pregnant without first consulting a physician. The risk to both mother and baby is greater from a major epileptic seizure than from taking medication. Even if phenytoin must be taken during the first trimester, the chance of having a normal baby is approximately 90 percent.
4. The use of anticonvulsant medications during pregnancy requires careful medical follow-up. Blood levels of the drugs should be checked frequently, generally monthly, to ensure that the dosage is effective and not toxic.
5. The pediatrician should be notified before delivery if anticonvul-

sants were prescribed during pregnancy so the baby can be checked immediately for any problems.

USE DURING BREASTFEEDING: Phenytoin is excreted into breast milk but does not appear to have an adverse effect on the newborn. The American Academy of Pediatrics considers phenytoin compatible with breastfeeding.

ALTERNATIVES TO MEDICATIONS: There is no nonpharmacologic alternative to phenytoin for the treatment of grand mal seizures. In some patients who have been free of seizures for several years the drug can be carefully withdrawn before pregnancy. However, phenytoin should not be discontinued without consulting your physician. All women with epilepsy should be careful to obtain adequate rest and to avoid alcohol.

GENERIC NAME: Pindolol

COMMON BRANDS: Visken

TYPE OF DRUG: (Prescription) Antihypertensive

FDA RISK CATEGORY FOR PREGNANCY: C

GENERAL INFORMATION: Pindolol is a member of a group of drugs called beta blockers. Beta blockers act by inhibiting a major chemical reaction in the nervous system. Each of these drugs is capable of slowing the heart rate and lowering blood pressure. Their uses in the general population include treatment of high blood pressure, control of abnormal rhythms of the heart, control of acute hyperthyroidism (overactive thyroid gland), relief of angina (heart pain), prevention of migraine headaches, and prevention of acute performance anxiety (stage fright).

POSSIBLE MATERNAL SIDE EFFECTS: Possible side effects include slow heart rate, fatigue, wheezing (in patients with asthma), and depression.

USE DURING PREGNANCY: Beta blockers cross the placenta, but they have not been linked to congenital malformations. A large study of the use of beta blockers during pregnancy revealed no evidence of abnormal fetal growth or development. They are now being used more frequently for the treatment of high blood pressure during pregnancy. Newborn infants of women who took pindolol near delivery should be checked closely in the newborn nursery for slow heart rate and low blood sugar.

USE DURING BREASTFEEDING: Beta blockers are excreted into breast milk and theoretically could slow the baby's heart rate. Nevertheless, the American Academy of Pediatrics considers pindolol and other beta blockers compatible with breastfeeding.

ALTERNATIVES TO MEDICATIONS: With a program of weight loss, mild salt restriction, exercise, and cessation of smoking many women can successfully decrease their blood pressure before pregnancy and remain off medications throughout at least the first trimester. However, if antihypertensive medication is necessary, another drug with a proven record of safety during pregnancy (such as methyldopa, p. 215) should be considered.

GENERIC NAME: Piperazine

COMMON BRANDS: Antepar, Vermizine

TYPE OF DRUG: (Prescription) Antihelmintic (antiworm)

FDA RISK CATEGORY FOR PREGNANCY: B

GENERAL INFORMATION: Piperazine is commonly used throughout the world for the treatment of intestinal infestations with roundworms and pinworms. Up to 75 percent of the drug is absorbed into the maternal circulation.

POSSIBLE MATERNAL SIDE EFFECTS: The most common side effects are nausea and vomiting. Weakness, dizziness, and unsteady gait can also occur.

USE DURING PREGNANCY: There have been very few reports of piperazine use during pregnancy. Consequently, its safety cannot be ensured.

USE DURING BREASTFEEDING: No information is available.

ALTERNATIVES TO MEDICATIONS: Treatment of most roundworm or pinworm infestations can safely be postponed until after pregnancy or at least until completion of the first trimester.

GENERIC NAME: Pneumococcal vaccine

COMMON BRANDS: Pneumovax 23, Pnu-Imune 23

TYPE OF DRUG: (Prescription) Vaccine

FDA RISK CATEGORY FOR PREGNANCY: C

GENERAL INFORMATION: Pneumococcal vaccine provides active immunity to infections (primarily pneumonia) caused by the bacteria *Streptococcus pneumoniae*. Only individuals with certain types of chronic medical disorders require vaccination with pneumococcal vaccine. Single vaccination provides lifetime immunity in most adults.

POSSIBLE MATERNAL SIDE EFFECTS: Side effects include soreness at the site of injection and low-grade fever.

USE DURING PREGNANCY: There have been no reports of fetal harm or birth defects from use of pneumococcal vaccine during pregnancy. Nevertheless, most women who require the vaccine should be vaccinated before pregnancy or wait until after delivery.

USE DURING BREASTFEEDING: No information is available.

ALTERNATIVES TO MEDICATIONS: There is no nonpharmacologic alternative to pneumococcal vaccine for the active prevention of pneumococcal pneumonia. Fortunately, protection from this disease is not necessary for most women.

GENERIC NAME: Potassium chloride

COMMON BRANDS: K-Dur, K-Lor, K-Lyte, K-Tab, Kaochlor, Kaon-Cl, KATO, Kay Ciel, Klor-Con, Klorvess, Klotrix, Micro-K, Slow-K, Ten-K

TYPE OF DRUG: (Prescription) Mineral

FDA RISK CATEGORY FOR PREGNANCY: C

GENERAL INFORMATION: Potassium is a naturally occurring constituent of human tissues and fluids. It is found in a variety of foods.

Supplements are usually not required unless there is excessive potassium loss due to prolonged vomiting, diarrhea, or treatment with a diuretic.

POSSIBLE MATERNAL SIDE EFFECTS: The most common side effect is nausea. However, excessive administration of potassium supplements can cause abnormal heart rhythms. Patients with chronic kidney disease are particularly vulnerable to excessive accumulation of potassium in the blood when given oral or intravenous supplements.

USE DURING PREGNANCY: Potassium chloride supplements are not necessary for most normal pregnant women since most normal diets provide adequate amounts. Women who do require additional potassium must be seen regularly by their physician in order to have their blood potassium level measured.

USE DURING BREASTFEEDING: Potassium chloride may be safely taken during breastfeeding.

ALTERNATIVES TO MEDICATIONS: Dietary sources of potassium include fresh citrus fruits, dried fruits (apricots, raisins, and dates), milk, and meat.

GENERIC NAME: Potassium iodide

COMMON BRANDS: Elixophyllin-Kl, Iodo-Niacin, Mudrane, Pediacof Cough Syrup, Pima Syrup, Quadrinal, SSKl

TYPE OF DRUG: (Prescription) Expectorant

FDA RISK CATEGORY FOR PREGNANCY: D

GENERAL INFORMATION: It is thought that potassium iodide decreases the viscosity (thickness) of mucus facilitating cough and removal of bronchial secretions. Several recent reports, however, have questioned its effectiveness.

POSSIBLE MATERNAL SIDE EFFECTS: The most common side effects are nausea and abdominal pain. Skin rashes are also common.

USE DURING PREGNANCY: Potassium iodide should not be used during pregnancy. The medication freely crosses the placenta and enters the fetal blood. Once in the fetal circulation iodide is taken up by the fetal thyroid gland and can cause a goiter (enlarged thyroid).

USE DURING BREASTFEEDING: Potassium iodide should not be used during breastfeeding. It can interfere with normal thyroid function in the newborn.

ALTERNATIVES TO MEDICATIONS: Steam or cool mist may be effective in loosening bronchial secretions so they can be removed by coughing.

GENERIC NAME: Prazepam

COMMON BRANDS: Centrax

TYPE OF DRUG: (Prescription) Antianxiety, sedative

FDA RISK CATEGORY FOR PREGNANCY: D

GENERAL INFORMATION: Prazepam is a member of a group of anti-anxiety medications called benzodiazepines. These drugs are used for the treatment of anxiety and insomnia. They work by relaxing skeletal muscles and by a direct action on the brain.

Benzodiazepines can be abused if taken indiscriminately or for a long period of time. Withdrawal symptoms including tremor, agitation, insomnia, muscle cramps, nausea, and seizures can occur if these drugs are discontinued abruptly after chronic use. Benzodiazepines should not be taken without careful medical supervision.

POSSIBLE MATERNAL SIDE EFFECTS: Common side effects with all benzodiazepines include sedation, depression, mental confusion, dizziness, unsteady gait, nightmares, fatigue, dry mouth, and low blood pressure. These drugs can interfere with the ability to safely drive a car or operate dangerous equipment. Physical and psychological dependence can occur with chronic use.

USE DURING PREGNANCY: All benzodiazepines rapidly cross the placenta and enter the fetal circulation. Blood levels in the fetus equal that of the mother's within one hour of taking a pill. Several studies have demonstrated a link between first-trimester use of benzodiazepines and birth defects. The most commonly reported malformations are cleft lip and cleft palate. Used near term benzodiazepines have been associated with lethargy, respiratory problems, and withdrawal symptoms in the newborn. Most authorities believe that it is best to avoid these medications during the first trimester and if possible throughout pregnancy.

USE DURING BREASTFEEDING: Benzodiazepines are excreted into breast milk in significant quantities. They can cause sedation in the newborn and should be avoided during breastfeeding.

ALTERNATIVES TO MEDICATIONS: Before using medications to control anxiety or stress consider the following strategy:

1. Identify the source of your anxiety. Worry often persists because of an inability to identify a problem and take action to solve it. Visualization can begin the process. Close your eyes and take a few deep breaths. Allow an image of the problem to arise.
2. Once you've defined the source of your anxiety, gather information. For example, if you are worried about the outcome of your pregnancy because of a possible hereditary problem or a medication you took before you knew you were pregnant, get information from your physician or a genetic counselor. In most cases what you discover will be very comforting.
3. After obtaining information, decide on a plan of action. Do what you can to deal with the problem, but once you've done all you can, change your focus and move on to other parts of life. Instead of worrying, concentrate on your life beyond the worry. Exercise or take walks. Plan how you will spend the evening or the weekend. Treat yourself to something pleasant, or think up a surprise for someone you care about. As your mind gets busy with other thoughts, you'll find that stress will begin to fade.
4. If anxiety persists despite your best efforts, see a therapist. Often only a few counseling sessions can effectively reduce anxiety and stress and eliminate the need for medication.

GENERIC NAME: **Prazosin**

COMMON BRANDS: Minipress, Minizide

TYPE OF DRUG: (Prescription) Antihypertensive

FDA RISK CATEGORY FOR PREGNANCY: C

GENERAL INFORMATION: Prazosin is a commonly used medication for the treatment of chronic hypertension. It works by relaxing and dilating arteries throughout the body. It is only available in an oral preparation.

POSSIBLE MATERNAL SIDE EFFECTS: Common side effects include drowsiness, dizziness, blurred vision, and dry mouth.

USE DURING PREGNANCY: Prazosin has not been extensively used during pregnancy. Consequently, its safety cannot be ensured. Other antihypertensives with a longer record of safe use during pregnancy are available.

USE DURING BREASTFEEDING: Small amounts of prazosin enter breast milk, but the effect on the newborn is not known.

ALTERNATIVES TO MEDICATIONS: With a program of weight loss, mild salt restriction, exercise, and cessation of smoking many women can successfully decrease their blood pressure before pregnancy and remain off medications throughout at least the first trimester. However, if antihypertensive medication is necessary, another drug with a proven record of safety during pregnancy (such as methyldopa, p. 215) should be considered.

GENERIC NAME: Primidone

COMMON BRANDS: Mysoline

TYPE OF DRUG: (Prescription) Anticonvulsant

FDA RISK CATEGORY FOR PREGNANCY: D

GENERAL INFORMATION: Primidone is chemically related to phenobarbital (p. 247). Like phenobarbital, it works by blocking nerve impulses in the brain to effectively reduce the risk of seizures in patients with epilepsy. Recently, several studies have suggested that generic forms of primidone may not be equally potent to brand preparations.

POSSIBLE MATERNAL SIDE EFFECTS: Side effects are similar to those associated with phenobarbital including drowsiness, lethargy, and confusion.

USE DURING PREGNANCY: The use of primidone during pregnancy remains controversial. It has been recognized that first-trimester use of the drug can cause a variety of fetal malformations. It is also acknowledged that epileptic seizures (possibly resulting from discontinuing anticonvulsant medication) can be associated with fetal death, birth defects, and harm to the mother.

With this dilemma in mind most authorities and the American College of Obstetricians and Gynecologists recommend the following:

1. All women with epilepsy whether or not they are taking anticonvulsant medication should consult their physician before attempting pregnancy or just as soon as pregnancy is suspected.
2. Women who have been free of seizures for several years should consult their physician to see whether medication can be discontinued before pregnancy. Some anticonvulsant medications are considered safer than others, and at least a change in medications may be appropriate.
3. Women with recurrent seizures should not stop taking their medications when they find out they are pregnant without first consulting a physician. The risk to both mother and baby is greater from a major epileptic seizure than from taking medication. Even if primidone must be taken during the first trimester, the chance of having a normal baby is approximately 90 percent.
4. The use of anticonvulsant medications during pregnancy requires careful medical follow-up. Blood levels of the drugs should be checked frequently, generally monthly, to ensure that the dosage is effective and not toxic.
5. The pediatrician should be notified before delivery if anticonvulsants were prescribed during pregnancy so the baby can be checked immediately for any problems.

USE DURING BREASTFEEDING: Primidone is excreted into breast milk in significant amounts and can cause sedation in the newborn. Although the American Academy of Pediatrics considers primidone (and phenobarbital) compatible with breastfeeding, careful follow-up of the baby is essential.

ALTERNATIVES TO MEDICATIONS: In some patients who have been free of seizures for several years the drug can be carefully withdrawn before pregnancy. However, primidone should not be discontinued without consulting your physician. All women with epilepsy should be careful to obtain adequate rest and to avoid alcohol.

GENERIC NAME: Probenecid

COMMON BRANDS: Benemid

TYPE OF DRUG: (Prescription) Antigout

FDA RISK CATEGORY FOR PREGNANCY: B

GENERAL INFORMATION: Probenecid has two major therapeutic uses. First, it is used to enhance the urinary excretion of uric acid, the substance responsible for gout. Second, it decreases the urinary excretion of penicillin (p. 244) and cephalosporin (p. 100), so that when it is given with these antibiotics higher blood levels are attainable.

POSSIBLE MATERNAL SIDE EFFECTS: Side effects are uncommon but occasionally nausea, diarrhea, and gas production occur.

USE DURING PREGNANCY: Probenecid has been used safely throughout pregnancy to enhance the effect of penicillin and cephalosporin antibiotics. No adverse effects have been reported.

USE DURING BREASTFEEDING: No information is available.

ALTERNATIVES TO MEDICATIONS: There is no nonpharmacologic alternative to probenecid.

GENERIC NAME: Prochlorperazine

COMMON BRANDS: Compazine

TYPE OF DRUG: (Prescription) Antinausea, antipsychotic

FDA RISK CATEGORY FOR PREGNANCY: C

GENERAL INFORMATION: Prochlorperazine alleviates nausea and vomiting by interrupting the nerve impulse from the stomach to the vomiting center in the brain. The drug's effect on the brain has also made it useful for the treatment of certain psychotic illnesses.

POSSIBLE MATERNAL SIDE EFFECTS: Use of prochlorperazine is frequently accompanied by side effects including dizziness, drowsiness,

262

dry mouth, and blurred vision. Rarely, the drug can cause a tempo-rary spastic tightening of the muscles of the neck, difficulty swallow-ing, and muscular problems similar to those seen in Parkinson's disease. These adverse effects sound very serious, but they usually go away promptly after the drug is stopped.

USE DURING PREGNANCY: It is felt that prochlorperazine can be safely used throughout pregnancy to control persistent nausea and vomiting. It should, however, be used only for a brief time and in the lowest possible dosage.

USE DURING BREASTFEEDING: It is not known if prochlorperazine is excreted into breast milk.

ALTERNATIVES TO MEDICATIONS: Nausea can often be controlled with the following measures:

- Avoid foods that appear or smell offensive to you. This may seem blatantly obvious, but the role of the psyche in nausea is a very important one.
- Avoid an empty stomach. Eat several small meals throughout the day rather than two or three larger ones. If a large meal is necessary, midday is probably the best time for it.
- Avoid greasy or fatty foods. Substitute foods rich in complex carbo-hydrates such as whole-grain breads, cereals, and pasta. Fresh green leafy vegetables may help alleviate nausea because they are rich in vitamin B_6.
- Eat a small snack at bedtime and save two crackers at the bedside. On awakening, eat the crackers before getting out of bed, and remain in bed for an additional few minutes.
- Drink plenty of fluids throughout the day to avoid dehydration.
- If nausea does occur, lie down. It helps. In fact, many women find that frequent rest periods forestall the discomfort.

GENERIC NAME: **Progestins**

COMMON BRANDS: Birth control pills, Delalutin, Provera

TYPE OF DRUG: (Prescription) Hormone

FDA RISK CATEGORY FOR PREGNANCY: D

GENERAL INFORMATION: Progestins are a group of synthetic hormones that act like the naturally occurring female sex hormone, progesterone. Progesterone causes the swelling of the uterus lining before pregnancy.

Synthetic progestins are used to initiate a menstrual period in some women who have been unable to have a spontaneous period due to a hormonal imbalance. They are also used in combination with estrogen in women who have completed menopause.

POSSIBLE MATERNAL SIDE EFFECTS: The most common side effect is nausea, which usually subsides after a few cycles.

USE DURING PREGNANCY: Since 1975 the FDA has issued a warning against the use of progestins during pregnancy because of reports of birth defects in a few infants exposed to the drug during the first trimester. Supported by new research, many physicians now dispute the need for this warning. A recent study demonstrated that there was no additional risk of birth defects beyond the baseline risk (approximately 3 percent of all pregnancies) when medroxyprogesterone (Provera) was taken during the first trimester.

Progestins are occasionally used to provide hormonal support during early pregnancy until the placenta can supply adequate hormone production.

USE DURING BREASTFEEDING: Progestins are not recommended for use during breastfeeding.

ALTERNATIVES TO MEDICATIONS: There are no nonpharmacologic alternatives to progestins.

GENERIC NAME: Propoxyphene

COMMON BRANDS: Darvocet, Darvon

TYPE OF DRUG: (Prescription) Analgesic

FDA RISK CATEGORY FOR PREGNANCY: C

GENERAL INFORMATION: Propoxyphene is a synthetic analgesic chemically related to methadone (p. 209) for relief of mild to moderate pain. The drug can be used alone or in a preparation combined with either aspirin (p. 82) or acetaminophen (p. 63). Chronic use of propoxyphene can lead to drug dependency.

POSSIBLE MATERNAL SIDE EFFECTS: The most common side effects are dizziness, sedation, nausea, and constipation.

USE DURING PREGNANCY: There have been three case reports of birth defects in infants whose mothers took propoxyphene during the first trimester. However, other drugs were used in each case. In a large study of 686 infants whose mothers took propoxyphene during the first trimester, no link between the drug and birth defects was noted. When propoxyphene is used regularly near term, infants should be carefully observed for narcotic withdrawal symptoms.

USE DURING BREASTFEEDING: Propoxyphene is excreted into breast milk, but there have been no reports of adverse effects in breastfed infants. Nevertheless, newborns exposed to the drug in breast milk should be observed for lethargy and poor feeding.

ALTERNATIVES TO MEDICATIONS: In many instances moderate pain can be controlled with biofeedback or relaxation techniques. If medication is needed, it is preferable to use acetaminophen (p. 63).

GENERIC NAME: **Propranolol**

COMMON BRANDS: Inderal, Inderide

TYPE OF DRUG: (Prescription) Antihypertensive

FDA RISK CATEGORY FOR PREGNANCY: C

GENERAL INFORMATION: Propranolol is a member of a group of drugs called beta blockers. Beta blockers act by inhibiting a major chemical reaction in the nervous system. Each of these drugs is capable of slowing the heart rate and lowering blood pressure. Their uses in the general population include treatment of high blood pressure, control of abnormal rhythms of the heart, control of acute hyperthyroidism (overactive thyroid gland), relief of angina (heart pain), prevention of migraine headaches, and prevention of acute performance anxiety (stage fright).

POSSIBLE MATERNAL SIDE EFFECTS: Possible side effects include slow heart rate, fatigue, wheezing (in patients with asthma), and depression.

USE DURING PREGNANCY: Beta blockers cross the placenta, but they have not been linked to congenital malformations. A large study

265

of the use of beta blockers during pregnancy revealed no evidence of abnormal fetal growth or development. They are now being used more frequently for the treatment of high blood pressure during pregnancy. Newborn infants of women who took propranolol near delivery should be checked closely in the newborn nursery for slow heart rate and low blood sugar.

USE DURING BREASTFEEDING: Beta blockers are excreted into breast milk and theoretically could slow the baby's heart rate. Nevertheless, the American Academy of Pediatrics considers propranolol and other beta blockers compatible with breastfeeding.

ALTERNATIVES TO MEDICATIONS: With a program of weight loss, mild salt restriction, exercise, and cessation of smoking many women can successfully decrease their blood pressure before pregnancy and remain off medications throughout at least the first trimester. However, if antihypertensive medication is necessary, another drug with a proven record of safety during pregnancy (such as methyldopa, p. 215) should be considered.

GENERIC NAME: **Propylthiouracil (PTU)**

COMMON BRANDS: PTU

TYPE OF DRUG: (Prescription) Antithyroid

FDA RISK CATEGORY FOR PREGNANCY: D

GENERAL INFORMATION: Propylthiouracil is used for the treatment of hyperthyroidism (overactive thyroid gland). It works by blocking the production of thyroid hormone in the thyroid gland (p. 212). The dosage of PTU must be carefully adjusted by measuring the level of thyroid hormone in the blood.

POSSIBLE MATERNAL SIDE EFFECTS: Excessive dosage of propylthiouracil may result in hypothyroidism (underactive thyroid gland). The drug can interfere with the production of white blood cells in the bone marrow. A complete blood count should be checked shortly after beginning therapy with propylthiouracil. Allergic reactions and skin rash can also occur.

USE DURING PREGNANCY: Propylthiouracil readily crosses the placenta to enter the fetal circulation. Once the drug is in the fetal blood, it is taken up by the thyroid gland and may cause a goiter (enlarged thyroid) in the baby. Nevertheless, it may be necessary to use propylthiouracil during pregnancy for some women with hyperthyroidism. In all cases only the lowest effective dosage of the drug should be used. Careful medical follow-up and regular thyroid function tests are necessary.

USE DURING BREASTFEEDING: Propylthiouracil enters breast milk and is easily absorbed by the breastfed infant. Only the lowest effective dosage of the drug should be used during breastfeeding and the infant should be checked by the pediatrician for signs of hypothyroidism.

ALTERNATIVES TO MEDICATIONS: Mild hyperthyroidism may not be a problem. Some women with mild hyperthyroidism may not require any medical therapy during pregnancy.

GENERIC NAME: **Pseudoephedrine**

COMMON BRANDS: Actifed, Afrinol, AllerAct, Benadryl Decongestant, Benylin Decongestant, Chlor-Trimeton Decongestant, Comtrex, Congestac, Contac Nighttime Cold Medicine, Deconamine, Drixoral, Fedahist, Neofed, Novafed, Novahistine DMX, PediaCare, Respaire SR, Sine-Off, Sinutab, Sudafed, Tylenol Cold Medication, Vicks Formula 44D Decongestant Cough Mixture, Vicks NyQuil Nighttime Colds Medicine

TYPE OF DRUG: (Over-the-counter and prescription) Decongestant

FDA RISK CATEGORY FOR PREGNANCY: C

GENERAL INFORMATION: Pseudoephedrine is a common component of many over-the-counter and prescription cold and allergy preparations. It works by shrinking swollen nasal mucous membranes and increases the patency of nasal airways. Nasal decongestion occurs within 30 minutes and lasts for 4 to 6 hours (up to 12 hours in the sustained-release preparations).

POSSIBLE MATERNAL SIDE EFFECTS: Side effects include mild stimulation, nervousness, insomnia, rapid heart rate, palpitations, dry mouth, and nausea.

USE DURING PREGNANCY: Preparations containing pseudoephedrine have been implicated in the cause of minor birth defects in animals but not in humans. It is important to bear in mind that most cold and allergy preparations containing pseudoephedrine also contain various other medications including antihistamines, other decongestants, aspirin, acetaminophen, and codeine. Before taking over-the-counter cold or allergy medications during pregnancy, consult your physician.

USE DURING BREASTFEEDING: Pseudoephedrine is probably excreted into breast milk and may cause restlessness and poor feeding in the infant.

ALTERNATIVES TO MEDICATIONS: As an alternative to decongestants for relieving a blocked nose, saline (salt water) spray or wash can liquify mucus.

GENERIC NAME: Psyllium

COMMON BRANDS: Alramucil, Cillium, Effer-Syllium, Fiberall, Hydrocil, Konsyl, Metamucil, Mucilose, Naturacil, Perdiem, Serutan

TYPE OF DRUG: (Prescription) Bulk laxative

FDA RISK CATEGORY FOR PREGNANCY: B

GENERAL INFORMATION: Psyllium is an indigestible, nonabsorbable form of fiber that absorbs water in the intestine and increases stool bulk. It stimulates peristalsis and bowel elimination and usually works within 12 hours.

POSSIBLE MATERNAL SIDE EFFECTS: Side effects are usually minimal, but increased gas and diarrhea can occur.

USE DURING PREGNANCY: Psyllium is safe for use during pregnancy. Although there are no special concerns about its use during pregnancy, psyllium laxatives should not be used in the presence of abdominal pain.

USE DURING BREASTFEEDING: Psyllium preparations may be used safely during breastfeeding.

ALTERNATIVES TO MEDICATIONS: Constipation is one of the most common gastrointestinal complaints during pregnancy even for women who were previously very regular. It is likely caused by the combined factors of pressure from the enlarging uterus and relaxation of intestinal muscle due to pregnancy hormones. Most women can control this problem by the following measures:

- Include some high-fiber cereal, prunes, or figs with breakfast. Do not, however, eat excessive amounts of fiber. It may be irritating to the stomach.
- Drink hot liquid with breakfast. This often has a stimulating effect on the colon.
- Allow plenty of time for appropriate bowel habits in the morning.

GENERIC NAME: Quinacrine

COMMON BRANDS: Atabrine

TYPE OF DRUG: (Prescription) Antimalarial, antiprotozoal, antiworm

FDA RISK CATEGORY FOR PREGNANCY: C

GENERAL INFORMATION: Quinacrine is used for treatment of malaria, tapeworms, and giardia. With newer, less toxic drugs available for the treatment of malaria and tapeworms, today quinacrine is primarily employed for the treatment of acute diarrhea due to giardia infestation.

POSSIBLE MATERNAL SIDE EFFECTS: Quinacrine can cause various skin rashes, blood problems, and gastrointestinal upset. In addition, the drug tends to accumulate in the body, causing yellow staining of the skin and blue or black pigmentation of the nails. In black patients with the condition called glucose-6-phosphate dehydrogenase (G-6-PD) deficiency, quinacrine can cause a sudden destruction of red blood cells (hemolytic anemia).

USE DURING PREGNANCY: Because quinacrine works by interfering with normal DNA synthesis in parasites, its effect on human DNA could theoretically alter normal cell development in the fetus during the first trimester. Animal studies, however, have not confirmed that the drug causes birth defects.

USE DURING BREASTFEEDING: Small amounts of quinacrine are excreted into breast milk. The effects on the newborn are not known.

ALTERNATIVES TO MEDICATIONS: Since acute diarrhea caused by giardia is not life-threatening or harmful to the baby, treatment with quinacrine can often be postponed until following delivery or at least until after the first trimester.

GENERIC NAME: Quinidine

COMMON BRANDS: Cardioquin, Duraquin, Quinaglute, Quinidex

TYPE OF DRUG: (Prescription) Antiarrhythmic

FDA RISK CATEGORY FOR PREGNANCY: C

GENERAL INFORMATION: Quinidine has long been used to treat abnormal rhythms of the heart. It works by altering the conduction of electrical impulses through certain parts of the heart. Careful medical follow-up is essential for patients treated with quinidine to ensure that the heart rhythm remains normal.

POSSIBLE MATERNAL SIDE EFFECTS: Common side effects include nausea, abdominal pain, decreased appetite, and diarrhea.

USE DURING PREGNANCY: There have been no reports linking the use of quinidine during pregnancy with birth defects. The drug does, however, cross the placenta and can cause a low platelet count in the newborn.

USE DURING BREASTFEEDING: Quinidine is excreted into breast milk but apparently does not harm the breastfed infant. The American Academy of Pediatrics considers quinidine compatible with breastfeeding.

ALTERNATIVES TO MEDICATIONS: There is no nonpharmacologic alternative to quinidine for the treatment of serious heart arrhythmias. There are, however, other available medications to control abnormal heart rhythms.

GENERIC NAME: Quinine

COMMON BRANDS: Quinamm, Quindan, Quine, Quinite

TYPE OF DRUG: (Over-the-counter and prescription) Antimalarial, muscle relaxant

FDA RISK CATEGORY FOR PREGNANCY: X

GENERAL INFORMATION: In the past quinine was used for the treatment of malaria. It has been replaced by more effective and less toxic medications. The drug is also available in a lower dosage, over-the-counter preparation for relief of muscle cramps.

POSSIBLE MATERNAL SIDE EFFECTS: The most common side effects include nausea and diarrhea. In black patients with the condition called glucose-6-phosphate dehydrogenase (G-6-PD) deficiency, quinine can cause a sudden destruction of red blood cells (hemolytic anemia).

USE DURING PREGNANCY: A variety of birth defects have been associated with the first-trimester use of quinine. Consequently, the drug should not be used during pregnancy.

USE DURING BREASTFEEDING: Quinine is excreted into breast milk, but no adverse effects have been reported in breastfed newborns.

ALTERNATIVES TO MEDICATIONS: Muscle cramps may be prevented by making sure to warm up slowly and completely before participating in vigorous exercise. Bedtime exercises designed to gently stretch the calf muscles may be helpful for preventing night-time cramps.

GENERIC NAME: **Rabies vaccine**

COMMON BRANDS: Imovax Rabies Vaccine

TYPE OF DRUG: (Prescription) Vaccine

FDA RISK CATEGORY FOR PREGNANCY: C

GENERAL INFORMATION: Rabies vaccine is made from a killed virus. It promotes active immunity against the rabies virus. The vaccine is usually given to individuals bitten by a wild or domestic animal suspected to have rabies.

POSSIBLE MATERNAL SIDE EFFECTS: Side effects are usually limited to pain at the site of injection.

USE DURING PREGNANCY: The vaccine is thought to be safe for use during pregnancy. Since the disease is nearly always fatal, the vaccine should not be withheld because of pregnancy in cases where there is any likelihood of acquiring rabies from an animal bite.

USE DURING BREASTFEEDING: The effect of rabies vaccine on the breastfed newborn is not known. Discontinuation of breastfeeding should be considered if vaccination is necessary.

ALTERNATIVES TO MEDICATIONS: There is no nonpharmacologic alternative to rabies vaccine. It should not be withheld because of pregnancy.

GENERIC NAME: Ranitidine

COMMON BRANDS: Zantac

TYPE OF DRUG: (Prescription) Antiulcer

FDA RISK CATEGORY FOR PREGNANCY: B

GENERAL INFORMATION: Ranitidine blocks the production of acid in the stomach and is used to treat gastric and duodenal (small intestine) ulcers.

POSSIBLE MATERNAL SIDE EFFECTS: Ranitidine is usually free of side effects.

USE DURING PREGNANCY: Ranitidine has not been studied extensively during human pregnancy, but birth defects have not been reported. When given in very high dosages to laboratory animals the drug has not been linked to birth defects.

USE DURING BREASTFEEDING: Ranitidine is excreted into breast milk and can reduce the production of gastric acid in the newborn. The American Academy of Pediatrics considers a similar drug, cimetidine (p. 110), unsafe for use during breastfeeding. Ranitidine should generally not be used during breastfeeding.

ALTERNATIVES TO MEDICATIONS: A program of dietary restriction alone is generally not adequate for treatment of stomach or intestinal ulcers. However, an alternative to cimetidine during pregnancy is the regular use of antacids (p. 78) between meals.

GENERIC NAME: Reserpine

COMMON BRANDS: Demi-Regroton, Diupres, Hydropres, Regroton, Salutensin, Ser-Ap-Es, Serpasil

TYPE OF DRUG: (Prescription) Antihypertensive

FDA RISK CATEGORY FOR PREGNANCY: C

GENERAL INFORMATION: Reserpine has been used in the past to treat chronic hypertension. There are now many newer antihypertensives available with fewer side effects.

POSSIBLE MATERNAL SIDE EFFECTS: Side effects include mental confusion, dizziness, depression, dry mouth, nasal stuffiness, nausea, and diarrhea.

USE DURING PREGNANCY: There have been several isolated reports of birth defects in infants whose mothers took reserpine during the first trimester. When used near term reserpine can cause nasal congestion and breathing problems in the newborn. Newer and safer medications for the treatment of hypertension should be used instead of reserpine during pregnancy.

USE DURING BREASTFEEDING: Reserpine is excreted into breast milk and can cause persistent nasal congestion in breastfed newborns.

ALTERNATIVES TO MEDICATIONS: With a program of weight loss, mild salt restriction, exercise, and cessation of smoking many women can successfully decrease their blood pressure before pregnancy and remain off medications throughout at least the first trimester. However, if antihypertensive medication is necessary, another drug with a proven record of safety during pregnancy (such as methyldopa, p. 215) should be substituted for reserpine.

GENERIC NAME: # Rho (D) immune globulin

COMMON BRANDS: Gamulin Rh, MICRhoGAM, Mini-Gamulin Rh, RhoGAM

TYPE OF DRUG: (Prescription) Immune serum

FDA RISK CATEGORY FOR PREGNANCY: C

GENERAL INFORMATION: The rhesus (Rh) factor is a protein substance found on the surface of red blood cells, named for a similar substance found on the red blood cells of rhesus monkeys. Most people are Rh-positive, meaning that their red blood cells carry the rhesus factor. About 15 percent of the population, however, does not have it and is said to be Rh-negative. Problems can arise when an Rh-negative woman becomes pregnant by an Rh-positive man. During a first pregnancy some of the baby's red blood cells can seep into the mother's circulation. If the fetal blood in a subsequent pregnancy is Rh-positive, maternal antibodies against Rh-positive red blood cells could cause severe anemia in the fetus.

To prevent Rh-incompatibility in a subsequent pregnancy, an injection of Rho (D) immune globulin is given to the mother during the third trimester and within 72 hours of delivery. The drug destroys the Rh-positive fetal red cells in the mother's circulation and thus antibodies that would affect subsequent pregnancies are not produced.

POSSIBLE MATERNAL SIDE EFFECTS: There is only minor soreness at the site of injection. All plasma used in the preparation of Rho (D) immune globulin is tested by an FDA approved method for the presence of HIV (AIDS virus) as well as for the hepatitis B virus, and all donors are carefully screened to eliminate those in high risk groups for disease transmission.

USE DURING PREGNANCY: Rho (D) immune globulin should be given to all Rh-negative women after every pregnancy, whether it goes to term or ends in a miscarriage or abortion. An injection of the drug should also be given at approximately 28 weeks of pregnancy to prevent occasional cases of sensitization during the third trimester.

USE DURING BREASTFEEDING: Rho (D) immune globulin is considered safe for injection during breastfeeding.

ALTERNATIVES TO MEDICATIONS: There is no nonpharmacologic alternative to Rho (D) immune globulin.

GENERIC NAME: Rifampin

COMMON BRANDS: Rifadin, Rifamate, Rimactane

TYPE OF DRUG: (Prescription) Antituberculosis

FDA RISK CATEGORY FOR PREGNANCY: C

GENERAL INFORMATION: Rifampin is used in combination with other antituberculous drugs for the treatment of active tuberculosis. The drug is rarely used alone.

POSSIBLE MATERNAL SIDE EFFECTS: The most common side effects are rash, fever, nausea, and vomiting. Rifampin can interfere with the action of birth control pills and lead to unwanted pregnancy.

USE DURING PREGNANCY: Rifampin has been shown to cross the placenta and enter the fetal circulation. It can cause malformations in mice and rats, but no link between the drug and birth defects has been demonstrated in humans.

USE DURING BREASTFEEDING: Rifampin is excreted into breast milk but does not appear to cause any harm to the newborn.

ALTERNATIVES TO MEDICATIONS: There is no nonpharmacologic alternative to rifampin for the treatment of active tuberculosis.

GENERIC NAME: Ritodrine

COMMON BRANDS: Yutopar

TYPE OF DRUG: (Prescription) Prevention of premature labor

FDA RISK CATEGORY FOR PREGNANCY: B

GENERAL INFORMATION: Ritodrine may halt premature labor by interfering with contractility of the uterus.

POSSIBLE MATERNAL SIDE EFFECTS: Side effects include restlessness, anxiety, headache, palpitations, elevated blood pressure, and rapid heart rate. Use of ritodrine may worsen blood sugar control in women with type I diabetes. It may also precipitate or worsen gestational diabetes.

USE DURING PREGNANCY: Ritodrine is approved for use during pregnancy to halt premature labor. It should not be used before the twentieth week of pregnancy and is usually discontinued after the thirty-sixth week.

USE DURING BREASTFEEDING: There is no approved use for ritodrine during breastfeeding.

ALTERNATIVES TO MEDICATIONS: In some cases complete bedrest will stop premature labor.

GENERIC NAME: Rubella vaccine

COMMON BRANDS: Biavax, Meruvax II

TYPE OF DRUG: (Prescription) Virus vaccine (live)

FDA RISK CATEGORY FOR PREGNANCY: X

GENERAL INFORMATION: Rubella vaccine is an attenuated live virus vaccine that provides active immunity against rubella (German measles) (p. 25). Women who have never had rubella or have not been immunized against the disease should receive the vaccine at a time when they are certain that they are not pregnant. A blood test can determine the status of immunity in an individual who is uncertain about her past history of the disease or prior immunization.

POSSIBLE MATERNAL SIDE EFFECTS: Side effects are usually limited to pain at the site of injection.

USE DURING PREGNANCY: Rubella vaccine should not be given during pregnancy because the live rubella virus could theoretically cause birth defects. Nonpregnant women who have been vaccinated should continue contraception and not attempt pregnancy for three months after the vaccination.

USE DURING BREASTFEEDING: Rubella vaccine is considered safe for administration during breastfeeding. In fact, the immediate postpartum period is considered an excellent opportunity to give rubella vaccine since pregnancy is very unlikely.

ALTERNATIVES TO MEDICATIONS: There is no nonpharmacologic alternative to rubella vaccine for obtaining active immunity to the disease. Since the vaccine should not be used during pregnancy, pregnant women should avoid contact with anyone suspected of having rubella.

GENERIC NAME: Scopolamine

COMMON BRANDS: Dallergy, Donnagel-PG, Donnatal, Ru-Tuss, Transderm Scōp

TYPE OF DRUG: (Over-the-counter and prescription) Antinausea, antimotion sickness

FDA RISK CATEGORY FOR PREGNANCY: C

GENERAL INFORMATION: Scopolamine is used in over-the-counter antinausea and allergy preparations. It is also effective in preventing motion sickness when administered by a transdermal (skin) patch.

POSSIBLE MATERNAL SIDE EFFECTS: Possible side effects include drowsiness, blurred vision, confusion, dry mouth, constipation, palpitations, and rapid heart rate.

USE DURING PREGNANCY: Scopolamine readily crosses the placenta. In two large studies no link could be established between first-trimester use of scopolamine and birth defects. However, chemically similar drugs have been associated with minor birth defects in pregnant rabbits given the drug intravenously during the first trimester. Used near term scopolamine may cause rapid heart rate in the fetus.

USE DURING BREASTFEEDING: No information is available.

ALTERNATIVES TO MEDICATIONS: Nausea can often be controlled with the following measures:

- Avoid foods that appear or smell offensive to you. This may seem blatantly obvious, but the role of the psyche in nausea is a very important one.
- Avoid an empty stomach. Eat several small meals throughout the day rather than two or three larger ones. If a large meal is necessary, midday is probably the best time for it.
- Avoid greasy or fatty foods. Substitute foods rich in complex carbohydrates such as whole-grain breads, cereals, and pasta. Fresh green leafy vegetables may help alleviate nausea because they are rich in vitamin B_6.
- Eat a small snack at bedtime and save two crackers at the bedside. On awakening, eat the crackers before getting out of bed, and remain in bed for an additional few minutes.
- Drink plenty of fluids throughout the day to avoid dehydration.
- If nausea does occur, lie down. It helps. In fact, many women find that frequent rest periods forestall the discomfort.

GENERIC NAME: **Senna**

COMMON BRANDS: Fletcher's Castoria, Genna, Gentlax-B, Gentle Nature, Nytilax, Senokot, Senolax

TYPE OF DRUG: (Over-the-counter) Laxative

FDA RISK CATEGORY FOR PREGNANCY: C

GENERAL INFORMATION: Senna has an irritant effect on the colon, which promotes bowel evacuation. It also enhances intestinal fluid accumulation thereby increasing the stool's moisture content.

POSSIBLE MATERNAL SIDE EFFECTS: The most common side effects are nausea and diarrhea. Chronic misuse can lead to drug dependence and malabsorption of important nutrients.

USE DURING PREGNANCY: Although senna has been approved for use during pregnancy, chronic use can lead to dependence on the drug and diarrhea with loss of important nutrients and minerals important for a healthy pregnancy. In most cases constipation can be effectively managed by appropriate dietary modifications without the use of laxatives. Occasionally, diarrhea due to senna can cause premature labor.

USE DURING BREASTFEEDING: Senna is excreted into breast milk and has been reported to cause diarrhea in the newborn. It should not be used during breastfeeding.

ALTERNATIVES TO MEDICATIONS: Constipation is one of the most common gastrointestinal complaints during pregnancy even for women who were previously very regular. It is likely caused by the combined factors of pressure from the enlarging uterus and relaxation of intestinal muscle due to pregnancy hormones. Most women can control this problem by the following measures:

- Include some high-fiber cereal, prunes, or figs with breakfast. Do not, however, eat excessive amounts of fiber. It may be irritating to the stomach.
- Drink hot liquid with breakfast. This often has a stimulating effect on the colon.
- Allow plenty of time for appropriate bowel habits in the morning.

GENERIC NAME: Simethicone

COMMON BRANDS: Gas-X, Mylanta II, Mylicon, Phazyme, Riopan Plus, Silain

TYPE OF DRUG: (Over-the-counter) Antigas

FDA RISK CATEGORY FOR PREGNANCY: C

GENERAL INFORMATION: Simethicone acts as a defoaming agent breaking up gas bubbles in the stomach and intestine. The drug is not absorbed from the intestinal tract.

POSSIBLE MATERNAL SIDE EFFECTS: None.

USE DURING PREGNANCY: Although there are no large studies confirming the safety of simethicone during pregnancy, the drug is not absorbed and is presumed safe.

USE DURING BREASTFEEDING: Simethicone poses no danger to breastfed infants.

ALTERNATIVES TO MEDICATIONS: Most abdominal gas pain during pregnancy results from excessive gas production in the colon (large intestine) where simethicone is unlikely to be effective. Dietary restriction of gas-forming foods is more likely to be helpful. Foods that commonly cause gas include beans, cabbage, dried fruits (apricots, raisins, dates), apples, apple juice, white breads, and other products made with all-purpose white flour. Since many of these foods are included in a well-balanced diet, it is helpful to consult a dietitian to help plan a diet designed to limit gas production.

GENERIC NAME: Spectinomycin

COMMON BRANDS: Trobicin

TYPE OF DRUG: (Prescription) Antibiotic

FDA RISK CATEGORY FOR PREGNANCY: B

GENERAL INFORMATION: Spectinomycin is an antibiotic given only by intramuscular injection. It is generally used for the treatment of gonorrhea in patients who are allergic to penicillin. The drug is not effective, however, against syphilis.

POSSIBLE MATERNAL SIDE EFFECTS: The only significant side effect is pain at the site of injection.

USE DURING PREGNANCY: Spectinomycin can be used during pregnancy for the treatment of acute gonorrhea in individuals allergic to penicillin. Use of the drug has not been linked with birth defects or fetal harm. It is important to also treat sexual partners.

USE DURING BREASTFEEDING: No information is available.

ALTERNATIVES TO MEDICATIONS: There is no nonpharmacologic alternative to antibiotics for the treatment of gonorrhea. Spectinomycin is usually reserved for patients allergic to penicillin.

GENERIC NAME: Spironolactone

COMMON BRANDS: Aldactazide, Aldactone

TYPE OF DRUG: (Prescription) Diuretic

FDA RISK CATEGORY FOR PREGNANCY: D

GENERAL INFORMATION: Spironolactone is a diuretic used for the treatment of hypertension and chronic edema (fluid retention). It should not be used for the relief of occasional fluid retention. Unlike other diuretics the drug does not usually cause the loss of potassium in the urine.

POSSIBLE MATERNAL SIDE EFFECTS: Spironolactone can cause excessive accumulation of potassium in the blood. The drug can also cause breast enlargement in men and breast soreness and menstrual irregularities in women.

USE DURING PREGNANCY: Spironolactone should not be used during pregnancy. The drug has been shown to cause malformations of the genital organs of male infants. If a diuretic must be used during pregnancy, hydrochlorothiazide (p. 170) or furosemide (p. 154) offer a safer alternative.

USE DURING BREASTFEEDING: The safety of spironolactone during breastfeeding cannot be ensured. Other, safer diuretics should be used in its place.

ALTERNATIVES TO MEDICATIONS: The use of diuretics during pregnancy is usually reserved for women with heart problems, chronic hypertension, or kidney disease. Mild edema (fluid retention) is a common occurrence during pregnancy and does not require treatment. If edema becomes uncomfortable, it can usually be relieved by

280

lying on your side for periods of 30 to 60 minutes. In some cases mild restriction of dietary salt intake may be necessary. Severe salt restriction, however, is not appropriate and may even be harmful. There is no evidence that so-called natural diuretics found in health food stores are effective, and their safety during pregnancy cannot be assured.

GENERIC NAME: Streptokinase

COMMON BRANDS: Kabikinase, Streptase

TYPE OF DRUG: (Prescription) Dissolves blood clots

FDA RISK CATEGORY FOR PREGNANCY: C

GENERAL INFORMATION: Streptokinase is a relatively new drug used only for the treatment of severe blood clots in the lung (pulmonary embolism) or in a large, deep vein of the leg (thrombophlebitis). Occasionally the drug is also used in the treatment of an acute heart attack. It can be given only by intravenous injection and must be carefully supervised by specialized medical personnel in an intensive care unit.

POSSIBLE MATERNAL SIDE EFFECTS: The most significant adverse effect is spontaneous hemorrhage which may be very difficult to control.

USE DURING PREGNANCY: There have been few reports of streptokinase use during pregnancy. Although the drug has been shown not to cross the placenta, it should be reserved only for patients with life-threatening blood clots. Used near term massive hemorrhage could complicate either vaginal or cesarean delivery.

USE DURING BREASTFEEDING: No information is available.

ALTERNATIVES TO MEDICATIONS: There is no nonpharmacologic alternative for treatment of severe life-threatening blood clots. In most cases, however, heparin (p. 166) can be used instead of streptokinase as an anticoagulant (blood thinner).

GENERIC NAME: Streptomycin

COMMON BRANDS: Streptomycin

TYPE OF DRUG: (Prescription) Antibiotic

FDA RISK CATEGORY FOR PREGNANCY: D

GENERAL INFORMATION: Today, the use of streptomycin is limited to the treatment of some patients with active tuberculosis.

POSSIBLE MATERNAL SIDE EFFECTS: The most serious adverse effect of streptomycin is nerve damage in the ear which may result in deafness.

USE DURING PREGNANCY: Streptomycin is known to cross the placenta and can cause nerve damage in the baby's ear and hearing loss. There are other safer drugs available for the treatment of active tuberculosis during pregnancy. There should rarely be any indication for streptomycin during pregnancy.

USE DURING BREASTFEEDING: Although streptomycin enters breast milk, it is poorly absorbed orally and should not adversely affect the newborn. Nevertheless, hearing loss is always a potential risk. Safer antibiotics are available in most cases.

ALTERNATIVES TO MEDICATIONS: Safer antibiotics are available for use during pregnancy.

GENERIC NAME: Sucralfate

COMMON BRANDS: Carafate

TYPE OF DRUG: (Prescription) Antiulcer

FDA RISK CATEGORY FOR PREGNANCY: B

GENERAL INFORMATION: Sucralfate is an oral medication used for the treatment of stomach and duodenal ulcers. Very little of the drug is absorbed from the gastrointestinal tract. The drug coats the ulcer crater and protects against damage from gastric acid.

POSSIBLE MATERNAL SIDE EFFECTS: Side effects are minimal, but constipation may occur. Sucralfate may inhibit absorption of other drugs and should be given two hours before or after other medications.

USE DURING PREGNANCY: There are only a few reports in the medi-

282

cal literature of sucralfate use during pregnancy. Because the drug is minimally absorbed from stomach or intestine, most authorities feel that it is safe for use during pregnancy. There have been no reports of birth defects or fetal harm.

USE DURING BREASTFEEDING: Sucralfate may be safely used during breastfeeding.

ALTERNATIVES TO MEDICATIONS: Dietary restriction and frequent antacids may provide an acceptable alternative to sucralfate. Women with stomach or duodenal ulcers should avoid alcohol, cigarettes, and aspirin or other drugs known to cause stomach irritation.

GENERIC NAME: Sulfasalazine

COMMON BRANDS: Azulfidine

TYPE OF DRUG: (Prescription) Antibiotic

FDA RISK CATEGORY FOR PREGNANCY: B

GENERAL INFORMATION: Sulfasalazine is a sulfa-type antibiotic (also see sulfonamides, p. 284) that is poorly absorbed from the gastrointestinal tract after oral administration. It is used primarily for the treatment of ulcerative colitis and Crohn's disease (inflammatory bowel disease) (p. 23). The mechanism by which it treats these diseases is not known.

POSSIBLE MATERNAL SIDE EFFECTS: The most common side effect of sulfasalazine is nausea, which can usually be minimized by taking the drug after meals. Rarely, the drug can cause a severe skin reaction called Stevens-Johnson syndrome. Patients who are known to be allergic to other sulfa antibiotics should avoid sulfasalazine.

USE DURING PREGNANCY: Sulfasalazine has been safely used during the first trimester of pregnancy. When used near term, however, all sulfa-containing antibiotics, including sulfasalazine, can theoretically interfere with the baby's ability to eliminate bile pigments (bilirubin) from the blood possibly resulting in jaundice. In patients with active inflammatory bowel disease it may be necessary to continue treatment with sulfasalazine despite the theoretical risk of jaundice in the newborn.

USE DURING BREASTFEEDING: Sulfa-containing antibiotics are excreted into breast milk in small amounts. There is a theoretical risk of jaundice in the breastfed infant. Several reports, however, have demonstrated that the risk is very small in healthy term babies. Premature infants may be at greater risk and should not be exposed to the drug through breast milk.

ALTERNATIVES TO MEDICATIONS: Inflammatory bowel disease may spontaneously improve to the extent that the dosage of sulfasalazine may be decreased or discontinued. However, the drug should not be stopped without consulting a physician.

GENERIC NAME: Sulfonamides

COMMON BRANDS: Azo Gantanol, Bactrim, Gantrisin, Pediazole, Septra

TYPE OF DRUG: (Prescription) Antibiotic

FDA RISK CATEGORY FOR PREGNANCY: B

GENERAL INFORMATION: Sulfonamides are sulfa-containing antibiotics primarily used for the treatment of uncomplicated urinary tract infections. Several preparations contain other antibiotics or active ingredients.

POSSIBLE MATERNAL SIDE EFFECTS: The most common side effect of sulfonamides is nausea, which can usually be minimized by taking the drug after meals. Rarely, these antibiotics can cause a severe skin reaction called Stevens-Johnson syndrome.

USE DURING PREGNANCY: Sulfonamides have been safely used during the first trimester of pregnancy for the treatment of urinary tract infections. When used near term, however, all sulfa-containing antibiotics can theoretically interfere with the baby's ability to eliminate bile pigments (bilirubin) from the blood possibly resulting in jaundice. Other, safer antibiotics are usually available for use near the time of delivery.

USE DURING BREASTFEEDING: Sulfonamides are excreted into breast milk in small amounts. There is a theoretical risk of jaundice in the breastfed infant. Several reports, however, have demonstrated that the risk is very small in healthy term babies. Premature infants may be at greater risk and should not be exposed to the drug through breast milk.

ALTERNATIVES TO MEDICATIONS: There is no nonpharmacologic alternative to antibiotics for the treatment of acute urinary tract infection. Penicillin-type antibiotics (p. 244) should be used in preference to sulfonamides whenever possible.

GENERIC NAME: # Sulindac

COMMON BRANDS: Clinoril

TYPE OF DRUG: (Prescription) Anti-inflammatory

FDA RISK CATEGORY FOR PREGNANCY: Not classified

GENERAL INFORMATION: Sulindac is a member of a class of drugs called nonsteroidal anti-inflammatory drugs (NSAIDs). It is indicated for the treatment of arthritis, muscle pain, headache, and pain associated with menstruation.

POSSIBLE MATERNAL SIDE EFFECTS: The most common side effects are nausea and abdominal pain. Rarely, sulindac can irritate the stomach and cause an ulcer or bleeding from the stomach.

USE DURING PREGNANCY: There have been no reports linking sulindac to birth defects when the drug was used during the first trimester. However, experience with the drug during early pregnancy is limited.

Used near term sulindac can have potential effects on pregnancy and the fetus. First, the drug can cause premature closure of an important blood vessel in the fetus called the ductus arteriosus. Normally, this blood vessel does not close until after delivery. Premature closure could result in a serious condition called pulmonary hypertension. Second, sulindac and other NSAIDs can inhibit labor and prolong pregnancy.

USE DURING BREASTFEEDING: Sulindac enters human breast milk, but its effect on the newborn is not known. The drug's safety during breastfeeding cannot be ensured.

ALTERNATIVES TO MEDICATIONS: Musculoskeletal pain can often be relieved with warm baths and massage. Painful arthritis can be alleviated by rest, heat, and physical therapy. Nonweight-bearing exercise such as swimming may offer some comfort while enhancing muscle tone. If medication is necessary, acetaminophen (p. 63) is probably the safest medication to take during pregnancy for relief of minor pain.

GENERIC NAME: Temazepam

COMMON BRANDS: Restoril

TYPE OF DRUG: (Prescription) Sedative

FDA RISK CATEGORY FOR PREGNANCY: D

GENERAL INFORMATION: Temazepam is a member of a group of antianxiety medications called benzodiazepines. These drugs are used for the treatment of anxiety and insomnia. They work by relaxing skeletal muscles and by a direct action on the brain. Benzodiazepines can be abused if taken indiscriminately or for a long period of time. Withdrawal symptoms including tremor, agitation, insomnia, muscle cramps, nausea, and seizures can occur if these drugs are discontinued abruptly after chronic use. Benzodiazepines should not be taken without careful medical supervision.

POSSIBLE MATERNAL SIDE EFFECTS: Common side effects with all benzodiazepines include sedation, depression, mental confusion, dizziness, unsteady gait, nightmares, fatigue, dry mouth, and low blood pressure. These drugs can interfere with the ability to safely drive a car or operate dangerous equipment. Physical and psychological dependence can occur with chronic use.

USE DURING PREGNANCY: All benzodiazepines rapidly cross the placenta and enter the fetal circulation. Blood levels in the fetus equal that of the mother's within one hour of taking a pill. Several studies have demonstrated a link between first-trimester use of benzodiazepines and birth defects. The most commonly reported malformations are cleft lip and cleft palate.

Used near term benzodiazepines have been associated with lethargy, respiratory problems, and withdrawal symptoms in the newborn. Most authorities believe that it is best to avoid these med-

286

ications during the first trimester and if possible throughout pregnancy.

USE DURING BREASTFEEDING: Benzodiazepines are excreted into breast milk in significant quantities. They can cause sedation in the newborn and should be avoided during breastfeeding.

ALTERNATIVES TO MEDICATIONS: Insomnia may be relieved by some of the following techniques:

- Generally, try to avoid daytime naps. However, for some women sleeping patterns change during pregnancy, and a nap may be necessary to supplement abbreviated nighttime sleep.
- Go to bed only when tired. Instead of lying in bed when you are wide awake, get up, do something, and then return to bed when you feel tired.
- Try to establish a regular sleep pattern. Recognize when you *are* able to sleep and build on that.
- Exercise daily. Even a 30-minute walk will aid relaxation.
- Learn techniques of progressive relaxation. These techniques are simple to learn and effective.
- Avoid stimulant drinks such as coffee, tea, and caffeine-containing colas. On the other hand, warm milk may help make you sleepy.
- Never use alcohol to induce sleep.
- If you awaken during the night, recall the dream just before you awoke. Reentering the dream can return you to sleep.
- Make love. Sex is relaxing and often ends with sleep.
- If you are lying awake because a problem is on your mind, talk it through with someone until it's resolved.

GENERIC NAME: Terbutaline

COMMON BRANDS: Brethaire, Brethine, Bricanyl

TYPE OF DRUG: (Prescription) Bronchodilator, premature labor inhibitor (tocolytic)

FDA RISK CATEGORY FOR PREGNANCY: B

GENERAL INFORMATION: Terbutaline acts directly on the muscle of the bronchial tubes to relieve bronchial spasm in individuals with asthma. It can be administered orally, by injection, or by aerosol inhaler. Side effects may be minimized when the drug is given by inhalation.

Terbutaline also has a direct effect on the muscles of the uterus. The drug relaxes uterine muscle and can reduce or prevent contractions.

POSSIBLE MATERNAL SIDE EFFECTS: Side effects include nervousness, tremors, insomnia, palpitations, and increased heart rate. Women with type I diabetes may note increased blood sugar levels during treatment with terbutaline. The drug can also precipitate gestational diabetes in some women.

USE DURING PREGNANCY: During pregnancy terbutaline can be used for the relief of wheezing due to asthma. There have been no reports of birth defects with first-trimester use.

Recently, the drug has also been used for the treatment of premature labor when the gestational age of the fetus is greater than 20 weeks and less than 36 weeks. When used for this purpose, terbutaline is administered by subcutaneous injection, pill, or by a small portable pump device capable of slowly infusing the drug subcutaneously throughout the day and night. It should be kept in mind, however, that for some women with premature labor, contractions will cease following bedrest without medications.

USE DURING BREASTFEEDING: Terbutaline is excreted into breast milk and may cause restlessness or poor feeding in the newborn.

ALTERNATIVES TO MEDICATIONS: In some cases asthma can be prevented by avoidance of known allergens, particularly animals. If you smoke, stop. It is generally a good rule, however, to use a bronchodilating inhaler at the earliest indication of wheezing. Often prompt effective relief of asthma can prevent minor episodes from becoming more severe and prolonged.

As an alternative to terbutaline for cessation of premature labor, complete bedrest is occasionally effective.

GENERIC NAME: **Terconazole**

COMMON BRANDS: Terazol 7 vaginal cream, Terazol 3 vaginal suppositories

TYPE OF DRUG: (Prescription) Antifungal

FDA RISK CATEGORY FOR PREGNANCY: C

GENERAL INFORMATION: Terconazole is available in cream or suppository for the treatment of yeast (candida) infections of the vagina and vulva. Often a vaginal discharge is mistakenly assumed to be caused by yeast infection. Since there are many other causes of acute vaginitis, treatment should not be begun without appropriate medical examination and laboratory confirmation.

POSSIBLE MATERNAL SIDE EFFECTS: Side effects are usually minimal, but vaginal burning and itching can occur.

USE DURING PREGNANCY: There has not been extensive experience with terconazole during pregnancy. However, in studies where rats were given the drug orally in a dosage 100 times the recommended intravaginal dose there was no evidence of birth defects. It remains possible that the fetus could be affected adversely by direct transfer of terconazole from the irritated vagina across amniotic membranes. In many cases treatment of vaginitis can be postponed until after pregnancy or at least until after the first trimester.

USE DURING BREASTFEEDING: It is not known whether terconazole is excreted into breast milk.

ALTERNATIVES TO MEDICATIONS: To help avoid vaginal yeast infections do not take antibiotics unnecessarily, wear loose cotton underwear, avoid harsh soaps and irritants, and be sure your partner does not have a chronic yeast infection. During pregnancy it is not always necessary to treat mild yeast infections.

GENERIC NAME: **Testosterone**

COMMON BRANDS: Andro 100, Andronaq-50, Andronate, Delatestryl, Depo-Testosterone, Duratest, Testone L.A., Testrin-P.A., Virilon

TYPE OF DRUG: (Prescription) Male hormone

FDA RISK CATEGORY FOR PREGNANCY: X

GENERAL INFORMATION: Testosterone is a male hormone used primarily in males to replace a deficiency of the hormone or to promote growth and development of male sexual organs in adolescents with a hormonal imbalance.

POSSIBLE MATERNAL SIDE EFFECTS: Side effects include masculinization when taken by women.

USE DURING PREGNANCY: Testosterone should not be used by pregnant women for any reason. The hormone can cause genital malformations in the baby.

USE DURING BREASTFEEDING: Testosterone should not be taken by lactating women. The hormone enters breast milk and will likely have an adverse effect on the baby.

ALTERNATIVES TO MEDICATIONS: There is no indication for testosterone or an alternative during pregnancy.

GENERIC NAME: Tetanus toxoid

COMMON BRANDS: Tetanus toxoid

TYPE OF DRUG: (Prescription) Tetanus immunization

FDA RISK CATEGORY FOR PREGNANCY: C

GENERAL INFORMATION: Tetanus toxoid provides immunity to tetanus, a potentially life-threatening illness. Individuals with a history of initial (primary) immunization and a booster within 10 years do not need tetanus toxoid following a clean wound.

POSSIBLE MATERNAL SIDE EFFECTS: Discomfort at the site of injection and a nodule that may persist for several weeks are both common. Patients may also develop low-grade fever and body aches for 24 to 48 hours.

USE DURING PREGNANCY: The American College of Obstetricians and Gynecologists recommends the use of tetanus toxoid during pregnancy for those women at risk who have not had primary immunization or a booster within 10 years.

USE DURING BREASTFEEDING: It is not known whether tetanus toxoid is excreted into breast milk.

ALTERNATIVES TO MEDICATIONS: There is no nonpharmacologic alternative to tetanus toxoid for individuals potentially exposed to the disease.

GENERIC NAME: Tetracycline

COMMON BRANDS: Achromycin, Cyclopar, Panmycin, SK-Tetracycline, Sumycin, Tetracap, Tetracyn, Tetrex

TYPE OF DRUG: (Prescription) Antibiotic

FDA RISK CATEGORY FOR PREGNANCY: Not classified

GENERAL INFORMATION: Tetracycline is a broad-spectrum antibiotic frequently used in nonpregnant individuals for the treatment of common respiratory infections, sexually transmitted diseases, and acne.

POSSIBLE MATERNAL SIDE EFFECTS: The most common side effect is nausea. Tetracycline may also cause an enhanced sensitivity to the burning effects of the sun.

USE DURING PREGNANCY: Tetracycline should not be used during pregnancy. The drug crosses the placenta and can stain the baby's teeth dark brown. Tetracycline can also interfere with normal bone growth.

Do not become alarmed if you inadvertently took tetracycline during the first trimester of pregnancy. Since teeth do not begin to form until the start of the second trimester, staining is unlikely if the drug was discontinued before the end of the first trimester. There is no reason to consider therapeutic abortion if tetracycline were mistakenly used during the first trimester.

USE DURING BREASTFEEDING: Tetracycline is excreted into breast milk in small amounts and could stain the baby's teeth. Other safer antibiotics should be used.

ALTERNATIVES TO MEDICATIONS: There is no nonpharmacologic alternative to antibiotics for the treatment of bacterial infections. However, several antibiotics known to be safe during pregnancy are available instead of tetracycline.

GENERIC NAME: Theophylline

COMMON BRANDS: Bronkodyl, Elixophyllin, Slo-bid, Slo-Phyllin, Sustaire, Theobid, Theo-Dur, Theolair, Theophyl, Theospan-SR, Theo-24, Theovent, Uniphyl

TYPE OF DRUG: (Prescription) Bronchodilator

FDA RISK CATEGORY FOR PREGNANCY: C

GENERAL INFORMATION: Theophylline may be taken on a daily basis for the prevention of wheezing in patients with asthma. Different preparations vary by their duration of action. Some must be taken four times daily while other sustained-release preparations need only be taken once each day. These drugs are relatively slow acting and are not as helpful for acute attacks of asthma as inhaled bronchodilators. In emergencies, however, theophylline can be given intravenously for more rapid action.

POSSIBLE MATERNAL SIDE EFFECTS: The most common side effects are nausea, loss of appetite, restlessness, tremor, insomnia, rapid heart rate, and palpitations. To minimize side effects avoid drinking caffeine-containing beverages and foods while taking theophylline. Blood levels of theophylline should be checked periodically to ensure the dosage is safe and effective.

USE DURING PREGNANCY: Several medical studies have shown that theophylline is safe for use during pregnancy. There has been no link between the drug and birth defects or fetal harm. The dosage of the drug may have to be changed as pregnancy progresses. Checking blood levels will help your physician determine the need for a change in dosage.

Theophylline also has a relaxing effect on the muscles of the uterus. The drug may be beneficial in reducing the strength and frequency of contractions in women with premature labor. Women treated with theophylline whose pregnancies extend beyond their due date may have to temporarily stop or decrease the dosage of the drug.

USE DURING BREASTFEEDING: Theophylline is excreted into breast milk and may cause irritability or poor feeding in the newborn, especially premature infants.

ALTERNATIVES TO MEDICATIONS: In some cases asthma can be prevented by avoidance of known allergens, particularly animals. If you smoke, stop. It is generally a good rule, however, to use a bronchodilating inhaler at the earliest indication of wheezing. Often prompt effective relief of asthma can prevent minor episodes from becoming more severe and prolonged.

GENERIC NAME: Thioridazine

COMMON BRANDS: Mellaril

TYPE OF DRUG: (Prescription) Major tranquilizer, antipsychotic

FDA RISK CATEGORY FOR PREGNANCY: C

GENERAL INFORMATION: Thioridazine is primarily used to treat psychoses such as schizophrenia. The drug acts on a portion of the brain called the hypothalamus. It affects parts of the hypothalamus that control metabolism, body temperature, alertness, muscle tone, and vomiting and may be used to treat problems related to any of those functions.

POSSIBLE MATERNAL SIDE EFFECTS: The most common side effect is drowsiness, especially during the first or second weeks of therapy. Less commonly thioridazine can cause jaundice (yellowing of the whites of the eyes and skin). Jaundice usually goes away when the drug is discontinued. The drug can also cause abnormal muscle spasms similar to Parkinson's disease. Any abnormal movements or muscle spasms should be reported to a physician immediately.

USE DURING PREGNANCY: There is only limited experience with the use of thioridazine during pregnancy. Although there have been no reports of birth defects attributable to the drug, thioridazine should be used during pregnancy only if necessary and in the lowest effective dosage.

USE DURING BREASTFEEDING: Thioridazine probably enters breast milk, but its effect on the newborn is not known. Caution should be exercised if the drug is used during breastfeeding.

ALTERNATIVES TO MEDICATIONS: Patients with major psychotic disorders often need medication to control abnormal behavior or obsessive thoughts. Occasionally, the drug dosage can be reduced with more frequent psychiatric counseling.

GENERIC NAME: Thyroid hormone

COMMON BRANDS: Armour Thyroid, Cytomel, Euthroid, Levothroid, Proloid, Synthroid, Thyrolar

TYPE OF DRUG: (Prescription) Hormone

FDA RISK CATEGORY FOR PREGNANCY: A

GENERAL INFORMATION: Thyroid hormone preparations are used to treat individuals with hypothyroidism (an underactive thyroid gland). The precise dosage can be determined by measuring the level of thyroid hormone in the blood. Normal thyroid hormone function is essential for metabolism, growth, and development.

POSSIBLE MATERNAL SIDE EFFECTS: There are no side effects of thyroid hormones unless they are given in an excessive dosage. Symptoms of an excessive dosage include nervousness, insomnia, tremor, rapid heart rate, headache, fever, sweating, and diarrhea.

USE DURING PREGNANCY: Although thyroid hormone may cross the placenta in small amounts, there is no evidence that this hormone has any detrimental effect on the baby. On the contrary, patients with untreated hypothyroidism may have difficulty becoming pregnant and are at increased risk of miscarriage. Thyroid hormone levels should be checked at least once each trimester to ensure that the dosage of thyroid hormone replacement is effective but not excessive.

USE DURING BREASTFEEDING: Minimal amounts of thyroid hormone are excreted into breast milk, but there have been no reports of adverse effects on the baby.

ALTERNATIVES TO MEDICATIONS: There is no nonpharmacologic alternative to thyroid hormone for women with hypothyroidism.

GENERIC NAME: Timolol

COMMON BRANDS: Blocadren, Timolide

TYPE OF DRUG: (Prescription) Antihypertensive

FDA RISK CATEGORY FOR PREGNANCY: C

GENERAL INFORMATION: Timolol is a member of a group of drugs called beta blockers. Beta blockers act by inhibiting a major chemical reaction in the nervous system. Each of these drugs is capable of slowing the heart rate and lowering blood pressure. Their uses in the general population include treatment of high blood pressure, control of abnormal rhythms of the heart, control of acute hyperthyroidism (overactive thyroid gland), relief of angina (heart pain), prevention of migraine headaches, and prevention of acute performance anxiety (stage fright).

POSSIBLE MATERNAL SIDE EFFECTS: Possible side effects include slow heart rate, fatigue, wheezing (in patients with asthma), and depression.

USE DURING PREGNANCY: Beta blockers cross the placenta, but they have not been linked to congenital malformations. A large study of the use of beta blockers during pregnancy revealed no evidence of abnormal fetal growth or development. They are now being used more frequently for the treatment of high blood pressure during pregnancy. Newborn infants of women who took timolol near delivery should be checked closely in the newborn nursery for slow heart rate and low blood sugar.

USE DURING BREASTFEEDING: Beta blockers are excreted into breast milk and theoretically could slow the baby's heart rate. Nevertheless, the American Academy of Pediatrics considers timolol and other beta blockers compatible with breastfeeding.

ALTERNATIVES TO MEDICATIONS: With a program of weight loss, mild salt restriction, exercise, and cessation of smoking many women can successfully decrease their blood pressure before pregnancy and remain off medications throughout at least the first trimester. However, if antihypertensive medication is necessary, another drug with a proven record of safety during pregnancy (such as methyldopa, p. 215) should be considered.

GENERIC NAME: Tobacco

COMMON BRANDS: Cigarettes, cigars, pipes

TYPE OF DRUG: (Over-the-counter) Nicotine

FDA RISK CATEGORY FOR PREGNANCY: Not classified

GENERAL INFORMATION: It is estimated that one-third of American women of childbearing potential smoke tobacco. As many as 25 percent of women smoke throughout pregnancy. Tobacco has no known therapeutic use.

POSSIBLE MATERNAL SIDE EFFECTS: The most important side effect is dependency. Long-term use clearly causes chronic lung disease, lung cancer, and heart disease and may contribute to other cancers as well.

USE DURING PREGNANCY: Nicotine, carbon monoxide, cyanide, and probably other components of cigarette smoke cross the placenta and appear in fetal blood in even higher concentrations than in maternal blood. The most consistently reported consequence of maternal smoking is a reduction in fetal growth rate. Smoking during pregnancy is also associated with an increased risk of premature birth, stillbirth, and neonatal death. All women who smoke should stop before attempting pregnancy.

USE DURING BREASTFEEDING: Several of the toxic substances from cigarette smoke enter breast milk. Furthermore, infants of mothers who smoke are at increased risk of more frequent respiratory infections from passive inhalation of cigarette smoke. Mothers should not expose their infants to cigarette smoke whether or not they breastfeed.

ALTERNATIVES TO MEDICATIONS: Women who smoke should make every effort to stop smoking before pregnancy. Most hospitals have medically supervised smoking cessation programs.

GENERIC NAME: Tolazamide

COMMON BRANDS: Tolinase

TYPE OF DRUG: (Prescription) Oral hypoglycemic agent (blood sugar–lowering drug)

FDA RISK CATEGORY FOR PREGNANCY: D

GENERAL INFORMATION: Tolazamide is one of several drugs effective for lowering blood sugar levels in patients with type II diabetes mellitus (adult-onset diabetes). Similar to other oral hypoglycemic agents, tolazamide acts by increasing the production of insulin in the pancreas and by enhancing the effect of insulin in the cells. The vast majority of individuals with type I diabetes (juvenile-onset) and some people with type II diabetes cannot achieve satisfactory control of their blood sugar levels with oral hypoglycemic agents and must take daily injections of insulin.

The most significant adverse effect of tolazamide is hypoglycemia—that is, a blood sugar level that is excessively low. Individuals allergic to sulfa-containing medications will likely be allergic to tolazamide.

USE DURING PREGNANCY: Like other oral hypoglycemic agents, tolazamide crosses the placenta. Other drugs in this class (sulfonylureas) have been shown to cause birth defects when given during the first trimester. When used near term oral hypoglycemic agents can cause severe hypoglycemia in the newborn immediately after delivery. Neither tolazamide nor any other oral hypoglycemic agents should be used during pregnancy. Women treated with these medications who are planning pregnancy should consult their physician and discontinue the drug before attempting to conceive. Some women will be able to satisfactorily control blood sugar levels with diet alone. Others will need to take daily injections of insulin. All patients who discontinue their diabetes medication will need frequent blood tests performed to ensure that blood sugars do not increase to dangerous levels.

USE DURING BREASTFEEDING: It is not known how much tolazamide enters breast milk. Because of the theoretical risk that even a small amount of the drug in breast milk could cause hypoglycemia in the newborn, tolazamide should generally be avoided during breastfeeding. Some patients can achieve adequate control of their blood sugars by careful diet. Other individuals, however, may require injections of insulin.

ALTERNATIVES TO MEDICATIONS: Some women with type II diabetes treated with tolazamide before pregnancy can satisfactorily control their blood sugars by following a strict diet. Most pregnant women, however, will have to take injections of insulin to maintain their blood sugar levels in the range appropriate for pregnancy.

GENERIC NAME: Tolbutamide

COMMON BRANDS: Orinase

TYPE OF DRUG: (Prescription) Oral hypoglycemic agent (blood sugar–lowering drug)

FDA RISK CATEGORY FOR PREGNANCY: D

GENERAL INFORMATION: Tolbutamide is one of several drugs effective for lowering blood sugar levels in patients with type II diabetes mellitus (adult-onset diabetes). Similar to other oral hypoglycemic agents, tolbutamide acts by increasing the production of insulin in the pancreas and by enhancing the effect of insulin in the cells. The vast majority of individuals with type I diabetes (juvenile-onset) and some people with type II diabetes cannot achieve satisfactory control of their blood sugar levels with oral hypoglycemic agents and must take daily injections of insulin.

The most significant adverse effect of tolbutamide is hypoglycemia—that is, a blood sugar level that is excessively low. Individuals allergic to sulfa-containing medications will likely be allergic to tolbutamide.

USE DURING PREGNANCY: Like other oral hypoglycemic agents, tolbutamide crosses the placenta. Other drugs in this class (sulfonylureas) have been shown to cause birth defects when given during the first trimester. When used near term oral hypoglycemic agents can cause severe hypoglycemia in the newborn immediately after delivery. Neither tolbutamide nor any other oral hypoglycemic agents should be used during pregnancy.

Women treated with these medications who are planning pregnancy should consult their physician and discontinue the drug before attempting to conceive. Some women will be able to satisfactorily control blood sugar levels with diet alone. Others will need to take daily injections of insulin. All patients who discontinue their diabetes medication will need frequent blood tests performed to ensure that blood sugars do not increase to dangerous levels.

USE DURING BREASTFEEDING: It is not known how much tolbutamide enters breast milk. Because of the theoretical risk that even a small amount of the drug in breast milk could cause hypoglycemia in the newborn, tolbutamide should generally be avoided during breastfeeding. Some patients can achieve adequate control of their blood sugars by careful diet. Other individuals, however, may require injections of insulin.

298

ALTERNATIVES TO MEDICATIONS: Some women with type II diabetes treated with tolbutamide before pregnancy can satisfactorily control their blood sugars by following a strict diet. Most pregnant women, however, will have to take injections of insulin to maintain their blood sugar levels in the range appropriate for pregnancy.

GENERIC NAME: # Tolmetin

COMMON BRANDS: Tolectin

TYPE OF DRUG: (Prescription) Anti-inflammatory

FDA RISK CATEGORY FOR PREGNANCY: C

GENERAL INFORMATION: Tolmetin is a member of a class of drugs called nonsteroidal anti-inflammatory drugs (NSAIDs). It is indicated for the treatment of arthritis, muscle pain, headache, and pain associated with menstruation.

POSSIBLE MATERNAL SIDE EFFECTS: The most common side effects are nausea and abdominal pain. Rarely, tolmetin can irritate the stomach and cause an ulcer or bleeding from the stomach.

USE DURING PREGNANCY: There have been no reports linking tolmetin to birth defects when the drug was used during the first trimester. However, experience with the drug during early pregnancy is limited.

Used near term tolmetin can have potential effects on pregnancy and the fetus. First, the drug can cause premature closure of an important blood vessel in the fetus called the ductus arteriosus. Normally, this blood vessel does not close until after delivery. Premature closure could result in a serious condition called pulmonary hypertension. Second, tolmetin and other NSAIDs can inhibit labor and prolong pregnancy.

USE DURING BREASTFEEDING: Tolmetin enters human breast milk, but its effect on the newborn is not known. The drug's safety during breastfeeding cannot be ensured.

ALTERNATIVES TO MEDICATIONS: Musculoskeletal pain can often be relieved with warm baths and massage. Painful arthritis can be alleviated by rest, heat, and physical therapy. Nonweight-bearing exercise such as swimming may offer some comfort while enhancing muscle tone. If medication is necessary, acetaminophen (p. 63) is probably the safest medication to take during pregnancy for relief of minor pain.

GENERIC NAME: Tranylcypromine

COMMON BRANDS: Parnate

TYPE OF DRUG: (Prescription) Antidepressant (Monoamine oxidase inhibitor p. 225)

FDA RISK CATEGORY FOR PREGNANCY: C

GENERAL INFORMATION: Some types of chronic depression are thought to originate from a chemical imbalance in the brain, possibly a deficiency of norepinephrine and serotonin. Tranylcypromine acts by inhibiting an enzyme called monoamine oxidase (MAO). Since MAO is responsible for the breakdown of norepinephrine and serotonin, any drug that inhibits MAO will increase levels of norepinephrine in the brain. In fact, MAO inhibitors such as tranylcypromine are very effective antidepressants.

POSSIBLE MATERNAL SIDE EFFECTS: Minor side effects of dizziness, fatigue, and dry mouth are common. More significant, however, is an unusual reaction between tranylcypromine (or any other MAO inhibitor) and certain foods that may result in a sudden elevation in blood pressure. Any patient treated with an MAO inhibitor should be given a detailed list of foods to avoid while taking this medication. Some foods to be avoided include beer, ale, sherry, red wine (especially chianti), aged cheese, sour cream, yogurt, herring, avocados, bananas, canned figs, raisins, dried sausages, meats prepared with tenderizers, soy sauce, and yeast extracts.

USE DURING PREGNANCY: Since experience with tranylcypromine during pregnancy is limited, its safety cannot be ensured. However, there have been no human or animal studies reporting a link between the drug and birth defects or fetal harm. The risk of hypertensive crisis (sudden elevation of blood pressure) from an MAO inhibitor and various foods (listed above) represents a special risk during pregnancy. Use of tranylcypromine during pregnancy requires expert medical supervision.

USE DURING BREASTFEEDING: No information is available.

ALTERNATIVES TO MEDICATIONS: Depression often gives rise to hopelessness, negativity toward oneself, and at times an inability to carry out normal activities of daily living. Some individuals may become intensely sad or grief-stricken over the loss of someone or something close to them. Others may suffer from chronic depression unrelated to a specific event. In many cases counseling is necessary to truly understand the cause and extent of depression. There are, however, a number of things you can do to deal with depression on your own:

1. Try to identify the specific situation or personal interaction that has caused your sense of hopelessness and negativity.
2. Make a fresh start at correcting the problem. Talk it through. If necessary, repair relationships with previously available support systems. Often family or close friends can serve to reduce your distress.
3. Realize that there are options for most situations. Seldom is there truly "no choice."
4. Understand some of the warning signs that indicate you have severe depression requiring professional counseling. Such signs include
   - Intense sadness, frequent bouts of crying, or depressed mood most of the day,
   - Uncharacteristically negative thoughts about yourself,
   - Markedly diminished interest or pleasure in most activities,
   - Diminished appetite and weight loss,
   - Chronic insomnia or sleeping excessively,
   - Feelings of worthlessness or guilt,
   - Persistent fatigue or lack of energy,
   - Inability to think or concentrate,
   - Thoughts or plans for suicide.
5. Patients with severe depression should not stop taking antidepressant medications without careful psychiatric supervision.

GENERIC NAME: **Trazodone**

COMMON BRANDS: Desyrel

TYPE OF DRUG: (Prescription) Antidepressant

FDA RISK CATEGORY FOR PREGNANCY: C

GENERAL INFORMATION: Trazodone is used for the treatment of chronic depression. It is thought to act by increasing the concentration of certain neurotransmitters (chemicals in the brain) known to be low in some patients with chronic depression. Depression related to a specific life event or loss is less likely to be alleviated with trazodone than chronic depression unrelated to a specific event.

POSSIBLE MATERNAL SIDE EFFECTS: Side effects include dizziness, sedation, fatigue, nightmares, blurred vision, dry mouth, rapid heart rate, and difficulty urinating.

USE DURING PREGNANCY: Experience with trazadone during pregnancy is limited. Chemically related antidepressants, called tricyclics, have been associated with a few reports of birth defects. There has been no clear link between trazodone and birth defects or fetal harm. Since trazodone has been shown to cross the placenta, it should be used only in cases of severe chronic depression and under careful medical supervision.

USE DURING BREASTFEEDING: Trazodone enters breast milk in small amounts, but its effect on the newborn is not known.

ALTERNATIVES TO MEDICATIONS: Depression often gives rise to hopelessness, negativity toward oneself, and at times an inability to carry out normal activities of daily living. Some individuals may become intensely sad or grief-stricken over the loss of someone or something close to them. Others may suffer from chronic depression unrelated to a specific event. In many cases counseling is necessary to truly understand the cause and extent of depression. There are, however, a number of things you can do to deal with depression on your own:

1. Try to identify the specific situation or personal interaction that has caused your sense of hopelessness and negativity.
2. Make a fresh start at correcting the problem. Talk it through. If necessary, repair relationships with previously available support systems. Often family or close friends can serve to reduce your distress.
3. Realize that there are options for most situations. Seldom is there truly "no choice."
4. Understand some of the warning signs that indicate you have severe depression requiring professional counseling. Such signs include:

- Intense sadness, frequent bouts of crying, or depressed mood most of the day,
- Uncharacteristically negative thoughts about yourself,
- Markedly diminished interest or pleasure in most activities,
- Diminished appetite and weight loss,
- Chronic insomnia or sleeping excessively,
- Feelings of worthlessness or guilt,
- Persistent fatigue or lack of energy,
- Inability to think or concentrate,
- Thoughts or plans for suicide.

5. Patients with severe depression should not stop taking antidepressant medications without careful psychiatric supervision.

GENERIC NAME: **Tretinoin**

COMMON BRANDS: Retin-A

TYPE OF DRUG: (Prescription) Antiacne

FDA RISK CATEGORY FOR PREGNANCY: B (see Use during Pregnancy)

GENERAL INFORMATION: Tretinoin is available as a cream or gel for the treatment of severe acne. Recently, the drug has also been used to smooth skin wrinkles due to aging. Patients who use tretinoin should follow specific instructions for application provided by a physician or the manufacturer. It must be used very sparingly.

POSSIBLE MATERNAL SIDE EFFECTS: Adverse reactions to tretinoin include skin peeling, blisters, changes in pigmentation, and marked sensitivity to the sun.

USE DURING PREGNANCY: Tretinoin is a derivative of vitamin A and is similar to other drugs known to cause birth defects when taken internally (see etretinate, p. 146, and isotretinoin, p. 187). Since tretinoin is only used topically, the risk of birth defects is thought to be very small. However, in view of even a theoretical risk it would be prudent to stop using tretinoin during pregnancy.

USE DURING BREASTFEEDING: It is not known if tretinoin applied to the skin enters breast milk.

ALTERNATIVES TO MEDICATIONS: Meticulous cleansing and limited exposure to sunlight may help prevent acne. Avoid heavy oil-based cosmetics.

GENERIC NAME: Triamcinolone

COMMON BRANDS: Azmacort

TYPE OF DRUG: (Prescription) Corticosteroid inhaler

FDA RISK CATEGORY FOR PREGNANCY: D

GENERAL INFORMATION: Triamcinolone inhaler is used for the treatment of chronic asthma. The drug is a form of corticosteroid (p. 119) effective for prevention of wheezing when used in a regular dosage twice each day. It is not effective for relief of acute wheezing.

POSSIBLE MATERNAL SIDE EFFECTS: Possible side effects include hoarseness, thrush (yeast infection of the mouth), and a dry, irritated throat.

USE DURING PREGNANCY: In recommended dosages triamcinolone has not been shown to cause malformations in humans. However, when given internally in extremely high dosages corticosteroids have been associated with an increased risk of cleft palate in laboratory rabbits and rats. Despite the FDA risk category, most authorities believe that corticosteroids given by inhalation are safe for use during pregnancy.

USE DURING BREASTFEEDING: It is not known if triamcinolone is excreted into breast milk.

ALTERNATIVES TO MEDICATIONS: In some cases asthma can be prevented by avoidance of known allergens, particularly animals. If you smoke, stop. It is generally a good rule, however, to use a bronchodilating inhaler at the earliest indication of wheezing. Often prompt effective relief of asthma can prevent minor episodes from becoming more severe and prolonged.

GENERIC NAME: Triamterene

COMMON BRANDS: Dyazide, Dyrenium, Maxzide

TYPE OF DRUG: (Prescription) Diuretic

FDA RISK CATEGORY FOR PREGNANCY: B

GENERAL INFORMATION: Triamterene is a diuretic used for the treatment of hypertension and for edema due to congestive heart failure, kidney failure, or liver failure. It should not be used for the relief of mild, self-limited fluid retention.

POSSIBLE MATERNAL SIDE EFFECTS: Unlike many other diuretics which cause the loss of potassium in the urine, triamterene causes the kidneys to retain potassium. Thus, if supplemental potassium or other drugs that cause potassium retention are combined with triamterene, hyperkalemia (excessive potassium in the blood) can occur. Hyperkalemia is a serious disorder that can produce abnormal, life-threatening arrhythmias (abnormal rhythms) of the heart. Patients treated with triamterene should have serum potassium levels determined periodically.

USE DURING PREGNANCY: No link between triamterene and birth defects has been reported in experimental animals. Nevertheless, experience with the drug during the first trimester of human pregnancy is limited. The drug should not be used for the relief of fluid retention commonly found during most normal pregnancies. Like other diuretics, triamterene can reduce normal maternal blood volume and diminish the flow of blood through the placenta to the baby. In some women with chronic heart or kidney disorders diuretics, including triamterene, may be necessary to control severe fluid retention.

USE DURING BREASTFEEDING: Triamterene has been shown to enter breast milk, but its effect on the newborn is not known.

ALTERNATIVES TO MEDICATIONS: The use of diuretics during pregnancy is usually reserved for women with heart problems, chronic hypertension, or kidney disease. Mild edema (fluid retention) is a common occurrence during pregnancy and does not require treatment. If edema becomes uncomfortable, however, it can usually be relieved by lying on your side for periods of 30 to 60 minutes. In some cases mild restriction of dietary salt intake may be necessary. Severe salt restriction, however, is not appropriate and may even be harmful. There is no evidence that so-called natural diuretics found in

305

health food stores are effective and their safety during pregnancy cannot be assured.

GENERIC NAME: Triazolam

COMMON BRANDS: Halcion

TYPE OF DRUG: (Prescription) Sedative

FDA RISK CATEGORY FOR PREGNANCY: D

GENERAL INFORMATION: Triazolam is a member of a group of anti-anxiety medications called benzodiazepines. These drugs are used for the treatment of anxiety and insomnia . They work by relaxing skeletal muscles and by a direct action on the brain. Benzodiazepines can be abused if taken indiscriminately or for a long period of time. Withdrawal symptoms including tremor, agitation, insomnia, muscle cramps, nausea, and seizures can occur if these drugs are discontinued abruptly after chronic use. Benzodiazepines should not be taken without careful medical supervision.

POSSIBLE MATERNAL SIDE EFFECTS: Common side effects with all benzodiazepines include sedation, depression, mental confusion, dizziness, unsteady gait, nightmares, fatigue, dry mouth, and low blood pressure. These drugs can interfere with the ability to safely drive a car or operate dangerous equipment. Physical and psychological dependence can occur with chronic use.

USE DURING PREGNANCY: All benzodiazepines rapidly cross the placenta and enter the fetal circulation. Blood levels in the fetus equal that of the mother's within one hour of taking a pill. Several studies have demonstrated a link between first-trimester use of benzodiazepines and birth defects. The most commonly reported malformations are cleft lip and cleft palate.

Used near term benzodiazepines have been associated with lethargy, respiratory problems, and withdrawal symptoms in the newborn. Most authorities believe that it is best to avoid these medications during the first trimester and if possible throughout pregnancy.

USE DURING BREASTFEEDING: Benzodiazepines are excreted into breast milk in significant quantities. They can cause sedation in the newborn and should be avoided during breastfeeding.

ALTERNATIVES TO MEDICATIONS: Insomnia may be relieved by some of the following techniques:

- Generally, try to avoid daytime naps. However, for some women sleeping patterns change during pregnancy, and a nap may be necessary to supplement abbreviated nighttime sleep.
- Go to bed only when tired. Instead of lying in bed when you are wide awake, get up, do something, and then return to bed when you feel tired.
- Try to establish a regular sleep pattern. Recognize when you *are* able to sleep and build on that.
- Exercise daily. Even a 30-minute walk will aid relaxation.
- Learn techniques of progressive relaxation. These techniques are simple to learn and effective.
- Avoid stimulant drinks such as coffee, tea, and caffeine-containing colas. On the other hand, warm milk may help make you sleepy.
- Never use alcohol to induce sleep.
- If you awaken during the night, recall the dream just before you awoke. Reentering the dream can return you to sleep.
- Make love. Sex is relaxing and often ends with sleep.
- If you are lying awake because a problem is on your mind, talk it through with someone until it's resolved.

GENERIC NAME: Trimethadione

COMMON BRANDS: Tridione

TYPE OF DRUG: (Prescription) Anticonvulsant

FDA RISK CATEGORY FOR PREGNANCY: D

GENERAL INFORMATION: Trimethadione is an anticonvulsant used in nonpregnant patients for the treatment of petit mal (minor) seizures. The drug is not effective for the treatment of grand mal (major motor) seizures. Today, trimethadione has largely been replaced by newer, less toxic drugs.

POSSIBLE MATERNAL SIDE EFFECTS: The drug commonly causes drowsiness and fatigue. In addition, trimethadione can cause severe skin reactions and can interfere with the ability of the bone marrow to produce red and white blood cells.

USE DURING PREGNANCY: Used during the first trimester trimethadione has a high likelihood of causing serious birth defects including mental retardation, speech difficulties, cleft lip or palate, heart malformations, urinary malformations, and growth retardation. Trimethadione should be discontinued before pregnancy or as soon as pregnancy is recognized and another, less toxic medication substituted.

USE DURING BREASTFEEDING: No information is available.

ALTERNATIVES TO MEDICATIONS: In some patients who have been free of seizures for several years the drug can be carefully withdrawn before pregnancy. However, trimethadione should not be discontinued without consulting your physician. All women with epilepsy should be careful to obtain adequate rest and to avoid alcohol.

GENERIC NAME: **Trimethobenzamide**

COMMON BRANDS: Tegamide, T-Gen, Ticon, Tigan, Tiject-20

TYPE OF DRUG: (Prescription) Antinausea

FDA RISK CATEGORY FOR PREGNANCY: C

GENERAL INFORMATION: Trimethobenzamide is a weak antihistamine primarily used for the relief of persistent nausea. It can be administered orally, by rectal suppository, or by intramuscular injection.

POSSIBLE MATERNAL SIDE EFFECTS: The most common side effects are drowsiness and dry mouth. When the drug is given by rectal suppository, some local irritation may occur.

USE DURING PREGNANCY: Trimethobenzamide has been used during pregnancy to control nausea. Several large studies have failed to demonstrate any link between use of the drug in normal dosages during the first trimester and birth defects. Severe or prolonged vomiting, however, may be a sign of serious stomach or intestinal problems and should be reported to a physician.

USE DURING BREASTFEEDING: Trimethobenzamide is excreted into breast milk, but no adverse effects have been demonstrated in breastfed infants.

ALTERNATIVES TO MEDICATIONS: Nausea can often be controlled with the following measures:

- Avoid foods that appear or smell offensive to you. This may seem blatantly obvious, but the role of the psyche in nausea is a very important one.
- Avoid an empty stomach. Eat several small meals throughout the day rather than two or three larger ones. If a large meal is necessary, midday is probably the best time for it.
- Avoid greasy or fatty foods. Substitute foods rich in complex carbohydrates such as whole-grain breads, cereals, and pasta. Fresh green leafy vegetables may help alleviate nausea because they are rich in vitamin B_6.
- Eat a small snack at bedtime and save two crackers at the bedside. On awakening, eat the crackers before getting out of bed, and remain in bed for an additional few minutes.
- Drink plenty of fluids throughout the day to avoid dehydration.
- If nausea does occur, lie down. It helps. In fact, many women find that frequent rest periods forestall the discomfort.

GENERIC NAME: **Trimethoprim**

COMMON BRANDS: Bactrim, Septra, Trimpex

TYPE OF DRUG: (Prescription) Antibiotic

FDA RISK CATEGORY FOR PREGNANCY: C

GENERAL INFORMATION: Trimethoprim is an antibiotic used for the treatment of uncomplicated urinary tract infections. Trimethoprim can be given alone or in a preparation combined with a sulfa antibiotic (see sulfonamides, p. 284).

POSSIBLE MATERNAL SIDE EFFECTS: Trimethoprim is usually well tolerated. Rarely, a severe skin reaction can occur.

USE DURING PREGNANCY: Trimethoprim has been used safely during the second and third trimesters. However, because the drug works by inhibiting the production of an essential chemical (folic acid) in bacteria, it could theoretically block the production of folic acid in the embryo during the first trimester. Other, safer antibiotics should generally be used during the first trimester of pregnancy.

USE DURING BREASTFEEDING: Trimethoprim is excreted into breast milk, but no adverse effects on breastfed infants have been reported. The American Academy of Pediatrics considers trimethoprim compatible with breastfeeding.

ALTERNATIVES TO MEDICATIONS: There is no nonpharmacologic alternative to antibiotics for the treatment of acute bacterial infection. However, another antibiotic should be substituted for trimethoprim during the first trimester.

GENERIC NAME: Triple sulfa cream (sulfathiazole, sulfacetamide, sulfabenzamide, urea)

COMMON BRANDS: Sultrin

TYPE OF DRUG: (Prescription) Vaginal antibiotic cream or tablet

FDA RISK CATEGORY FOR PREGNANCY: C

GENERAL INFORMATION: Triple sulfa cream or tablet is used for the topical treatment of vaginal infection caused by bacteria called Gardnerella.

POSSIBLE MATERNAL SIDE EFFECTS: Generally side effects are limited to vaginal irritation. Sulfa creams can be absorbed from the vagina and cause allergic reactions in individuals sensitive to sulfa.

USE DURING PREGNANCY: Sulfa antibiotics have been safely used during the first trimester of pregnancy. When used near term, however, all sulfa-containing antibiotics, including triple sulfa cream or tablets, can theoretically interfere with the baby's ability to eliminate bile pigments (bilirubin) from the blood possibly resulting in jaundice.

USE DURING BREASTFEEDING: Sulfa-containing antibiotics are excreted into breast milk in small amounts. There is a theoretical risk of jaundice in the breastfed infant. Several reports, however, have demonstrated that the risk is very small in healthy term babies.

Premature infants may be at greater risk and should not be exposed to the drug through breast milk.

ALTERNATIVES TO MEDICATIONS: Treatment of mild vaginal infections can often be postponed until after delivery.

GENERIC NAME: Tuberculosis skin test

COMMON BRANDS: Aplitest, PPD, Tine test

TYPE OF DRUG: (Prescription) Diagnostic skin test for tuberculosis

FDA RISK CATEGORY FOR PREGNANCY: C

GENERAL INFORMATION: Tuberculosis (TB) skin tests use tuberculin, a protein isolated from cultures of the organism that causes TB, to identify individuals who have been exposed to the disease. The test is performed by injecting 5 units of purified tuberculin (PPD) under the skin. The test is considered positive if a surrounding hard area larger than 10 mm occurs within 48 hours. It is usually necessary for a qualified health-care professional to interpret the test 48 hours after it has been applied.

POSSIBLE MATERNAL SIDE EFFECTS: Individuals who have active TB or are highly sensitive to tuberculin may respond to the test with a large area of redness and inflammation. In some cases, individuals who are suspected of having TB are given a small "test dose" of PPD to avoid a major skin reaction.

USE DURING PREGNANCY: Tuberculosis skin tests have been used safely during human pregnancy. Because TB can be transmitted to the infant at birth, it is important to identify mothers at risk of the disease during pregnancy.

USE DURING BREASTFEEDING: Tuberculosis skin tests can be safely applied during breastfeeding.

ALTERNATIVES TO MEDICATIONS: A tuberculosis skin test can be safely applied during pregnancy and should not be withheld in women suspected of having tuberculosis.

GENERIC NAME: Typhoid vaccine

COMMON BRANDS: Typhoid Vaccine

TYPE OF DRUG: (Prescription) Vaccine (inactivated)

FDA RISK CATEGORY FOR PREGNANCY: C

GENERAL INFORMATION: Typhoid vaccine promotes active immunity to typhoid fever in 70 to 90 percent of individuals vaccinated.

POSSIBLE MATERNAL SIDE EFFECTS: Side effects include pain, redness, and swelling at the site of injection. Low-grade fever and mild muscle aches can also occur.

USE DURING PREGNANCY: Typhoid vaccine is a killed bacteria vaccine. The risk to the fetus from the vaccine is unknown. However, typhoid fever is a serious infectious disease with a high mortality for both mother and fetus. The American College of Obstetricians and Gynecologists recommends vaccination during pregnancy for women exposed to typhoid through travel to high-risk areas of the world. Such high-risk areas can be identified by contacting the Centers for Disease Control in Atlanta, Georgia.

USE DURING BREASTFEEDING: It is not known whether typhoid vaccine is excreted into breast milk.

ALTERNATIVES TO MEDICATIONS: The only alternative to typhoid vaccine is avoiding travel to areas where the disease is known to be prevalent.

GENERIC NAME: Urokinase

COMMON BRANDS: Abbokinase

TYPE OF DRUG: (Prescription) Dissolves blood clots

FDA RISK CATEGORY FOR PREGNANCY: C

GENERAL INFORMATION: Urokinase is a relatively new drug used only for the treatment of severe blood clots in the lung (pulmonary embolism) or in a large, deep vein of the leg (thrombophlebitis). Occasionally the drug is also used in the treatment of an acute heart attack. It can be given only by intravenous injection and must be carefully supervised by specialized medical personnel in an intensive care unit.

POSSIBLE MATERNAL SIDE EFFECTS: The most significant adverse effect is spontaneous hemorrhage, which may be very difficult to control.

USE DURING PREGNANCY: There have been few reports of urokinase use during pregnancy. Although the drug has been shown not to cross the placenta, it should be reserved only for patients with life-threatening blood clots. Used near term massive hemorrhage could complicate either vaginal or cesarean delivery.

USE DURING BREASTFEEDING: No information is available.

ALTERNATIVES TO MEDICATIONS: There is no nonpharmacologic alternative for treatment of severe life-threatening blood clots. In most cases, however, heparin (p. 166) can be used instead of streptokinase as an anticoagulant (blood thinner).

GENERIC NAME: Valproic acid

COMMON BRANDS: Depakene

TYPE OF DRUG: (Prescription) Anticonvulsant

FDA RISK CATEGORY FOR PREGNANCY: Not classified

GENERAL INFORMATION: Valproic acid is an anticonvulsant used to control grand mal (major motor) seizures in nonpregnant individuals with epilepsy. The drug is often employed when other anticonvulsants have not been effective. It is often used in combination with another anticonvulsant such as phenobarbital (p. 247) or carbamazepine (p. 98).

POSSIBLE MATERNAL SIDE EFFECTS: Valproic acid can cause prolonged bleeding, sedation, depression, headache, hallucinations, nausea, and liver damage.

USE DURING PREGNANCY: If possible, valproic acid should be avoided during pregnancy. First-trimester use has been clearly implicated in the cause of various malformations including microcephaly, cleft lip and palate, heart defects, and lumbosacral meningocele. Although no anticonvulsant is completely free of risk during pregnancy, others appear to be associated with less risk to the baby than valproic acid. Patients with epilepsy should not discontinue use of

313

their medication without consulting a physician, since uncontrolled seizures are also known to harm the fetus.

USE DURING BREASTFEEDING: Valproic acid is excreted into breast milk in small amounts. Its effect on the newborn is not known.

ALTERNATIVES TO MEDICATIONS: In some patients who have been free of seizures for several years the drug can be carefully withdrawn before pregnancy. If possible, another anticonvulsant should be substituted for valproic acid before pregnancy, but no change in medication should be made without consulting a physician.

GENERIC NAME: Vancomycin

COMMON BRANDS: Vancocin, Vancoled, Vancor

TYPE OF DRUG: (Prescription) Antibiotic

FDA RISK CATEGORY FOR PREGNANCY: C

GENERAL INFORMATION: Vancomycin is a potent antibiotic usually reserved for treatment of serious infections in patients allergic to penicillin, or for treatment of a severe diarrheal illness called pseudomembranous colitis.

POSSIBLE MATERNAL SIDE EFFECTS: When vancomycin is administered intravenously, it can cause fever, chills, and redness at the base of the neck. An excessively high dosage can result in hearing loss. The drug is poorly absorbed when given by mouth and usually does not cause any side effects.

USE DURING PREGNANCY: Vancomycin has been safely used during pregnancy. It is usually reserved, however, for the prevention of bacterial endocarditis (infection on a heart valve) in patients allergic to penicillin with known heart valve abnormalities. Women with valvular heart disease are usually given antibiotics before delivery.

USE DURING BREASTFEEDING: No information is available.

ALTERNATIVES TO MEDICATIONS: There is no nonpharmacologic alternative to antibiotics for the treatment of bacterial infections. However, vancomycin is generally reserved for treatment of serious infections in patients allergic to penicillin.

GENERIC NAME: Verapamil

COMMON BRANDS: Calan, Isoptin

TYPE OF DRUG: (Prescription) Antihypertensive, antiarrhythmic

FDA RISK CATEGORY FOR PREGNANCY: C

GENERAL INFORMATION: Verapamil is a member of a class of medication known as calcium-channel blockers. Calcium-channel blockers are used to treat hypertension (high blood pressure), abnormal rhythms of the heart, and angina pectoris (heart pain). These drugs are also capable of suppressing spontaneous contractions of the uterus.

POSSIBLE MATERNAL SIDE EFFECTS: The most common side effects are constipation, drowsiness, headache, and fatigue. Blood pressure must be checked frequently to ensure that it does not fall too low.

USE DURING PREGNANCY: Verapamil and other calcium-channel blockers have not been used extensively during pregnancy in the United States. Other antihypertensive medications that have been used for many years during pregnancy are usually given in preference to this newer class of drugs. Verapamil can be given intravenously for rapid reduction of high blood pressure in patients with preeclampsia. In addition, recent studies have suggested that calcium-channel blockers may be useful for treatment of premature labor.

USE DURING BREASTFEEDING: Experience with calcium-channel blockers in breastfeeding is limited. However, there are no reports of adverse effects.

ALTERNATIVES TO MEDICATIONS: With a program of weight loss, mild salt restriction, exercise, and cessation of smoking many women can successfully decrease their blood pressure before pregnancy and remain off medications throughout at least the first trimester. However, if antihypertensive medication is necessary, another drug with a proven record of safety during pregnancy (such as methyldopa, p. 215) should be considered.

GENERIC NAME: Vitamin A (Retinol)

COMMON BRANDS: Aquasol A

TYPE OF DRUG: (Over-the-counter) Fat-soluble vitamin

FDA RISK CATEGORY FOR PREGNANCY: A (Risk factor X if used in dosages greater than the recommended dietary allowance (RDA).

GENERAL INFORMATION: Vitamin A is an essential component of normal vision and maintenance of mucous membranes. Deficiency can result in night blindness or even more profound loss of vision. **POSSIBLE MATERNAL SIDE EFFECTS:** Adverse effects occur only with toxic dosages (hypervitaminosis A).

USE DURING PREGNANCY: Vitamin A intake during pregnancy should be increased only about 20 percent to approximately 1,000 retinol units per day. This modest increase in the intake of vitamin A allows for the extra storage of the vitamin by the fetus. No effects on the fetus from low levels of vitamin A have been reported.

Vitamin A supplements should be used with the same caution during pregnancy as any other drug. Large supplements of vitamin A have been shown to cause birth defects in experimental animals, and isotretinoin (p. 187), a drug similar to vitamin A, has been linked to several major malformations in humans. The amount of vitamin A found in most prenatal vitamin preparations is adequate and safe for pregnancy.

USE DURING BREASTFEEDING: Breast milk usually contains sufficient vitamin A for the newborn. The effect of large maternal doses of vitamin A on breastfeeding infants is not known.

ALTERNATIVES TO MEDICATIONS: Dietary sources of vitamin A include carrots, liver, spinach, and cantaloupe.

GENERIC NAME: # Vitamin B₁ (Thiamine)

COMMON BRANDS: Betaline S

TYPE OF DRUG: (Over-the-counter) Water-soluble vitamin

FDA RISK CATEGORY FOR PREGNANCY: A

GENERAL INFORMATION: Vitamin B_1 is an essential component of carbohydrate metabolism. Deficiency of thiamine is common in alcoholics and patients who suffer from chronic malnutrition. Dietary deficiencies may be seen in countries where unenriched white rice or white flour are the mainstays of the diet. Severe vitamin B_1 deficiency may lead to a condition called beriberi.

POSSIBLE MATERNAL SIDE EFFECTS: There are no significant side effects associated with vitamin B_1.

USE DURING PREGNANCY: The requirement for vitamin B_1 (thiamine) increases in early gestation. The recommended dietary allowance (RDA) increases from approximately 1.0 to 1.4 mg per day. Severe deficiency, which is extremely rare in the United States, can result in an infant born with congenital beriberi.

USE DURING BREASTFEEDING: In amounts that do not exceed the RDA, vitamin B_1 is safe to take during breastfeeding. It is excreted into breast milk and fulfills a nutritional requirement of the infant.

ALTERNATIVES TO MEDICATIONS: Dietary sources include brewer's yeast and whole-grain cereals.

GENERIC NAME: Vitamin B_2 (riboflavin)

COMMON BRANDS: B-C Bid, Glutofac, Mega-B, Ribo-2, Therabid, Vicon-C

TYPE OF DRUG: (Prescription) Water-soluble vitamin

FDA RISK CATEGORY FOR PREGNANCY: A

GENERAL INFORMATION: Vitamin B_2 is a water-soluble vitamin important for the manufacture of proteins. Deficiency of vitamin B_2 can lead to cracking of the lips and a dry irritation of the tongue.

POSSIBLE MATERNAL SIDE EFFECTS: There are no side effects when the RDA is not exceeded.

USE DURING PREGNANCY: The RDA during pregnancy is 1.5 mg per day. There have been no reports of human malformations caused by a deficiency of vitamin B_2. Severe deficiency in late gestation has reportedly been associated with premature birth and stillbirth.

USE DURING BREASTFEEDING: Vitamin B_2 may be supplemented during breastfeeding in amounts that do not exceed the RDA.

317

ALTERNATIVES TO MEDICATIONS: Dietary sources include liver, milk, yogurt, and cottage cheese.

GENERIC NAME: Vitamin B$_3$ (Niacin)

COMMON BRANDS: Niac, Nicobid, Nicolar, Nicotinex

TYPE OF DRUG: (Over-the-counter) Water-soluble vitamin

FDA RISK CATEGORY FOR PREGNANCY: A

GENERAL INFORMATION: Vitamin B$_3$ is a water-soluble vitamin important for several essential biochemical reactions in the body. Severe deficiency of vitamin B$_3$ can lead to a disease called pellagra characterized by severe skin rash and dementia.

POSSIBLE MATERNAL SIDE EFFECTS: Side effects occur only with large dosages and may include hot flashes, nausea, vomiting, sweating, and palpitations.

USE DURING PREGNANCY: The RDA for pregnant women is 15 mg per day. There have been no reports of fetal harm from deficiency or excess of vitamin B$_3$.

USE DURING BREASTFEEDING: Vitamin B$_3$ may be supplemented during breastfeeding in amounts that do not exceed the RDA.

ALTERNATIVES TO MEDICATIONS: Dietary sources include liver, nuts, chicken, and whole grains.

GENERIC NAME: Vitamin B$_6$ (Pyridoxine)

COMMON BRANDS: Bee six, Hexa-Betalin, Pyroxine

TYPE OF DRUG: (Prescription) Water-soluble vitamin

FDA RISK CATEGORY FOR PREGNANCY: A

GENERAL INFORMATION: Vitamin B$_6$ is a water-soluble vitamin that acts as an essential coenzyme in the metabolism of proteins.

POSSIBLE MATERNAL SIDE EFFECTS: There are no side effects when the RDA is not exceeded.

USE DURING PREGNANCY: During pregnancy a 25 percent increase of vitamin B_6, to 2.6 mg per day, is recommended. Neither deficiency or excess of the vitamin has been linked to fetal malformations in humans.

USE DURING BREASTFEEDING: Supplementation with vitamin B_6 is not necessary during breastfeeding. Large doses of the vitamin may actually interfere with milk production by suppressing production of the hormone prolactin.

ALTERNATIVES TO MEDICATIONS: Dietary sources include liver, meat, fish, chicken, and whole-grain breads.

GENERIC NAME: Vitamin B_9 (folic acid)

COMMON BRANDS: Folvite

TYPE OF DRUG: (Prescription) Water-soluble vitamin

FDA RISK CATEGORY FOR PREGNANCY: A

GENERAL INFORMATION: Vitamin B_9 is a water-soluble vitamin important for the normal production of red blood cells. Deficiency may lead to anemia.

POSSIBLE MATERNAL SIDE EFFECTS: There are no side effects when the RDA is not exceeded.

USE DURING PREGNANCY: Vitamin B_9 (folic acid) deficiency during pregnancy is common among undernourished women and women not receiving vitamin supplements. Some reports have suggested that deficiency of the vitamin may result in a smaller than expected baby. The recommended daily allowance during pregnancy is 0.8 mg per day. Some medications such as phenytoin (p. 252) are known to decrease levels of folic acid and require additional supplements. Standard multiple vitamin preparations may not contain enough vitamin B_9 for many pregnant women. Women who are anemic or women who take anticonvulsant medications should consult their physician to see whether additional supplements are required.

USE DURING BREASTFEEDING: Vitamin B_9 is excreted in breast milk. Supplementation with 0.5 to 0.8 mg per day is appropriate for breastfeeding.

ALTERNATIVES TO MEDICATIONS: Dietary sources include brewer's yeast, peanuts, liver, green leafy vegetables, and beets.

GENERIC NAME: Vitamin B_{12} (Cobalamin)

COMMON BRANDS: Betalin 12, Cobex, Cyanoject, Cyomin, Sytobex, Vibal

TYPE OF DRUG: (Prescription) Water-soluble vitamin

FDA RISK CATEGORY FOR PREGNANCY: A

GENERAL INFORMATION: Vitamin B_{12} is a water-soluble vitamin important for the production of red blood cells and normal nerve cells. Deficiency may result in anemia.

POSSIBLE MATERNAL SIDE EFFECTS: There are no side effects when the RDA is not exceeded.

USE DURING PREGNANCY: Mild deficiency of vitamin B_{12} is common during pregnancy but does not pose a significant risk to mother or baby. Severe deficiency may result in anemia. The required daily allowance during pregnancy is 4 micrograms per day.

USE DURING BREASTFEEDING: Vitamin B_{12} is excreted into breast milk. Breastfeeding women should take 4 micrograms per day.

ALTERNATIVES TO MEDICATIONS: Dietary sources include meat, eggs, liver, and shellfish.

GENERIC NAME: Vitamin C (Ascorbic acid)

COMMON BRANDS: Arco-Cee, Ascorbicap, Cebid, Cemill, Cetane, Cevi-Bid, Ce-Vi-Sol, Cevita, C-Span, Vitacee

TYPE OF DRUG: (Over-the-counter and prescription) Water-soluble vitamin

GENERAL INFORMATION: Vitamin C is a water-soluble vitamin essential for the formation of collagen. Since humans are not capable of synthesizing vitamin C, daily intake is important. Deficiency of vitamin C can lead to scurvy, a condition marked by degenerative changes in the capillaries, bone, and connective tissue. There has been considerable controversy about the value of high doses of vitamin C for prevention of the common cold. Studies have not consistently shown this practice to be effective.

POSSIBLE MATERNAL SIDE EFFECTS: There are no side effects when the RDA is not exceeded. Excessive amounts can cause diarrhea.

USE DURING PREGNANCY: Vitamin C levels progressively decline during pregnancy. Mild vitamin C deficiency does not appear to pose any risk for the fetus. On the other hand, vitamin C is an essential component of good maternal nutrition. The RDA during pregnancy is 80 mg per day.

There has been some theoretical concern that large doses of vitamin C during pregnancy may condition the fetus to high levels and lead to a condition called infantile scurvy despite a diet that contains the usual amount of vitamin C. Because of this theoretical concern, amounts of the vitamin in excess of the RDA are not recommended during pregnancy.

USE DURING BREASTFEEDING: Vitamin C is excreted into breast milk. The RDA for vitamin C during breastfeeding is 90 to 100 mg per day. Maternal supplementation up to the RDA is needed only in women with poor nutrition.

ALTERNATIVES TO MEDICATIONS: Dietary sources include citrus fruits and juices, broccoli, turnip greens, and brussel sprouts.

GENERIC NAME: **Vitamin D**

COMMON BRANDS: Calciferol, Vitamin D capsules

TYPE OF DRUG: (Over-the-counter) Fat-soluble vitamin

FDA RISK CATEGORY FOR PREGNANCY: C

GENERAL INFORMATION: Vitamin D is a fat-soluble vitamin that acts to regulate the serum concentration of calcium by affecting absorption from the gastrointestinal tract, excretion from the kidneys, and resorption from bone. Deficiency of vitamin D can lead to abnormalities of bone strength—rickets in children and osteomalacia in adults.

POSSIBLE MATERNAL SIDE EFFECTS: There are no side effects when the RDA is not exceeded. Excessive dosage may cause high serum calcium levels, kidney stones, nausea and vomiting, and calcifications of soft tissues.

USE DURING PREGNANCY: The RDA for adult pregnant women is 400 to 600 international units (IV) per day. For pregnant teenagers the RDA is increased to 600 to 800 IU per day to allow for the mother's own skeletal growth. Deficiency of vitamin D during pregnancy can lead to low serum calcium levels, muscle cramps, defective tooth enamel, or rickets in the newborn.

On the other hand, excessive administration can also cause problems in the baby. Excessive doses of vitamin D have been implicated in malformations of the face and skull. It is best to limit vitamin D intake to the RDA during pregnancy. One quart of fortified milk provides 400 IU of vitamin D.

USE DURING BREASTFEEDING: The RDA for vitamin D during breastfeeding is 400 to 600 IU per day. Vitamin D supplements are recommended for lactating women whose dietary intake of the vitamin is inadequate or if the infant lacks sufficient exposure to sunlight.

ALTERNATIVES TO MEDICATIONS: Common dietary sources include milk, liver oils, and egg yolk.

GENERIC NAME: Vitamin E (Alpha tocopherol)

COMMON BRANDS: Aquasol E, E-Ferol, Eprolin Gelseals, E-Vital, Tocopher-Caps, Vita-Plus E

TYPE OF DRUG: (Over-the-counter) Fat-soluble vitamin

FDA RISK CATEGORY FOR PREGNANCY: A

GENERAL INFORMATION: Daily vitamin E intake is essential for good health, although its exact biological function is not known.

POSSIBLE MATERNAL SIDE EFFECTS: There are no side effects when the RDA is not exceeded.

USE DURING PREGNANCY: The RDA for vitamin E during pregnancy is 10 to 15 mg per day. There are no known adverse fetal effects from deficiency or excessive vitamin E during pregnancy.

USE DURING BREASTFEEDING: Maternal supplementation is recommended only if diet does not provide sufficient vitamin E to meet the RDA (15 mg per day).

ALTERNATIVES TO MEDICATIONS: Dietary sources include vegetable oils and dark green leafy vegetables.

GENERIC NAME: Vitamin K (Phytonadione)

COMMON BRANDS: AquaMEPHYTON

TYPE OF DRUG: (Prescription) Fat-soluble vitamin

FDA RISK CATEGORY FOR PREGNANCY: C

GENERAL INFORMATION: Phytonadione is a synthetic, fat-soluble substance identical to vitamin K, the natural vitamin found in a variety of foods. It is required for the production of several blood clotting factors. Deficiency of vitamin K may result if intestinal bacteria are reduced by prolonged antibiotic therapy. Problems with normal blood clotting may result.

POSSIBLE MATERNAL SIDE EFFECTS: There are no side effects when the RDA is not exceeded.

USE DURING PREGNANCY: Since vitamin K is manufactured in the intestine, most women do not require supplements during pregnancy. However, it has been suggested that women treated with anticonvulsants, particularly phenytoin (p. 252), be given oral supplements of vitamin K during the last two weeks of gestation to prevent bleeding problems in the newborn. This form of treatment remains unproven. Other physicians suggest giving vitamin K by injection to newborns whose mothers took anticonvulsants and to infants thought to be at special risk of bleeding problems.

USE DURING BREASTFEEDING: Vitamin K is not excreted into breast milk. Therefore, infants at risk of bleeding problems must be given supplements by injection.

ALTERNATIVES TO MEDICATIONS: Dietary sources of vitamin K include turnip greens, broccoli, and green tea. Vitamin K is also produced by bacteria in the intestine.

GENERIC NAME: Yellow fever vaccine

COMMON BRANDS: YF-VAX

TYPE OF DRUG: (Prescription) Vaccine

FDA RISK CATEGORY FOR PREGNANCY: D

GENERAL INFORMATION: Yellow fever vaccine is a live attenuated virus vaccine that promotes active immunity to yellow fever. Use of the vaccine is generally restricted to travelers to areas of the world known to be endemic for the disease. Yellow fever is a serious, potentially fatal infectious disease.

POSSIBLE MATERNAL SIDE EFFECTS: Adverse effects include pain at the site of injection, low-grade fever, and muscle aches.

USE DURING PREGNANCY: Because the vaccine is produced from a live virus, it should be avoided during pregnancy unless exposure to the disease is unavoidable.

USE DURING BREASTFEEDING: It is not known whether yellow fever vaccine enters breast milk or whether there is any adverse effect on the newborn.

ALTERNATIVES TO MEDICATIONS: Travel to regions of the world where the risk of yellow fever is high should be avoided during pregnancy.

GENERIC NAME: Zidovudine (AZT)

COMMON BRANDS: Retrovir

TYPE OF DRUG: (Prescription) Antiviral

FDA RISK CATEGORY FOR PREGNANCY: C

GENERAL INFORMATION: Zidovudine interferes with replication of viruses and has been shown to be active against the human immunodeficiency virus (HIV) responsible for AIDS. Use of the drug for the treatment of AIDS remains experimental and should be carefully supervised by a physician experienced in the management of patients with HIV-related diseases.

POSSIBLE MATERNAL SIDE EFFECTS: The most serious adverse effect is suppression of red and white blood cell production in the bone marrow. Severe anemia requiring transfusion can result for therapy.

USE DURING PREGNANCY: There has not been sufficient experience with zidovudine during pregnancy to ensure its safety. Preliminary studies in rats, using dosages up to 20 times the human dosage, have revealed no evidence of harm to the fetus. Since AIDS is a fatal disease, use of this new medication during pregnancy may be necessary.

USE DURING BREASTFEEDING: It is not known whether zidovudine is excreted into breast milk.

ALTERNATIVES TO MEDICATIONS: There is no nonpharmacologic alternative to zidovudine for the treatment of AIDS. Since the human immunodeficiency virus can be transmitted to the baby, termination of pregnancy should be considered.

❧ SELECTED REFERENCES

1. Abrams, R.S. Handbook of medical problems during pregnancy. Norwalk: Appleton & Lange, 1989.
2. American Academy of Pediatrics. The transfer of drugs and other chemicals into human breast milk. *Pediatrics*, 1983. 72:375–83.
3. Berkowitz, R.L., Coustan D. R., Mochizuki T.K. Handbook for prescribing medications during pregnancy. 2nd ed. Boston: Little, Brown, 1986.
4. Briggs, G.G. , Freeman R.K., Yaffe S.J. Drugs in pregnancy and lactation. 2nd ed. Baltimore: Wiliams and Wilkins, 1986.
5. Briggs, G.G., Freeman R.K., Yaffe S.J. Drugs in pregnancy and lactation, Update. Baltimore: Williams and Wilkins, 1988–1989.
6. Cunnigham, F.G., MacDonald P.C., Gant N.F. Williams Obstetrics. Norwalk: Appleton & Lange, 1989.
7. Gilman, A.G., Goodman L.S., Gilman A. The pharmacological basis of therapeutics. 7th ed. New York: Macmillan, 1985.
8. Heinonen, O.P., Slone D., Shapiro S. Birth defects and drugs in pregnancy. Littleton: Publishing Sciences Group, 1977.
9. Niebyl, J.R. Drug use in pregnancy, 2nd ed. Philadelphia: Lea & Febiger, 1988.
10. Office of technology assessment task force. Reproductive health hazards in the workplace. Philadelphia: J.B. Lippincott Company, 1988.
11. Physician's desk reference. Oradell: Medical Economics Company, Inc., 1990.
12. Physician's desk reference for nonprescription drugs. Oradell: Medical Economics Company, Inc., 1990.
13. Rayburn, W.F., Zuspan F.P. Drug therapy in obstetrics and gynecology. 2nd edition. Norwalk: Appleton and Lange, 1986.
14. Shardein, J.L. Chemically induced birth defects. New York: Marcel Dekker, 1985.
15. Shepard, T.H. Catalog of teratogenic agents. Baltimore: Johns Hopkins University Press, 1989.

⚘ INDEX

Generic drug names are indicated by **bold type.**

330

Aralen, 105–6
Arco-Cee, 320–21
A. R. M. Allergy Relief Medicine, 80, 251–52
Arm & Hammer pure baking soda, 78–79
Armour Thyroid, 294
Arsenic, 51
Arthritis
  drug treatment for, 82–84, 173–74
  rheumatoid, 35
Arthritis Pain Formula, 82–84
Artificial sweeteners, 44, 45, 81–82
Ascorbic acid, 320–21
Ascorbicap, 320–21
Ascriptin, 82–84
Aspartame, 45, 81–82
Aspartate, 45
Aspirin, 35, 82–84, 161, 243, 264
Aspirin with Codeine, 118–19
Astemizole, 79
Asthma, 18–20
  drug treatment for, 122, 142–43 (see also Bronchodilator drugs; Corticosterioid drugs, oral inhalers)
Atabrine, 269–70
Atenolol, 84–85
Ativan, 196–97
Atropine, 135–36
Atrovent, 184–85
Attenuvax, 202–3
Augmentin, 74–75
Autoimmune diseases, 34
Axid, 235–36
Azatadine, 80
Azathioprine, 85–86
Azmacort, 304
Azo Gantanol, 284–85
AZT (Ziodovudine), 324–25
Azulfidine, 283–84

Bacterial infections, 31–32
Bactrim, 284–85, 309–10
Barbita, 247–49
Barbiturates, 86–88
Basaljel, 78–79
Bayer, 82–84
Bayer Children's Cough Syrup, 251–52
Baytussin, 163
Beclomethasone, 88
Beclovent, 88
Beconase, 88
Beer, 45, 67–68
Bee six, 318–19

Belladenal, 89
Belladonna, 89, 174
Bellaspaz, 89, 174–75
Bellergal, 89
Bellergal-S, 143–44
Benadryl, 80
Benadryl Decongestant, 267–68
Bendectin, 21, 80
Benemid, 262
Bentectin, 21, 80
Benylin, 80, 127–28, 163
Benylin Decongestant, 267–68
Benzedrine, 75–76
Benzene, 50
Benzodiazepines, 69–71, 104–5, 113–14, 115–16, 128–29, 152–53, 164, 196–97, 221–22, 240–41, 258, 286–87, 306–7
Beta blockers, 84–85, 219, 228–29, 254–55, 265–66, 294–95
Betaline S, 316–17
Betalin 12, 320
Betamethasone, 119–20
Bicillin, 244–45
Birth control pills, 89–90, 145, 263–64. See also Contraceptive devices
Birth defects
  cause and frequency of, 6–7
  caused by environmental hazards (see Environmental hazards)
  caused by mother's medical problems (see Medical problems in pregnancy)
  threshold level of drugs causing, 5
Bisacodyl, 90–91
Biscolax, 90–91
Bismuth subsalicylate, 91–92
Bisodol, 78–79
Blocadren, 294–95
Blood-clots, 18, 121, 166–67, 281, 312–13. See also Phlebitis; Anticoagulant drugs
Blood disorders, 32–34
  anemia, 32–33, 103, 153, 185–86
  bleeding and clotting problems, 17–18, 33–34
  Von Willebrand's disease, 34
Blood pressure, elevated, 15–16
Blood sugar-lowering drugs, 157–58, 160–61, 296–97, 297–99
Blood sugar-raising drugs, 159–60
Bonine, 80
Bowel. See Irritable bowel syndrome

332

Chlorpheniramine, 80
Chlorpromazine, 106–7
Chlorpropamide, 12, 107–8
Chlorthalidone, 108–9
Chlor-Trimeton, 80, 81
Chlor-Trimeton Decongestant, 267–68
Chocolate, 96–97
Choledyl, 241–42
Cholestasis of pregnancy, 109
Cholesterol-lowering drugs, 109–10,
    156–57, 197–98
Cholestyramine, 109–10
Chooz, 78–79
Chromagen, 185–86
Cibalith-S, 193–94
Cigarettes, 44, 114, 233–34, 295–96
Cigars, 295–96
Cillium, 268–69
Cimetidine, 23, 110, 272
Cipro, 110–11
Ciprofloxacin, 110–11, 231, 237
Civil Rights Act of 1964, 42
Claforan, 100–102
Cleaners, hazards of chemical, 50–51
Clemastine, 80
Cleocin, 111–12
Clindamycin, 111–12
Clinoril, 285–86
Clomid, 112
Clomiphene, 112
Clonazepam, 113–14
Clonidine, 114–15
Clorazepate, 115–16
Clotrimazole, 116–17
Cobalamin, 320
Cobex, 320
Cocaine, 117–18
Codan Syrup, 171–72
Codeine, 37, 118–19
Codimal DH, 171–72
Coffee, 96–97
Cola, 96–97
Colace, 136–37
Colitis, 23
Collaborative Perinatal Project, 62
Colrex Expectorant, 163
Combipres, 108–9, 114–15
Compazine, 262–63
Comtrex, 80, 127–28, 267–68
Congenital rubella syndrome, 25
Congestac, 267–68
Conjugated estrogens, 145
Constipation, 22, 90–91, 199–200. See
    also Laxatives

Contac, 80, 127–28, 251–52
Contac Cough Formula, 163
Contac Nighttime Cold Medicine, 267–
    68
Contraceptive device, 182–83
Contraceptive drugs, 89–90, 236–37,
    263–64
Convulsions in pregnancy, 37. See also
    Anticonvulsive drugs; Sedatives
Copper, 51
Corgard, 228–29
Coricidin, 80, 251–52
Correctol, 136–37, 249–50
Corticosteroids, 20, 23, 34, 35, 119–20
    oral inhalers, 88, 149–50, 304
Corzide, 228–29
Co-Tylenol, 80, 127–28
Cough suppressants, 118–19, 127–28,
    171–72
Cough syrups, 67–68
Coumadin, 18, 121
Coumarin anticoagulants, 121
Cremacoat, 127–28
Cremacoat 2, 163
Crohn's disease, 23, 283
Cromolyn, 20, 121
C-Span, 320–21
Cu–7, 182–83
Cyanoject, 320
Cyclizine, 80
Cyclobenzaprine, 122–23
Cycloheximide fungicide, 52
Cyclopar, 291
Cyclophosphamide, 123–24
Cyclosporine, 124–25
Cyomin, 320
Cyproheptadine, 80
Cytomegalovirus (CMV), 25, 48
Cystospaz-M, 174–75
Cytomel, 294
Cytotec, 225
Cytoxan, 123–24

Dallergy, 276–77
Dalmane, 152–53
Danazol, 125
Danocrine, 125
Darvocet, 264–65
Darvon, 264–65
Datril, 63–64
DDE insecticide, 52
DDT insecticide, 52
Decadron, 119–20
Deca-Durabolin, 77–78

use frequency of, in pregnancy, 1–2
use of this book to understand, 2–4
Dulcolax Pills and Suppositories, 90–91
Durabolin, 77–78
Duranest, 194–95
Duraquin, 270
Duratest, 289–90
Duricef, 100–102
Dyazide, 304–6
Dyes, 178–79
Dynapen, 130–31, 244–45
Dyrenium, 304–6

Ecotrin, 82–84
Edema, 16. *See also* Diuretic drugs
E. E. S., 144–45
E-Ferol, 322–23
Effer-Syllium, 268–69
Elavil, 73–74
Elixophyllin, 292–93
Elixophyllin-KI, 183–84, 257–58
Empirin, 82–84
Empirin #3, 118–19
E-Mycin, 144–45
Enalapril, 140
Encainide, 141
Endep, 73–74
Endocarditis, 17
Endometriosis, 125
Enkaid, 141
Entex, 251–52
Entuss, 171–72
Environmental hazards, 4, 41–43
    air pollution, 43–44
    food additives/contaminants, 44–47
    heavy metals, 51–52
    hospital and health-care hazards, 48–
        50
    hyperthermia (excessive heat), 47–48
    pesticides, 52–54
    physical exertion, 54–55
    radiation, microwaves, and
        ultrasound, 55–58
    solvents and cleaners, 50–51
Ephedrine, 141–42
Epilepsy, 37, 231, 247–49, 252–54, 260–
    61. *See also* Anticonvulsant drugs;
    Convulsions in pregnancy;
    Sedatives
Epinephrine, 20, 80, 142–43
Epi-Pen, 142–43
Eprolin Gelseals, 322–23
Equagesic, 82–84, 207–8
Equal artificial sweetener, 81–82

Equanil, 207–8
Ergomar, 143–44
Ergostat, 143–44
Ergotamine, 36–37, 143–44
ERYC, 144–45
Ery Ped, 144–45
Ery-Tab, 144–45
Erythema infectiosum, 27
Erythrocin, 144–45
Erythromycin, 30, 144–45
Esgic with Codeine, 118–19
Esidrix, 170–71
Eskabarb, 86–88
Eskalith, 193–94
Estrogens, 89–90, 145
Ethanol, 67–68
Ethosuximide, 37, 146
Ethylene oxide fungicide, 52
Etidocaine, 194–95
Etraton, 73–74
Etretinate, 146–47, 303
Euthroid, 192, 294
Eutonyl, 225–27
Evac-U-Lax, 249–50
E-Vital, 322–23
Excedrin, 82–84, 96–97
Exercise, hazards of excessive, 54–55
Ex-Lax, 249–50
Expectorant, 163, 183–84, 257–58
Extra Gentle Ex-Lax, 136–37

Famotidine, 147–48
Fat-lowering drugs, 156–57
Fedahist, 80, 163, 267–68
Feen-A-Mint, 136–37, 249–50
Femiron, 185–86
Femstat, 95–96
Fenoprofen, 148–49
Fentanyl, 149
Feosol, 185–86
Feostat, 185–86
Fergon, 185–86
Fero-Folic–500, 153–54, 185–86
Ferrous fumarate, 185–86
Ferrous gluconate, 185–86
Ferrous sulfate, 185–86
Fertility drugs, 112, 205–6
Fetal alcohol syndrome, 67
Fetus
    birth defects in, 5, 6–7, 13
    development of, 7–8
    effects of drugs on, 5 (*see also* name
        of specific drug)
    effects of mother's medical problems

Headaches, 36–37
  anti-migraine drug treatment, 143–44, 217–18
Health-care hazards during pregnancy, 48–50
Heartburn, 21–22
Heart drugs, 133–34. *See also* Antiarrhythmic drugs; Antihypertensive drugs; Digoxin
Heart problems during pregnancy, 16–17
Heat (see hyperthermia)
Heavy metals, 51–52
Hemaspan, 185–86
Hemocyte, 185–86
Hemorrhoids, 22
Heparin, 18, 166–67, 281, 313
Hepatitis, 27–29, 48
  hepatitis A, 27–28
  hepatitis B, 28–29
  hepatitis B vaccine, 167–68
  mononucleosis, 29
Hep-B-Gammagee, 177–78
Heptachlorepoxide insecticide, 52
Heptavax B, 167–68
Herbicides, 46, 52–54
Heroin, 168–69
Herpes, genital, 30–31
  drug treatment for, 65
Hexa-Betalin, 318–19
Hiprex and Urex (methenamine hippurate), 211–12
Hismanal, 79
HIV (human immunodeficiency virus), 24. *See also* AIDS (acquired immunodeficiency syndrome) virus
Hold, 127–28
Hormones, 97–98, 125, 132–33, 145, 181–82, 192, 263–64, 289–90, 294
Hospital hazards encountered during pregnancy, 48–50
Humibid, 163
Humulin, 181–82
Hycodan, 171–72
Hycomine, 171–72
Hycotuss, 171–72
Hydralazine, 169–70
Hydrocet, 171–72
Hydrochlorothiazide (HCTZ), 170–71, 280
Hydrocil, 268–69
Hydrocodone, 171–72
Hydrocortisone, 119–20
HydroDIURIL, 170–71

Hydromorphone, 172–73
Hydropres, 272–73
Hydroxychloroquine, 173–74
Hygroton, 108–9
Hyoscyamine sulfate, 174–75
Hyperactive behavior, drug treatment for, 216–17
Hyperemesis gravidarum, 21
Hyperetic, 170–71
Hyperstimulation syndrome, 206
Hypertension, 15–16. *See also* Antihypertensive drugs
Hyperthermia during pregnancy, 47–48
Hyperthyroidism, 15, 212, 266
Hypoglycemia
  agent for inducing, 157–58, 160–61, 296–97, 297–99
  as drug side effect, 107
  treatment for, 159–60
Hypothyroidism, 14, 212, 266
Hytuss, 163

Iberet, 185–86
Iberet-Folic, 153–54
Ibuprofen, 35, 175–76
Idiopathic thrombocytopenic purpura (ITP), 34
Iletin, 181–82
Illicit drugs, 77–78, 117–18, 168–69, 198–99, 201–2, 246
Ilosone, 144–45
Imipramine, 176–77
Immune globulins, 26, 177–78, 202, 273
  for viral hepatitis, 27, 28–29
Immune serum, 177–78, 273–74
Immunizations, 32, 290. *See also* Vaccines
Immunosuppressive drugs, 85–86, 124–25
Imodium, 195–96
Imovax Rabies Vaccine, 271–72
Imuran, 35, 85–86
Inderal, 265–66
Inderide, 265–66
Indigo carmine, 178–79
Indocin, 179–80
Indomethacin, 35, 179–80
Infections, 23–32
  bacterial, 31–32
  common viral/influenza, 23–24
  hospital, 48
  other serious viral, 24–29
  sexually transmitted, 24, 29–31

Infertility drugs, 92–93
Inflammation treatment. *See* Anti-
    inflammatory drugs
Inflammatory bowel disease, 23, 283
Influenza virus, 23–24, 48
    vaccine for, 24, 180–81
INH, 186–87
Innovar, 149
Insecticides, 52–54
Insomnia, alternatives to medication
    for, 102–3, 152–53, 211, 249, 287,
    307. *See also* Sedatives
Insulin, 6, 11–12, 181–82
Insulin resistance, 12
Intal, 121
Intestinal and digestive disorders, 20–
    23
Intrauterine device (IUD), 182–83
Iodide, 183–84
    radioactive, 15
Iodo-Niacin, 183–84
Ipratropium, 184–85
Iron supplements, 33, 185–86
Irospan, 185–86
Irritable bowel syndrome, 89, 174
Isoclor, 163
Isoniazid (INH), 186–87
Isoptin, 315
Isotretinoin, 36, 187–88, 303, 316
IUD (interuterine device), 182–83

Janimine, 176–77
Jaundice, 283, 284, 310

Kabikinase, 281
Kanamycin, 72–73
Kandremul, 222–23
Kantrex, 72–73
Kaochlor, 256–57
Kaolin and pectin mixtures, 188–89
Kaon-Cl, 256–57
Kaopectate, 188–89
Kapectolin, 188–89
Kasof, 136–37
KATO, 256–57
Kay Ciel, 256–57
K-Dur, 256–57
Keflex, 100–102
Keflin, 100–102
Keftabs, 100–102
Ketoconazole, 189–90
Ketoprofen, 190–91
Kewlcof, 171–72
Kidney disorders, 108, 170

Kido-Niacin, 257–58
Kinesed, 89
Klonopin, 113–14
K-Lor, 256–57
Klor-Con, 256–57
Klorvess, 256–57
Klotrix, 256–57
K-Lyte, 256–57
Konsyl, 268–69
K-P, 188–89
K-Pec, 188–89
K-Tab, 256–57
Kwell, 155–56

Labetalol, 191–92
Laniazid, 186–87
Lanoxicaps, 133–34
Lanoxin, 133–34
Larotid, 74–75
Lasix, 154–55
Laxatives, 22, 69, 90–91, 136–37, 199–
    200, 222–23, 249–50, 268–69, 277–
    78
Lead, hazards of, 51–52
Levelen, 89–90
Levothroid, 192, 294
Levothyroxine, 192
Levsin, 174–75
Levsinex Timecaps, 174–75
Librax, 104–5
Librium, 104–5
Lice, 155–56
Lidocaine, 194–95
Limbitrol, 73–74
Lindane insecticide, 52, 53, 155–56
Linea nigra, 36
Lipid (fat) lowering drugs, 156–57
Lippes Loop, 182–83
Liquiprin, 63–64
Liquor, 45, 67–68
Lisinopril, 192–93
Lithane, 193–94
Lithium, 193–94
    hazards, 51
Lithobid, 193–94
Lithonate, 193–94
Lithotabs, 193–94
Local anesthetics, 194–95
Loestrin, 89–90
Lomotil, 135–36
Loniten, 224–25
Lo/Oural, 89–90
Loperamide, 195–96
Lopid, 156–57

338

346